AF588104

Marginal Donors

Takehide Asano • Norihide Fukushima
Takashi Kenmochi • Naoto Matsuno
Editors

Marginal Donors

Current and Future Status

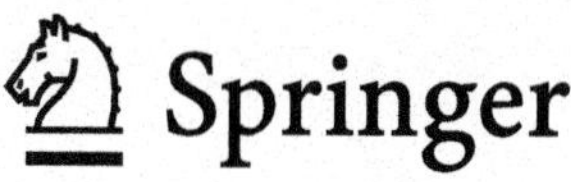

Editors
Takehide Asano
Department of Surgery and Clinical Research Center
Chiba-East National Hospital
Chiba, Japan

Takashi Kenmochi
Department of Organ Transplant Surgery
Fujita Health University
Aichi, Japan

Norihide Fukushima
Department of Therapeutics for End-Stage Organ Dysfunction
Osaka University Graduate School of Medicine
Osaka, Japan

Naoto Matsuno
Division for Innovative Surgery and Transplantation
National Center for Child Health and Development
Tokyo, Japan

ISBN 978-4-431-54483-8 ISBN 978-4-431-54484-5 (eBook)
DOI 10.1007/978-4-431-54484-5
Springer Tokyo Heidelberg New York Dordrecht London

Library of Congress Control Number: 2014930158

Printed on acid-free paper

Springer is part of Springer Science+Business Media (www.springer.com)

Preface

Organ procurement from brain-dead donors was not socially accepted for a long time in Japan. For that reason, organ transplantation in this country involved accumulating experience in using organs from donors after circulatory death (DCDs) and from living donors, adhering for the most part to criteria that exceeded the usual standards for organ donation.

It was first shown by Yoji Iwasaki and his colleagues in the 1960s that kidneys procured from uncontrolled DCDs could be transplanted safely [Iwasaki Y et al (1969) Cadaveric renal transplantation (I): patient selection and transplantation method. J Jpn Soc Transpl 4(1):72–78 (in Japanese); Iwasaki Y et al (1969) Cadaveric renal transplantation (II): post-transplantation course and care. J Jpn Soc Transpl 4(1):79–84 (in Japanese)]. Following their initial success, they continued with other cases and established clinical standards for renal transplantation from uncontrolled DCDs. [Iwasaki Y (ed) Cadaveric renal transplantation (1974) Igaku Shoin, Tokyo]. Also in Japan, some organ-preservation solutions and new preservation methods were developed, and their clinical applications were carried out widely. Research on viability assay methods was also productive. There were numerous groundbreaking results and satisfying clinical performances with organ transplants from marginal donors.

In Europe and the United States, where the use of brain-dead donors was widely accepted, transplants from DCDs were not performed except during the dawn of the transplant era. There were wide differences in the concept of the "marginal donor." In 1995, the Maastricht Classification was advocated. There remained, however, a wide discrepancy between their practices and ours regarding the actual conditions of DCDs.

In 2001, from the results of a kidney transplantation, an extended criteria donor (ECD) was defined by the United Network for Organ Sharing (UNOS) as a donor who has one or more factors influencing the results of a transplant—factors such as advanced age, cerebrovascular disorders, hypertension, and/or organ functional disorders. This concept was accepted widely and classified marginal donors into DCDs and ECDs, with further categorization into controlled and uncontrolled DCDs. Discussion of marginal donors thus has become more intelligible and can now be debated as a common topic.

Recently, donations from DCDs not only for kidney but also for pancreas and lung transplantation have been clinically achieved. Even with liver and heart transplantation, although still in the experimental–trial stage, aggressive research has been reported as organ shortages have become much more apparent. Factors and standards for grading DCDs and ECDs are different for each organ, and transplant results still vary. This situation is expected to change with an increase in knowledge from clinical and experimental studies. Improvement in the usability of marginal donors would be a boon for patients who have suffered organ failure.

This book is the first compilation of information about marginal donors. It mainly describes the history of the concept of marginal donors and the standard and current views of DCDs, standard criteria donors (SCDs), and ECDs for each organ. We regret that many of our predecessors' achievements have not yet been introduced Publication of this book has been made possible by Springer, Japan. The book was written and edited by the members of the Japanese Society for Organ Preservation and Medical Biology and reflects the results of their work. We express our profound gratitude to them.

Chiba, Japan Takehide Asano

Contents

Part I
History of Marginal Donors in the World

Chapter 1
History of Marginal Donors in the World

Norihide Fukushima

1.1 Introduction

Cadaver organ transplantation was started with donation after cardiac death (DCD). As determination of brain death was not established until 1968, the first liver transplant by Starzl et al. [1] in 1963 and the first heart transplant by Barnard [2] in 1967 were performed with DCD donors whose organs were procured under cardiopulmonary support (CPB). After the Harvard ad hoc committee [3] published the Harvard criteria for brain death in June 1968, organ donation from brain-dead persons has become the main current of cadaver organ transplantation. However, in Japan, only uncontrolled DCD kidney transplantation has been done since the 1960s, because brain-dead organ transplantation was not permitted for a long time.

As organ transplantation rapidly increased and organ shortage became more remarkable, DCD have been widely introduced in the clinical practice and the use of organs, especially kidneys, from DCD donors has been reported in multiple series [4] since the late 1980s in the developed countries. At that time, controlled DCD was the main current. Therefore, organs were harvested after cardiac death induced by extubation of the donor.

As percutaneous cardiopulmonary support (PCPS) was introduced in the clinical settings in the late 1980s, uncontrolled DCD using PCPS was initiated in Spain [5]. In 2000, Steen et al. [6] started uncontrolled DCD lung transplantation in Sweden (Table 1.1).

N. Fukushima (✉)
Department of Therapeutics for End-Stage Organ Dysfunction, Osaka University Graduate School of Medicine, 2-2 Yamada-oka, Suita, Osaka 565-0871, Japan
e-mail: nori@surg1.med.osaka-u.ac.jp

T. Asano et al. (eds.), *Marginal Donors: Current and Future Status*,
DOI 10.1007/978-4-431-54484-5_1,

Table 1.1 History of organ transplantation

	Animal experiment and xenotransplant	Clinical experiences in the world	Clinical experiences in Japan
1902	Ullmann (Austria): animal experiments of RTx		
1905	Carrel (USA): animal experiments of HTx and RTx		
1906	Jaboulay (France): renal xenograft (sheep and pigs)		
1910	Sainai (Kyoto University): animal experiments of RTx January 5 Unger: renal xenotransplant (primates)		
1923	Neuhof: renal xenotransplant (lambs)		
1933		April 3 Voronoy (Ukraine): DCD RTx	
1940s	Medawar (USA): elucidation of mechanism of rejection		
1952	Dausset (USA): elucidation of human leukocytes antigens		
1954		December 23 Merrill and Murray (USA): successful RTx between identical twins	
1956			Kusunoki, Inoue (Niigata University): living RTx
1959		January 24 Merrill and Murray (USA): successful allogeneic RTx	
1961		March Calne (UK), Murray (USA): use of azathioprine in RTx	
1962		April 6 Murray (USA): successful DCD RTx	
1963	Reemtsma (USA): renal xenotransplant (chimpanzees and baboons)	March 1 Starzl (USA): lung Tx from uncontrolled DCD donor using CPB June 3 Alexandre (Belgium): first RTx from brain-dead donor June 11 Hardy (USA): lung Tx from uncontrolled DCD donor	

1964	Hardy (USA): heart xenotransplant (chimpanzees) Starzl (Ж): renal xenotransplant (chimpanzees and baboons)		March 20 Nakayama (Chiba University): heterotopic liver Tx from uncontrolled DCD donor March 27 Kimoto (Tokyo University): living RTx for chronic renal failure
1965	Lower (USA): long-term canine survival after HTx		June 25 Shinonoi (Tokyo Medical College): partial lobe lung Tx
1966		December 17 Lillihei (USA): pancreas Tx from uncontrolled DCD donor using CPB	
1967	Terasaki (USA): studies of HLA serotyping in RTx	December 3 Barnard (South Africa): HTx from uncontrolled DCD donor using CPB December 6 Kantrowitz (USA): HTx from an anencephalic baby	
1968	Cooley (USA): heart xenotransplant (sheep)	January 6 Shumway (USA): HTx from controlled DCD donor	August 8 Wada (Sapporo Medical College): first HTx
1969	Starzl (USA): liver xenotransplant (chimpanzees and baboons)		
1978		Calne (USA): use of cyclosporine in RTx	
1980	Reitz (USA): heart and lung Tx (primates)		
1981		March 9 Reitz (USA): heart and lung Tx	
1984	Bailey (USA): newborn heart xenotransplant (baboon)		September 25 Fukao (Tsukuba University): pancreas/kidney Tx from brain-dead donor
1988		Cooper (USA): bilateral lung transplantation	
1989		December 8, 1988 Raia (Brazil): living liver Tx Starzl, Todo (USA): use of tacrolimus in RTx and liver Tx	January 19 Ohta (Tokyo Women Medical College): ABO-incompatible RTx November 3 Nagasue (Shimane Medical College): living liver Tx
1990	Groth (Sweden): pancreas xenotransplant (pig)	Starnes (USA): living lobar lung Tx Grant (USA): simultaneous intestine/liver Tx Valero (Spain): RTx from uncontrolled DCD donors using PCPS	June 15 Ozawa (Kyoto University): living liver Tx

(continued)

Table 1.1 (continued)

	Animal experiment and xenotransplant	Clinical experiences in the world	Clinical experiences in Japan
1991	Czaplicki (Porland): heart xenotransplant (Pig)		
1992		Sollinger (USA): use of mycophenolate mofetil in RTx Starzl (USA): restart liver Tx from controlled DCD donors	
1993	Mokowka (USA): liver xenotransplant (Pig)	Love (USA): lung Tx from controlled DCD donor	October 22 Sugimachi (Kushu University): liver Tx from uncontrolled DCD donor
1994	Starzl (USA): liver xenotransplant (baboons)		
1995		Bunnapradist (USA): use of Neoral in RTX	
1996		Appel (Germany): use of everolimus in RTx	July 9 Tanaka (Kyoto University): living intestine Tx
1997			October 17 Japanese organ transplant act
1998			October 28 Shimizu, Date (Okayama University): living lobar lung Tx
1999		Shapiro (Canada): long-term graft after survival from pancreatic islet Tx	February 28 First heart, liver, and kidney Tx from a brain-dead donor: HTx (Osaka University), liver Tx (Shinshu University), RTx (Tohoku University, National Nagasaki Central Hospital) Tanaka (Kyoto University): living domino liver Tx
2000		October Steen (Sweden): lung Tx from uncontrolled DCD donor	March 29 Single lung Tx from a brain-dead donor (Osaka and Tohoku University) April 25 Pancreas/kidney Tx from a brain-dead donor (Osaka University)
2001		Budds (USA): use of FTY720 in RTx	March 19 Bilateral lung Tx from a brain-dead donor (Osaka University), intestine Tx from a brain-dead donor (Kyoto University)
2004			January 7 Living pancreas/kidney Tx (National Sakura University)
2009			January 17 Heart and lung Tx (Osaka University)

1.2 The Dawn of Organ Transplantation from DCD Donors

On April 3, 1963, Voronoy et al. [7] did the first allogeneic kidney transplantation in Ukraine. The recipient was a 25-year-old woman with acute renal failure by intake of mercuric chloride. The donor was a 60-year-old man who died of basilar fracture. His kidney was procured 6 h after cardiac arrest. Although she urinated soon after transplantation, urination stopped and she died on the second posttransplant day (POD).

In April 1962, Murray et al. [8] successfully performed DCD kidney transplantation in Boston. The recipient was a 23-year-old man. The donor was a 30-year-old man. As cardiopulmonary bypass could not be removed because of severe cardiac failure after open cardiac surgery, his body temperature was cooled down to 20 °C by CPB and his kidney was procured and transplanted. Total ischemic time (TIT) was 2 h. The graft started to function 5 days after transplantation and the recipient was given azathioprine (AZP) and survived for more than a year.

On March 1, 1963, Starzl et al. [1] did the first liver transplant in Denver. The recipient was a 3-year-old boy with biliary atresia. His thymus was excised on February 12 and he was given AZP for 14 days prior to transplantation. The donor was a 3-year-old boy whose heart arrested during the surgery of brain tumor. After cardiopulmonary resuscitation was tried for 45 min, he was pronounced dead. CPB was installed by putting the cannulae into the femoral artery and vein. After the body temperature was cooled down to 15 °C, his liver was procured. He died of massive bleeding. In the second and third case, CPB was started soon after cardiac arrest to shorten TIT. CPB time was 375, 98, and 126 min, respectively. TIT was 465, 152, and 192 min, respectively. The second case died of pneumonia on the 22nd POD and the third case died of gastrointestinal bleeding on the 7th POD. Starzl did the first successful liver transplantation from controlled DCD, as did Shumway's first heart transplantation.

On December 3, 1967, Barnard [2] did the first allogeneic heart transplantation from a DCD donor. After the donor was moved to the operating room with a coroner, she was extubated; 5 min after the heart stopped, she was pronounced dead by the coroner. Her chest was opened soon and CPB was installed. After the body was cooled down, her heart and kidneys were procured. The recipient died on the 18th POD.

On January 6, 1968, Shumway and Stinson et al. [9] did the first heart transplantation from a controlled DCD donor. After the donor was diagnosed as brain dead by neurologists and pronounced dead, he was extubated and the heart was procured.

The first brain-dead organ transplantation (kidney) was done by Alexandre et al. [10] in Belgium in 1963. As the concepts of brain death were not established yet then, brain-dead organ donation became the main current in the early 1970s after the Harvard criteria was published.

1.3 Marginal Donors in Brain-Dead Organ Donation

In the early 1970s when brain-dead organ donation was started, outcomes of cadaver organ transplantation were very poor, because the organ preservation technique was immature and the optimal organ donor criteria and the safe and efficient immunosuppressive regimen were not established. After good preservation solution, such as the UW solution, was developed and safe and efficient immunosuppressive regimen using cyclosporine and so on was established in the early 1980s, the outcomes of organ transplantation became satisfactory.

As the outcomes of organ transplantation were improved, organ donor criteria have been gradually modified. And then, the so-called standard criteria were established. As organ transplantation rapidly increased and donor shortage became severer, the criteria of organ donors were reevaluated and the extended criteria were made for each organ. As the extended criteria were different among organs and countries, please see details of the extended criteria in the chapter of each organ.

In order to save more patients who need organ transplantation, we need to increase organs transplanted per donor (OTPD) by intensively managing the donor. Antidiuretic hormone (ADH) and thyroid hormones have been used to stabilize hemodynamics of the donor in the developed countries since the late 1990s.

As donor shortage is extremely severe in Japan because of very strict Organ Transplantation Act, special strategies for maximizing organ transplant opportunities should be established. Since November in 2002, special transplant management doctors were sent to donor hospitals in order to assess donor's organ function and to identify which organ could be transplanted. They also intensively cared for the donor to stabilize hemodynamics and to improve cardiac and lung function by intravenously giving ADH and pulmonary toileting by bronchofiberscope. In Japan, OTPD has been 5.5 organs in consecutive 100 brain-dead organ procurement since February 1999 [11].

1.4 Organ Transplantation from Controlled DCD Donors

In the late 1980s, organ shortage became more remarkable. DCD was paid attention again. As the outcomes of DCD organ transplantation in the dawn of organ transplantation in the late 1960s were very poor, many animal experiments were done in many institutes to establish DCD organ preservation technique. In the 1990s, DCD have been widely introduced in the clinical practice and the use of kidneys and livers from controlled DCD donors has been reported in multiple series [4].

However, in the Catholic countries, such as Spain, cessation of mechanical respiratory support means suicide and is not permitted, unless family consent for brain death is obtained. Therefore, controlled DCD is not permitted in such countries. The time after cardiac arrest for considering personal death is different among countries. In most countries, the time is about 5 min, but 15 min in Italy.

1.5 Organ Transplantation from Uncontrolled DCD Donors: Multiple Organ Transplantation from Uncontrolled DCD Donors in Spain

As PCPS was introduced in the clinical settings in the late 1980s, uncontrolled DCD using PCPS was initiated in Spain. Koyama et al. [12] did the first experiment of DCD using PCPS. Under PCPS, the body temperature of the donor animals was cooled down and the kidneys were procured and transplanted. The author of this chapter [13] also did several animal experiments of multiple organ transplantation (heart, lung, and kidneys) using PCPS.

In Spain, PCPS was first used in the clinical settings of uncontrolled DCD donors [5]. In the 1990s, they cooled donor body temperature from 15 to 20 °C, and normothermic recirculation trough CPB was used since 1997.

The donor criteria for multiple organ transplantation [14, 15] from uncontrolled DCD donors in Spain included, in addition to the general criteria for donor selection, an age under 65 and a warm ischemia time lower than 150 min with a period of warm ischemia without cardiopulmonary resuscitation maneuvers less than 30 min. Only I and IV Maastricht NHBD categories were considered. Currently kidneys, liver, and lungs were transplanted from uncontrolled DCD donors.

1.6 Lung Transplantation from Uncontrolled DCD Donors in Sweden

In 2000, Steen et al. [6] started uncontrolled DCD lung transplantation in Sweden. After cardiac arrest, the chest tubes were inserted and the body was topically cooled. Since then, uncontrolled DCD lung transplantation was started in Australia [16] and the outcomes became comparable to those of lung transplantation from brain-dead donors.

1.7 Increased Roles of "Normothermic" Perfusion Techniques on Organ Preservation [17]

Preservation injury is an important factor not only in the short-term but also in the long-term outcome of transplantation, and success rates are directly related to the duration of cold ischemia. In recent years, the increasing discrepancy between transplant waiting lists and the supply of cadaveric donor organs has led to the transplantation of increasingly marginal organs. This group is characterized by particularly poor tolerance of the various injuries that occur during the process of preservation and transplantation.

Although cooling reduces the metabolic rate of biological tissue, continued cellular processes lead to depletion of ATP and accumulation of metabolic products. When the organ is rewarmed and reperfused with oxygenated blood, the rapid metabolism of metabolic products within an organ depleted of energy stores leads to ischemia-reperfusion injuries. The use of marginal donor organs and, particularly, those from DCD donors exacerbates the problems of preservation and ischemia-reperfusion injury. This is a limiting factor in the use of such donor organs.

The use of hypothermic machine perfusion has been shown to improve the immediate function rate of stored kidneys, but does not enable normal cellular metabolic function or prevent depletion of energy stores or prevent all the deleterious direct effects of cooling. Cold preservation is now seen as an important limiting factor in the further expansion of transplantation.

The principle of normothermic perfusion is to recreate the physiological environment by maintaining normal temperature and providing the essential substrates for cellular metabolism, oxygen, and nutrition. In addition to a reduction in ischemia-reperfusion injury, a further potential advantage of normothermic perfusion is the assessment of viability, because the organ is metabolically active, and it is possible to measure function and to predict posttransplant outcome before subjecting the patient to surgery. This is an increasingly important issue as more marginal organs are used.

To date the only uses of normothermic perfusion in a clinical environment have been in heart and lung transplantation. As the utility and potential benefits of normothermic preservation are more recognized, we may expect to see further clinical trials in other areas of transplantation.

References

1. Starzl TE, Marchioro TL, Vonkaulla KN, et al. Homotransplantation of the liver in humans. Surg Gynecol Obstet. 1963;117:659–76.
2. Barnard CN. The operation — A human cardiac transplant: an interim report of a successful operation performed at Groote Schuur Hospital, Cape Town. S Afr Med J. 1967;41:1271–4.
3. Ad Hoc Committee of the Harvard Medical School. A definition of irreversible coma: report of the Ad Hoc Committee of the Harvard Medical School to examine the definition of brain death. JAMA. 1968;205:337–40.
4. Abt PL, Desai NM, Crawford MD, et al. Survival following liver transplantation from non-heartbeating donors. Ann Surg. 2004;239:87–92.
5. Valero R, Cabrer C, Oppenhaimer F, et al. Normothermic recirculation reduces primary graft dysfunction of kidneys obtained from non-heart-beating donors. Transpl Int. 2000;13:303–10.
6. Steen S, Sjoberg T, Pierre L, et al. Transplantation of lungs from a non-heart-beating donor. Lancet. 2001;357:825–9.
7. Matevossian E, Kern H, Hüser N, et al. Surgeon Yurii Voronoy (1895–1961) – a pioneer in the history of clinical transplantation: in memoriam at the 75th anniversary of the first human kidney transplantation. Transpl Int. 2009;22:1132–9.
8. Murray JE, Merrill JP, Harrison JH, et al. Prolonged survival of human-kidney homografts by immunosuppressive drug therapy. N Engl J Med. 1963;268:1315–23.

9. Stinson EB, Dong Jr E, Schroeder JS, et al. Initial clinical experience with heart transplantation. Am J Cardiol. 1968;22:791–803.
10. Squifflet JP. The history of transplantation at the Catholic University of Louvain, Belgium 1963–2003. Acta Chir Belg. 2003;103:10–20.
11. Fukushima N, Ono M, Nakatani T, et al. Strategies for maximizing heart and lung transplantation opportunities in Japan. Transplant Proc. 2009;41:273–6.
12. Koyama I, Hoshino T, Nagashima N, Adachi H, Ueda K, Omoto R. A new approach to kidney procurement from non-heart-beating donors: core cooling on cardiopulmonary bypass. Transplant Proc. 1989;21:1203–5.
13. Fukushima N, Shirakura R, Chang JC, et al. Successful experimental multiorgan transplant from non heart beating donors using percutaneous cardiopulmonary support. ASAIO J. 1998;44:M525–8.
14. Fondevilaa C, Hessheimera AJ, Ruiz A, et al. Liver transplant using donors after unexpected cardiac death: novel preservation protocol and acceptance criteria. Am J Transpl. 2007;7:1849–55.
15. Gamez P, Cordoba M, Ussetti P, et al. Lung transplantation from out-of-hospital non-heart-beating lung donors. One-year experience and results. J Heart Lung Transplant. 2005; 24:1098–110.
16. Snell GI, Levvey BJ, Oto T, et al. Early lung transplantation success utilizing controlled donation after cardiac death donors. Am J Transplant. 2008;8:1282–9.
17. Reddy SP, Brockmann J, Friend PJ. Normothermic perfusion: a mini-review. Transplantation. 2009;87:631–2.

Part II
Management of Extended Criteria Donors

Chapter 2
Management of Extended Criteria Donors

Norihide Fukushima

2.1 Introduction

Only about 20 % of brain-dead donors in Japan have been fitted in a so-called standard criteria donor for all organs including the heart, lung, liver, pancreas, and kidney. Therefore, it is very important for us to maximize the number of transplantable organs in order to resolve severe donor shortage in Japan [1]. From these aspects, the purposes of donor management are not only to stabilize donor's hemodynamics until organ procurement surgery but also to maximize donor organ availability and to improve function of extended criteria donor organs. If organ availability is increased, more patients can be saved by organ transplantation. Maximizing donor organ availability is also the last wish of donors and donor families. However, if a transplant recipient died due to a very marginal donor organ, the donor family feels the loss of their loved one again. Therefore, the prevention of primary graft dysfunction (PGD) is essential for the donor family as well as for recipients.

Full-scale donor management begins after the patient is pronounced brain dead and his or her family agrees to donate the organ(s), especially in Japan. In general, donor management is based on the treatment of cardiac and respiratory dysfunction resulting in the improvement of hemodynamics, oxygen supply, and finally other organ function. The targets of hemodynamic parameters are systemic blood pressure >90 mmHg, central venous pressure (CVP) of 6–10 mmHg, urine output of 100 mL/h (0.5–3 mL/kg/h), and heart rate of 80–120 beats/min. As organ procurement surgery begins within 12 h after full-scale donor management is started, it is very different from the usual intensive care to stabilize hemodynamics and to maintain and improve organ function as much as possible in a short period. Moreover, it is important for the physicians who perform donor management to recognize the pathophysiology of brain death from the beginning to completion period.

N. Fukushima (✉)
Department of Therapeutics for End-Stage Organ Dysfunction, Osaka University Graduate School of Medicine, 2-2 Yamada-oka, Suita, Osaka 565-0871, Japan
e-mail: nori@surg1.med.osaka-u.ac.jp

T. Asano et al. (eds.), *Marginal Donors: Current and Future Status*,
DOI 10.1007/978-4-431-54484-5_2, © Springer Japan 2014

2.2 Pathophysiology of Brain Death

2.2.1 Physiological Changes at Completion of Brain Death

Novitzky et al. reported animal experiments of brain death in baboons, induced by placing a Foley catheter in the subdural space through a burr hole and instilling 20–30 mL of saline [2]. This resulted in acute intracranial hypertension leading to brain stem herniation and brain death. During and following the agonal period there was a short-lived, but devastating, catecholamine "storm" [2, 3], which was the result of endogenous catecholamine release from postganglionic sympathetic nerve endings. Novitzky et al. reported that serum concentration of noradrenaline (NAD), adrenaline (AD), and dopamine (DOA) elevated to approximately 1,600, 1,100, and 450 pg/mL, respectively, 5 min after balloon inflation in this baboon model. The hemodynamic response was a significant elevation of the systemic vascular resistance (SVR), resulting in systemic hypertension, acute left ventricular failure, fall in cardiac output, and acute transient mitral valve regurgitation, leading to a rise in left atrial pressure. These events led to blood volume displacement into the venous compartment, with pulmonary volume overloading. The electrocardiogram (ECG) showed multiple arrhythmias plus ischemic changes in all animals.

However, when the intracranial pressure is increased slowly, the animals underwent a lesser hyperdynamic response and experienced only approximately 25 % of the rise in epinephrine levels seen in animals undergoing sudden brain death. In the human clinical situation, there is a broad spectrum of adverse hemodynamic instability that is observed, which may, in part, reflect the speed at which brain death is induced.

After the initial outpouring of catecholamines following the onset of brain death, catecholamine levels rapidly returned to control levels and subsequently to levels below baseline, when endocrine changes, reflecting pituitary failure, developed.

In clinical settings, brain death is associated with a massive increase in catecholamine levels (the sympathetic/autonomic storm), sometimes resulting in increased heart rate, systemic blood pressure, cardiac output, and SVR. The consequences of autonomic storm are an imbalance between myocardial oxygen demand and supply, which triggers metabolic functional alterations and sometimes anatomical heart damage (myocytolysis and micronecrosis) [4]. Electrocardiographic signs of myocardial ischemia, conduction abnormalities, and arrhythmia are also common during this period.

Histological examination of cardiac tissue exposed to autonomic storm shows changes typical of widespread ischemic damage and necrosis, and profound end-organ vasoconstriction has been demonstrated in animal models [5]. However, this period of intense catecholamine release is short-lived (typically minutes) and self-limited and may require no treatment. Nevertheless, many experimental studies and recent clinical observations suggest that treatment of autonomic storm (short-acting β-blocker drugs or nitroprusside) is a viable strategy to attenuate myocardial dysfunction and increase the number and success rate of heart procurements and cardiac transplantation [6–8].

Regardless of whether the systemic arterial pressure is low or high, the donor is usually hypovolemic. Brain death-induced physiological changes lead to an increase in capillary permeability and create a functional intravascular hypovolemia. In addition, absolute or relative hypovolemia is commonly present in these patients because of increased fluid loss (i.e., mannitol, glycerol, other diuretic therapy, or diabetes insipidus). This hypovolemic state is difficult to assess without monitoring CVP or pulmonary capillary wedge pressure (PCWP).

Severely brain-injured patients develop acute lung injury (ALI) and/or adult respiratory distress syndrome (ARDS) in 15–20 % of cases. In addition, lung function can be impaired through different mechanisms including neurogenic pulmonary edema, aspiration, hemo-pneumothorax, atelectasis, and later on pneumonia. The presence of pulmonary dysfunction in acute brain injury is well known and has previously been attributed to hydrostatic phenomenon induced by a massive increase in sympathetic activity. However, an acute systemic inflammatory response also appears to play an integral role in the development of such injury by initiating infiltration of activated neutrophils into the lungs. Moreover, severe brain injury resulting in brain stem death is characterized by the release of proinflammatory mediators into the systemic circulation. This inflammatory response may determine the preclinical lung injury present in the potential lungs, which together with the ischemia-reperfusion injury may affect primary graft dysfunction. Indeed Follette et al. reported that the administration of high-dose steroids after brain death improved oxygenation and increased lung donor utilization by limiting the cytokine-mediated cellular injury [9].

2.2.2 *Absent or Decreased Secretion of Antidiuretic Hormone After Brain Death*

Antidiuretic hormone (ADH) is formed in the supraoptic and paraventricular nuclei of the hypothalamus by cleavages of a preprohormone of 168 amino acids and then a prohormone, vasopressin, is transported to the posterior lobe of the pituitary gland which stores it. Its release depends primarily on two factors, hyperosmolality and blood volume, and in addition on the effects of certain drugs.

The effects of vasopressin result from stimulation of V1 and V2 receptors, V1 mainly responsible for vasoconstriction, V2 for the antidiuretic effect.

V1 receptors are coupled by G protein to phospholipase C. Its activation elicits the hydrolysis of PIP2 in IP3 and DAG, which induces an increase of intracellular calcium concentration, responsible for the vasoconstriction. With doses higher than those which are necessary to induce water retention, ADH induces vasoconstriction. The plasma concentration of vasopressin can be sufficient to increase peripheral resistance and arterial pressure. The decrease in cutaneous blood flux seen in smokers could be the consequence of an increase in the secretion of vasopressin under the influence of nicotine.

V2 receptors are coupled by G protein to adenylcyclase. Its activation elicits an increase in cAMP which, via protein kinases, induces the activation of aqueous channels called aquaporins of type 2 or AQP2 mainly located in the renal collecting duct. Under the influence of vasopressin AQP2 migrate from the cytoplasm to the apical membrane. In nephrogenic diabetes insipidus there are AQP2 alterations. The ADH increases water permeability of collecting ducts in the cortical and medullary part of the kidney. It induces the incorporation of aquaporins in the apical membrane of collecting ducts and induces their opening, which allows water reabsorption.

The effects of brain death on the hypothalamic-hypophyseal axis are profound. The most frequent and almost immediate manifestation is diabetes insipidus due to loss of ADH secretion secondary to supraventricular and paraventricular hypothalamic nuclei ischemia. ADH was undetectable within 6 h. As ADH is secreted from the peripheral tissues, undetectable levels of ADH have been noted in 75 % of brain death. As antidiuretic action of ADH is decreased, the kidneys are unable to concentrate urine and excrete large amounts (4 mL/kg/h) of dilute urine (specific gravity <1.005 and urine osmolality <200 mOsm/L). Polyuria may lead to hypernatremia (>145 mEq/mL, which is common and sometimes severe and worsening), associated with rising serum osmolality and hypovolemia. As the vasoconstrictive effect of ADH is decreased, the vascular tone of systemic arteries is decreased, leading to hypovolemic shock. Therefore, absent or decreased secretion of ADH after brain death is associated with hemodynamic instability and compromised transplantable organ function.

Low-dose arginine vasopressin, in addition to treating diabetes insipidus, results in reduced inotropic requirements and has been associated with good kidney, liver, and heart graft function [2, 8, 10–12]. Pure vasopressors, like ADH, are less likely to cause metabolic acidosis or pulmonary hypertension and may be more appropriate than NAD for the vasoplegic shock phase.

2.2.3 *Decrease in Anterior Pituitary Function After Brain Death*

Anterior pituitary function (blood supply via hypophyseal extradural arteries) is usually preserved, but viable deficiency of hormones regulated by the anterior pituitary including thyroid hormone [triiodothyronine (T3) and free thyroxine (T4)], adrenocorticotropic hormone, thyroid-stimulating hormone (TSH), and growth hormone has been described. This striking and acute hormonal depletion was very common and has been implicated in hemodynamic derangement seen after brain death in experimental animal models.

Cortisol levels were increased at 5 min and then declined progressively to sub-baseline levels [13]. Plasma levels of free T3 and T4 fell to 50 % of control levels within 1 h after brain death and became undetectable within 9 and 16 h, respectively, but TSH showed no significant change. Insulin levels declined to 50 %

within 3 h and to 20 % within 13 h [14]. Prompted by these results, the Cape Town group evaluated hormone replacement therapy, first in brain-dead animals [15] and then in brain-dead human organ donors [2].

However, this striking and acute hormonal depletion is not certain and questionable in clinical practice. Although a rapid decline in plasma levels of free T3 is seen after brain death as a result of impaired TSH secretion and peripheral conversion of T4, attempts to thyroid disturbances in organ donors have produced conflicting data [2]. Moreover, there has been inconsistent improvement or conflicting results in the assessed physiological parameters after replacement of these hormones in both animals and humans [16].

The studies by the Cape Town group on the benefits of hormonal therapy did not achieve rapid universal acceptance, in part because of published studies that failed to confirm low levels of T3, T4, cortisol, and insulin after brain death [17, 18] and/or published studies that failed to demonstrate any beneficial cardiac and circulatory effect of T3/T4 administration [19, 20]. This may have been for a number of reasons: not all brain-dead donors have total absence of anterior pituitary function (and therefore some have measurable T3 levels), some groups failed to measure free T3, not all donors are hemodynamically unstable [21–23] and the benefit from T3/T4 therapy might not be seen, and an inadequate dosage of T3/T4 may have been administered. However, in many countries, such as the USA, Canada, and Australia, hormone resuscitation strategies (ADH, T4, and methylprednisolone) are recommended to manage brain-dead donors [8].

The optimal dose of i.v. methylprednisolone for the brain-dead donor remains uncertain. High doses have been recommended [24, 25] and the UNOS study [8] indicated a beneficial effect on the heart when it was the sole hormone administered. Because the half-life of i.v. methylprednisolone is short [26], we believe that it is desirable to repeat the dosage when organ retrieval is delayed.

2.2.4 Cessation of Autonomic Nerve Regulations on Circulation

After brainstem ischemia and necrosis, the brain-heart connections are definitively disrupted. Brain death results in complete cessation of normal variations of the autonomic cardiovascular centers and a cessation of the baroreflex function [27]. Rapenne et al. [28] described that as soon as the diagnosis of brain death was clinically suggested, the heart rate variability (HRV) analysis demonstrated a lack of control of the sympathetic and parasympathetic components of the autonomic nerve system on cardiovascular regulation. A very small LF power spectrum could be found in these patients; free from regulation by the higher centers, the sympathetic nerves of the spinal cord continue to generate small autonomic impulses to control vasomotor tone.

Disrupted brain-heart connections, the so-called denervation, are also observed in heart transplant recipients. The authors described that transplanted hearts could not augment cardiac performance rapidly in response to acute decrease in the preload due to loss of the brain-heart connection [29]. In normal hearts, if a preload of the heart rapidly decreases, autonomic sympathetic nerves are activated through vagal reflexes, resulting in an increase in heart rate and cardiac contractility. However, the transplanted hearts do not increase their rate or contractility by autonomic response to a rapid decrease in preload. The augmentation of cardiac performance of the transplanted hearts has been thought to depend mainly on an increase in AD secretion from the adrenal gland. Thus, the transplanted heart has been thought to be unable to rapidly enhance performance in response to a rapid decrease in the preload, such as sudden hemorrhage or occlusion of inferior vena cava.

As shown in heart transplant recipients, the hemodynamics of brain-dead persons is also unstable. For example, a decrease in blood return to the heart due to hemorrhage, putting pressure on the upper abdomen, or postural change may easily cause hypotension. After a few minutes of hypotension, AD is secreted from the adrenal glands due to spinal reflex and hypertension usually up to 150 mmHg and tachycardia may be observed. In uncontrolled brain-dead persons, systemic blood pressure and heart rate may rise and fall. This phenomenon is usually seen in a patient with hypovolemia due to diabetes insipidus. An increase in AD secretion may reduce a density of beta-adrenergic receptors (BAR) on the vessels and the myocardium.

2.2.5 *Absent Cough Reflex*

After brainstem ischemia and necrosis, the cough reflex is lost as seen in lung transplant recipients. This change probably influences susceptibility to respiratory infection and the consequences of atelectasis. As it is very difficult to aspirate deep sputa, bronchofiberscopy (BFS), by clearance of secretions and blood clots and correction of endotracheal tube malposition, may improve lung function.

2.2.6 *Alteration of BAR Systems*

Various changes in BAR systems occur during and after brain death. D'Amico et al. [30] reported a decrease in BAR density during brain death in adult and pediatric pigs. Deterioration of myocardial performance after brain death correlated temporally with desensitization of the myocardial BAR signal transduction pathway. Authors have previously reported that myocardial BAR may be depressed by the large doses of catecholamines (CAs) used to maintain donor hemodynamics after brain death [31]. The authors also revealed a significant inverse correlation between BAR density and serum AD level, but not between Bmax and serum NAD or DA levels [32]. Bmax values in patients treated with AD were significantly lower than those in patients treated without AD; there was a significant inverse correlation between Bmax and the administered dose of AD. These data suggest that exogenous AD reduces BAR density in brain-dead patients and support the conventional criteria in which retrieval of cardiac grafts is restricted to donors who can be managed with minimal to moderate levels of inotropic support.

2.3 Donor Assessment and Management

In order to manage a donor properly, hemodynamics, respiratory function, infection, and other organ functions of the donor should be undertaken precisely. As there are no specific strategies for liver or renal dysfunction, cardiopulmonary management to improve organ perfusion and blood gas and metabolic management are the main therapeutic strategies for management of extended criteria donors.

2.3.1 Role of Echocardiography and Circulatory Management

The aggressive assessment and optimal management of donor left ventricular (LV) dysfunction offer a tremendous potential to increase cardiac donor utilization as a significant proportion of hearts are declined for reasons of "poor ventricular function." However, strong evidence indicates that grafts from younger donors with left ventricular dysfunction can completely recover to normal function over time in the donor and following transplantation into a recipient [33]. Although echocardiography is very effective in screening for anatomical, especially valvular, anomalies of the heart, the use of a single echo examination in terms of a "snapshot assessment" of pump function to determine the physiological suitability of a donor graft is not well supported by evidence.

Instead, better physiological assessment and donor management of LV dysfunction are achieved by Swan-Ganz catheterization (SGC) investigations, which have led to favorite long-term outcomes [34]. By serial SGC investigations, specific physiological targets such as mean blood pressure >60 mmHg, CVP <12 mmHg, pulmonary capillary wedge pressure <12 mmHg, and left ventricular stroke work index >15 g m/m^2 while on only one single inotrope can be achieved, resulting in specified hemodynamic categories [34].

In the presence of LV underfilling, the LV seems to be hypertrophic or to have suitable LV systolic function. Therefore, circulatory blood should be estimated by CVP, PCWP, or the size and respiratory movement of the inferior vena cava (IVC) as well as doses of inotropes prior to undergoing echocardiography to assess cardiac function.

The goals of hemodynamic management are to achieve euvolemia, to adjust vasoconstrictors and vasodilators to maintain a normal afterload, and to optimize cardiac output without relying on high doses of beta-agonists or other inotropes, which increase myocardial oxygen demands, deplete the myocardium of high-energy phosphates, and decrease the density of BAR in the vessels and the myocardium. The target levels of hemodynamic parameter are as follows: systemic blood pressure >90 mmHg, CVP of 6–10 mmHg, urine output of 100 mL/h (or 0.5–3 mL/kg/h), and heart rate of 80–120 beats/min.

2.3.2 *Role of Bronchofiberscopy (BFS) and Respiratory Management*

A ventilatory strategy with high tidal volumes is potentially harmful and may exacerbate donor lung injury already triggered by the systemic inflammatory response. The use of low-tidal-volume ventilation was shown to be beneficial in a randomized controlled study for ALI and ARDS when compared to traditional tidal volumes. No such a trial has been performed to look if one ventilatory mode is superior to another in the care of the brain-dead organ donor. However, given similarities in the pathophysiological changes occurring in ARDS and lung injury after brain death, we might expect that beneficial management strategies can be extrapolated.

Recruitment maneuvers are an important component of donor optimization, especially when the oxygenation is subnormal and pulmonary abnormalities are visible on chest x-ray. Atelectasis is a common finding in the lung of cadaveric donors due to prolonged ventilation in the supine position. Prevention of atelectasis will reduce the development of atelectrauma by cyclic closing and reopening of the collapsed lung regions. Recruitment strategies include pressure-controlled ventilation with an inspiratory pressure of 25 cm H_2O (should be less than 30 cm H_2O) and a positive end-expiratory pressure of 15 cm H_2O for a short interval (2 h) before turning to conventional volume-controlled ventilation with a tidal volume of 10 mL/kg and positive end-expiratory pressure (PEEP) of 5 cm H_2O. To prevent loss of alveolar recruitment, higher levels of PEEP should be used immediately after these maneuvers. Bronchoscopy should be routinely (6–8 h interval) performed on all potential lung donors to assess for airway damage and visible signs of infection. Regular suctioning of retained secretions through a closed ventilator circuit may be beneficial to improve gas exchange. Target ranges of partial pressure of oxygen and carbon dioxide in arterial blood (PaO_2 and $PaCO_2$) are 70–10 mmHg and 30–35 mmHg, respectively. To protect the lungs, inspired fraction in oxygen (FiO_2) should be kept as low as possible.

Postural change and air tract aspiration may cause hypotension due to a decrease in blood return to the heart in brain-dead persons. From these aspects, it is very important to stabilize hemodynamics by using ADH. If one side of the lung was not suitable to be transplanted due to pneumonia, the other side of the thorax is held up to prevent purulent sputa coming into the healthy lung.

2.3.3 Administration of ADH

Low-dose arginine vasopressin, in addition to treating diabetes insipidus, results in reduced inotropic requirements and has been associated with good kidney, liver, and heart graft function as shown previously. As ADH is also effective to improve vascular tone and BAR system, ADH should be given even in patients with low urine output. ADH may improve hemodynamics and renal function resulting in an increase in urine output as shown in patients with postcardiotomy or septic shock [35].

Desmopressin is beneficial primarily for the treatment of diabetes insipidus in organ donors and is not usually associated with the reduction of inotrope requirements [36]. Furthermore, there is one report indicating that desmopressin may be associated with a higher incidence of human pancreatic graft thrombosis [37].

ADH should be given through CVP line with a continuous dose of 0.01–0.02 U/Kg/h or 0.5–1 U/h after an initial bolus dose of 0.5–1 U [1, 24, 25]. If hemodynamics improves, NAD and then AD should be tapered off rapidly in favor of DOA or DOB [1, 24, 25]. If internal and external adrenaline approaches a normal range, heart rate is usually in a range of 90–120 beats/min. ADH should be given until cannulation of all procured organs become ready and heparin is given to keep stable hemodynamics during procurement operation [1].

Diabetes insipidus may cause high urine output, high serum sodium, low serum potassium, high serum osmolality, reduced circulatory blood volume, and reduced intracellular fluid, resulting in liver or renal dysfunction and arrhythmia. To prevent or treat these consequences, ADH administration is also important for donor management [1].

Adjustments of serum sodium (135–150 mEq/L) [38] and potassium (3.8–4.5 mEq/L), hematocrit (>30 %), blood sugar (120–180 mg/dL), and body temperature (35.5–36.5 °C) are also important.

References

1. Fukushima N, Ono M, Nakatani T, et al. Strategies for maximizing heart and lung transplantation opportunities in Japan. Transplant Proc. 2009;41(1):273–6.
2. Novitzky D, Cooper DK, Rosendale JD, Kauffman HM. Hormonal therapy of the brain-dead organ donor: experimental and clinical studies. Transplantation. 2006;82(11):1396–401.
3. Mascia L, Mastromauro I, Viverti S, et al. Management of optimize organ procurement in brain dead donors. Minerva Anestesiol. 2009;75:125–33.
4. Wood KE, Becker BN, McCartney JG, et al. Current concepts: care of potential organ donor. N Engl J Med. 2004;351:2730–9.
5. Wilhalem MJ, Pratschke J, Laskowski IA, et al. Brain death and its impact on the donor heart-lessons from animal models. J Heart Lung Transplant. 2000;19:414–8.

6. Audibert G, Charpentier C, Sequim-Devaux C, et al. Improvement of donor myocardial function after treatment of autonomic storm during brain death. Transplantation. 2006;82:1031–6.
7. Ryan JB, Hicks M, Cropper JR, et al. Functional evidence of reversible ischemic injury immediately after the sympathetic storm associated with experimental brain death. J Heart Lung Trasnplant. 2003;22:922–8.
8. Rosendale JD, Kauffman HM, McBride MA, et al. Hormonal resuscitation yields more transplanted hearts, with improved early function. Transplantation. 2003;5(8):1336–41.
9. Follette DM, Rudich SM, Babcock WD. Improved oxygenation and increased lung donor recovery with high-dose steroid administration after brain death. J Heart Lung Transplant. 1998;17:423–9.
10. Pennefether SH, Bullock RE, Mantle D, Dark JH. Use of low dose arginine vasopressin to support brain-dead organ donors. Transplantation. 1995;59:58.
11. Kinoshita Y, Okamoto K, Yahata K, et al. Clinical and pathological changes of the heart in brain death maintained with vasopressin and epinephrine. Pathol Res Pract. 1990;186(1):173–9.
12. Iwai A, Sakano T, Uenishi M, et al. Effects of vasopressin and catecholamines on the maintenance of circulatory stability in brain-dead patients. Transplantation. 1989;48(4):613–7.
13. Novitzky D, Wicomb WN, Cooper DKC, et al. Electrocardiographic, haemodynamic and endocrine changes occurring during experimental brain death in the chacma baboon. J Heart Transplant. 1984;4:63.
14. Wicomb WN, Cooper DKC, Lanza RP, et al. The effects of brain death and 24 hours storage by hypothermic perfusion on donor heart function in the pig. J Thorac Cardiovasc Surg. 1986;91:896.
15. Novitzky D, Wicomb WN, Cooper DKC, Tjaalgard MA. Improved cardiac function following hormonal therapy in brain dead pigs: relevance to organ donation. Cryobiology. 1987;24:1.
16. Kutsogiannis DJ, Pagliarello G, Doig C, Ross H, Shemie SD. Medical management to optimize donor organ potential: review of the literature. Can J Anaesth. 2006;53(8):820–30.
17. Powner DJ, Hendrich A, Lagler RG, et al. Hormonal changes in brain dead patients. Crit Care Med. 1990;18:785.
18. Gramm HJ, Meinhold H, Bickel U, et al. Acute endocrine failure after brain death? Transplantation. 1992;54:851.
19. Randell TT, Hockerstedt KAV. Triiodothyronine treatment in brain-dead multiorgan donors. Transplantation. 1992;54:736.
20. Goarin JP, Cohen S, Riou B, et al. The effects of triiodothyronine on hemodynamic status and cardiac function in potential heart donors. Anesth Analg. 1996;83:41.
21. Wheeldon DR, Potter CDO, Oduro A, et al. Transforming the "unacceptable" donor: outcomes from adoption of a standardized donor management technique. J Heart Lung Transplant. 1995;14:734.
22. Jeevanandam V. Triiodothyronine: spectrum of use in heart transplantation. Thyroid. 1997;7:139.
23. Salim A, Vassiliu P, Velmahos GC, et al. The role of thyroid hormone administration in potential organ donors. Arch Surg. 2001;136:1377–80.
24. Zaroff JG, Rosengard BR, Armstrong WF, et al. Consensus conference report: maximizing use of organs recovered from the cadaver donor: cardiac recommendations. Circulation. 2002;106:836.
25. Zaroff JG, Rosengard BR, Armstrong WF, et al. Maximizing use of organs recovered from the cadaver donor: cardiac recommendations. J Heart Lung Transplant. 2002;21:1153.
26. Keller F, Hemmen T, Schoneshofer M, et al. Pharmacokinetics of methylprednisolone and rejection episodes in kidney transplant patients. Transplantation. 1995;60:330.
27. Conci F, Di Rienzo M, Castiglioni P. Blood pressure and heart rate variability and baroreflex sensitivity before and after brain death. J Neurol Neurosurg Psychiatry. 2001;71:621–31.
28. Rapenne T, Moreau D, Lenfant F, Boggio V, Cottin Y, Freysz M, et al. Could heart rate variability analysis become an early predictor of imminent brain death? A pilot study. Anesth Analg. 2000;91:329–36.
29. Fukushima N, Shirakura R, Nakata S, et al. Failure of rapid autonomic augmentation of cardiac performance in transplanted hearts. Transplant Proc. 1998;30(7):3344–6. No abstract available.

30. D'Amico TA, Buchanan SA, Lucke JC, et al. The preservation of cardiac function after brain death: a myocardial pressure-dimension analysis. Surg Forum. 1990;41:277–9.
31. Sakagoshi N, Shirakura R, Nakano S, et al. Serial changes in myocardial beta-adrenergic receptor after experimental brain death in dogs. J Heart Lung Transplant. 1992;11:1054–8.
32. Fukushima N, Sakagoshi N, Ohtake S, et al. Effects of exogenous adrenaline on the number of the beta-adrenergic receptors after brain death in humans. Transplant Proc. 2002;34:2571–4.
33. Milano A, Livi U, Casula R, et al. Influence of marginal donors on early results after heart transplantation. Transplant Proc. 1993;25:3158.
34. Stoica SC, Satchithananda DK, Charman S, et al. Swan-Ganz catheter assessment of donor hearts: outcome of organs with borderline hemodynamics. J Heart Lung Transplant. 2002;21:615.
35. Ranger GS. Antidiuretic hormone replacement therapy to prevent or ameliorate vasodilatory shock. Med Hypotheses. 2002;59(3):337–40.
36. Guesde R, Barrou B, Leblanc I, et al. Administration of desmopressin in brain-dead donors and renal function in kidney patients. Lancet. 1998;352:1178.
37. Marques RG, Rogers J, Chavin KD, et al. Does treatment of cadaveric organ donors with desmopressin increase the likelihood of pancreas graft thrombosis? Results of a preliminary study. Transplant Proc. 2004;36:1048.
38. Hoefer D, Ruttmann-Ulmer E, Smits JM, Devries E, Antretter H, Laufer G. Donor hypo- and hypernatremia are predictors for increased 1-year mortality after cardiac transplantation. Transpl Int. 2010;23(6):589–93.

Part III
Heart Transplantation

Chapter 3
DCD for Heart Transplantation

Norihide Fukushima

3.1 Introduction

The history of human organ transplantation had begun in 1954 [1], when Joseph Murray, later a Nobel Laureate, and his team carried out a human organ transplant, taking a kidney from an identical twin. In 1962, Murray performed the first successful cadaveric kidney transplant [2]. In 1963, Starzl [3] achieved the first human liver transplant and Hardy [4] performed the first lung transplant. In those days, the surgical team brought a brain-dead donor into the operating room with the recipient for the removal; the respirator was then stopped, and everyone waited for the donor's heart to cease to beat. Technically, therefore, these donors were donation after cardiac death (DCD) donors.

Although this has not been well known by the general public as well as many physicians, the first heart transplantation (HTx) by Barnard [5] on 3 December 1967 was also performed from a DCD donor. A 54-year-old man dying of end-stage ischemic heart disease received the heart from a motor vehicle accident victim who had suffered severe brain injury. The donor's ventilator was switched off. Her heart would stop beating naturally from hypoxia within 10–12 min. She was certified dead 5 min upon absence of ECG activity, spontaneous respirations, and reflexes and placed on cardiopulmonary bypass, and the heart was resuscitated. The graft was perfused with the cardiopulmonary bypass machine in a fashion of Marcus' "interim parabiotic perfusion" technique and transplanted using a Lower–Shumway technique. The recipient, diabetic and undergoing treatment for *Pseudomonas* cellulitis of the legs, recovered, but died of *Pseudomonas* pneumonia after 18 days.

N. Fukushima (✉)
Department of Therapeutics for End-Stage Organ Dysfunction, Osaka University Graduate School of Medicine, 2-2 Yamada-oka, Suita, Osaka 565-0871, Japan
e-mail: nori@surg1.med.osaka-u.ac.jp

T. Asano et al. (eds.), *Marginal Donors: Current and Future Status*,
DOI 10.1007/978-4-431-54484-5_3, © Springer Japan 2014

On 6 January 1968, Shumway and Stinson et al. did the first heart transplantation from a controlled DCD donor. After the donor was diagnosed as brain dead by neurologists and declared dead, he was extubated and the heart was procured.

Until the first set of criteria for brain death (BD) was issued by the Ad Hoc Committee of the Harvard Medical School in July 1968 [6], many HTxs were performed from DCD donors. Even after the number of HTxs from brain-dead (BD) donor increased, outcomes of HTx had not been satisfactory until cyclosporine was introduced. However, as donor shortage from BD donors had been severe at that time, many investigators had studied HTx from DCD donors, but their results were poor. Then the number of animal experiments of HTx from DCD donors was gradually declined as BD donors increased after then.

In the late 1980s, Shirakura et al. [7, 8] and Gundry et al. [9] separately reported that administration of steroid, prostaglandin, and calcium blocker arrested the heart without ventricular fibrillation after asphyxia and that function of the cardiac graft transplanted from such a DCD donor was as good as that of heart-beating donor hearts. The author of this chapter had worked with these two investigators and studied HTx from DCD and multiple organ transplantation from DCD using percutaneous cardiopulmonary bypass (PCPS) [9] as described later in basic researches.

Finally three infant HTxs from DCD donors were preformed in Denver Children's Hospital between 2004 and 2006 [10]. This chapter would introduce the protocol of HTx from DCD donors as a representative protocol, because they were only the recent cases of HTxs from DCD donors in the world.

3.2 Donor Criteria

As the heart is very susceptible to warm ischemia, HTxs from DCD donors were only performed under Maastricht Category III (withdrawal of life-supporting therapy, the so-called controlled DCD). Before the donor's ventilator was discontinued, cardiac function was assessed carefully and donor care was provided under the direction of the intensive care team.

3.3 Harvest and Preservation [10]

The withdrawal of life-supporting ventilation is performed in the operating room by the intensivist and the primary nurse. The donor is prepared for surgery and monitored with the use of electrocardiography and pulse oximetry. The femoral venous and arterial sheaths are placed with the use of local anesthesia, and an initial heparin bolus of 100 U/kg of body weight is given intravenously. Comfort care is given by the intensive care team and included sedation and analgesia typical for withdrawal of life support: fentanyl at a mean dose of 4 μg/kg and lorazepam at a mean dose of 0.1 mg/kg.

Extubation is performed, followed by an additional intravenous dose of 300 U of heparin/kg. The attending physician in the critical care unit monitored the patient for evidence of cardiocirculatory function by means of auscultation and observation for arterial pulsation. When cardiocirculatory function ceased, the first patient was observed for 3 min before death was declared and the organ-donation process initiated.

On the basis of recommendations of the ethics committee, for the other two donors, the observation period was shortened to 1.25 min. If death occurs within 30 min after extubation, the patient is considered to be a candidate for donation, and cold preservation fluid (30–50 mL/kg) is infused through the distal port of a balloon arterial catheter placed in the ascending aorta. At the same time, a median sternotomy is performed, and topical cooling is begun. The inferior vena cava is immediately opened. In the second and third donors, venous-blood withdrawal was performed simultaneously with aortic infusion to prevent cardiac distention. After organ donation, the family of the donor was offered the choice of spending time with their child.

3.4 Viability Assay

Although several attempts of viability assay for cardiac graft from DCD donors have been studied, no viability assay has been used clinically yet.

In the future, there will be some possibilities to permit ex vivo donor heart assessment including identification of occult pathologic condition such as DCD donor hearts as well as donor coronary disease using ex vivo perfusion machine, such as the "Organ Care System" developed by the TransMedics company.

3.5 Outcomes of Infant HTx from DCD (Three Cases)

Orthotopic HTx involving donors who died from cardiocirculatory causes was performed in three recipients at a mean age of 2.2 months in Denver Children's Hospital [10]. The diagnosis leading to transplantation was complex congenital heart disease in two patients (one with a double-outlet right ventricle, transposition of the great vessels, a ventricular septal defect, and coarctation and the other with a hypoplastic left ventricle, mitral stenosis, aortic stenosis, and severely restricted atrial–septal communication) and, in the third patient, severe dilated cardiomyopathy requiring continuous intravenous inotropic support.

Time to cardiac arrest after withdrawal of life support was 18.3 ± 8.3 min, and total ischemic time was 162 ± 51 min. Although serum troponin I level increased after HTx, all three recipients survived more than 6 months (Table 3.1.).

Table 3.1 Characteristics of heart transplantation involving three DCD donors

Donor	Time to death after withdrawal of life support (min)	Total ischemic time (min)	Troponin I level before withdrawal of life support (in donor) (ng/mL)	Troponin I level after transplantation (in recipient) (ng/mL)	Recipient outcome at 6 months
1	11.5	221	0.2	30	Alive
2	27.5	127	0.5	23	Alive
3	16.0	139	0.3	127	Alive
	18.3 ± 8.3	162 ± 51	0.3 ± 0.2	60 ± 58	

Plus–minus values are means ± SD

3.6 Basic Research

3.6.1 *Animal Experiments of HTx from DCD Donors*

The myocardium of agonally arrested hearts is damaged by hypoxia during antemortem shock, anoxia during asphyxia, and warm ischemia from the moment of cardiac arrest until the initiation of preservation. To utilize an asphyxiated cadaver heart as a donor organ depends upon countering the several factors causing myocardial damage. A series of experimental studies were designed to establish the optimum method to preserve agonally arrested cadaver hearts for orthotopic HTx.

To protect the myocardium against agonal asphyxia and warm ischemia until cardiac arrest, donor animals were pretreated with 30 ng/kg of a prostacyclin analogue (OP41483; PGI2A), 0.05 mg/kg verapamil, and 0.05 mg/kg propranolol intravenously for 20 min [7]. Selective coronary perfusion was performed through an aortic balloon catheter placed in the aortic root prior to thoracotomy, a 10-min perfusion with warm blood cardioplegia to resuscitate the myocardium, previously described as the so-called warm induction and using cold crystalloid cardioplegia to minimize the warm ischemic time. These hearts were preserved in University of Wisconsin (UW) solution for 24 h and transplanted orthotopically. Prior to aortic unclamping, leukocyte-depleted terminal blood cardioplegia was given antegrade for about 10 min, as described previously.

In those studies all animals were weaned easily from cardiopulmonary bypass, and their hemodynamics were stable during the 1-h observation period following bypass without the use of catecholamine after orthotopic HTx. The left ventricular function after discontinuation of cardiopulmonary bypass was not different from that before asphyxia. The myocardial content of adenosine triphosphate (ATP) was restored by warm induction and terminal blood cardioplegia [7], which probably play a role in preserving cardiac function.

3.6.2 *Animal Experiments of Multiple Organ Procurement from DCD Donors Using PCPS*

Those methods to preserve the hearts were at the expense of other organs. Thus, we have also studied methods to reanimate and preserve multiple organs from asphyxiated DCD donors and have reported excellent graft function. In the previous series, the thoracotomy was made to measure cardiac function and to apply cardiopulmonary bypass, and the animals were exsanguinated during asphyxia.

In the clinical setting, no intervention that is not aimed to treat the patients can be done before cardiac arrest. Thus, thoracotomy or exsanguination cannot be done before cardiac arrest. In the present study, PCPS was applied to avoid thoracotomy, and no exsanguination was done during asphyxia until PCPS was started.

Thirteen beagles were used as donors and another 8 beagles as heart, 5 as lung, and 5 as kidney recipients [8]. The donor beagles were asphyxiated with pancuronium bromide with cessation of respiratory support after giving 30 ng/kg of prostacyclin analogue (OP41483; PGI2A), 0.05 mg/kg verapamil, 0.05 mg/kg propranolol, and 1 mg/kg nafamostat mesilate (FUT) intravenously for 20 min. All hearts were arrested within 20 min without ventricular fibrillation. The organs were kept in the dead body for 30 min, an interval established as the period likely to expire while the donor's family recognized the donor's death, took their farewell, and consented. Then perfusion and drainage cannulae were inserted into the femoral artery and vein: the total body was reperfused by PCPS at a perfusion flow of 100 mL/kg/min and at perfusion blood temperature of 26 °C for 1 h, which was accepted as the time for the donor to be transported to the operating room and prepared for harvesting.

Priming fluid for PCPS consisted of the four drugs mentioned above and 30 mL/L of KCl to produce cardiac arrest. The serum potassium level was kept at about 8 mEq/L by continuous administration of KCl. After 40 min of perfusion using PCPS, a bilateral horizontal thoracotomy was performed through the fourth intercostal space. After placing perfusion cannulae into the aortic root and the pulmonary trunk, PCPS was stopped. The donor hearts and lungs were perfused with cold crystalloid cardioplegia (ROE solution; 10 mL/kg) and modified Collins solution (MCS; 20 mL/kg), respectively, after clamping the ascending aorta. The heart and the left lung were excised. The abdominal organs were perfused with UW solution (50 mL/L) through a cannula placed in the femoral artery at a pressure of 40 mmHg, and the right kidney was excised.

The eight donor hearts were immersed in UW solution for 24 h and transplanted orthotopically through the left thoracotomy as previously described. The heart was reperfused with leukocyte-depleted blood cardioplegia (60 mL/kg) prior to aortic unclamping, as shown previously, which contained 600 ng/L of PGI2A to reduce reperfusion injury. The five left donor lungs were immersed in modified MCS prior to orthotopic transplantation. After placing the blood sampling tube into the pulmonary veins of the right recipient lung and the donor lung, the chest was closed in the usual fashion. Oxygen saturation levels of the pulmonary veins were measured daily after transplantation. The three kidneys were immersed in UW solution and transplanted heterotopically in the left groin. After placing the urine sampling tube, the groin was closed.

During pretreatment, no changes in heart rate and blood pressure were observed. All transplanted hearts beat spontaneously after aortic unclamping. All heart recipients could be weaned from cardiopulmonary bypass without any intravenous catecholamine; the chest was closed under stable hemodynamic condition for more than 6 h. The procured hearts showed no intracellular edema or myocyte necrosis. In lung-recipient animals, the oxygen and carbon dioxide pressures of pulmonary vein blood from the donor lung were not different from those of the recipient (control) right lung. All animals survived until the lung was rejected. The procured lung showed no intracellular edema histologically. All transplanted kidneys made urine soon after reperfusion, with more than 1 mL/kg/h of urine output. Creatinine clearance of the donor kidney was 120 ± 21 mg/mL/min.

References

1. Merrill JP, Murray JE, Harrison JH, Guild WR. Successful homotransplantations of the human kidney between identical twins. JAMA. 1956;160:277–82.
2. Merrill JP, Murray JE, Takacs FJ, Harger EB, Wilson RE, Dammin GJ. Successful transplantation of kidney from a human cadaver. JAMA. 1963;185:347–53.
3. Starzl TE, Marchioro TL, Vonkaulla KN, Hermann G, Brittain RS, Waddell WR. Homotransplantation of the liver in humans. Surg Gynecol Obstet. 1963;117:659–76.
4. Hardy JD, Webb WR, Dalton Jr ML, Walker Jr GR. Lung homotransplantations in man. JAMA. 1963;186:1065–74.
5. Barnard CN. The operation. A human cardiac transplant: an interim report of a successful operation performed at Groote Schuur Hospital, Cape Town. S Afr Med J. 1967;41:1271–4.
6. Ad Hoc Committee. A definition of irreversible coma. Report of the Ad Hoc Committee of the Harvard Medical School to examine the definition of brain death. JAMA. 1968;205:337–40.
7. Shirakura R, Matsuda H, Nakano S, et al. Cardiac function and myocardial performance of 24-hour-preserved asphyxiated canine hearts. Ann Thorac Surg. 1992;53:440–4.
8. Fukushima N, Shirakura R, Ohtake S, et al. Studies of the multiorgan procurement system from non-heart-beating donors. Transplant Proc. 2000;32(2):281–4.
9. Gundry SR, Fukushima N, Eke CC, Hill AC, Zuppan C, Bailey LL. Successful survival of primates receiving transplantation with "dead", nonbeating donor hearts. J Thorac Cardiovasc Surg. 1995;109:1097–102.
10. Boucek MM, Mashburn C, Dunn S, et al. Pediatric heart transplantation after declaration of cardiocirculatory death. N Engl J Med. 2008;359(7):709–14.

Chapter 4
ECD for Heart Transplantation

Norihide Fukushima

4.1 Introduction

In October 1997, the Japanese Organ Transplant Act was issued and we needed to successfully start the first heart transplantation (HTx) in Japan. For this reason, very strict criteria for the donor heart were established by the task force committee for heart transplantation in the Ministry of Health, Labour and Welfare. These criteria were comparable to the so-called standard criteria for the donor heart in the world.

On February 28, 1999, the first HTx was successfully performed in Japan [1] and 127 HTx were done up to the end of August 2012. Although many efforts to shorten the transportation time of the heart were done, mean transportation and total ischemic time (TIT) were about 2 and 3 h, respectively. On the other hand, as the Japanese Organ Transplant Act was very strict, brain-dead organ donation was extremely limited in Japan and only 184 brain-dead donors were available for 13 years after the Act was issued. In order to respond to the will of the donor and donor families, we needed to transplant the heart as much as possible. For these reasons, more hearts should be transplanted from the extended criteria donor (ECD) in Japan than other developed countries.

Since brain-dead organ transplantation was started in 1999, every organ procurement team has taken their own skillful physicians to the procurement hospital [2]. They evaluated the condition of donor organs by echocardiography and flexible bronchofiberscopy (BFS) by themselves in the intensive care unit (ICU), before procurement operation [2].

Since November of 2002, special transplant management doctors (a medical consultant, MC) have been sent to the procurement hospital. They assessed donor organ function and identified which organs were useful for transplantation.

N. Fukushima (✉)
Department of Therapeutics for End-Stage Organ Dysfunction, Osaka University Graduate School of Medicine, Suita, Osaka, Japan
e-mail: nori@surg1.med.osaka-u.ac.jp

T. Asano et al. (eds.), *Marginal Donors: Current and Future Status*,
DOI 10.1007/978-4-431-54484-5_4, © Springer Japan 2014

They also intensively cared for the donor, stabilized the donor hemodynamics by giving antidiuretic hormone (ADH) and reducing the dose of intravenous catecholamine as much as possible, and improved donor cardiac and lung function by preventing and treating lung infection before procurement teams arrived at the donor hospital.

Out of 184 brain-dead donors, 136 heart, 1 heart–lung, 143 lung, 159 liver, 1,311 pancreas, and 12 small bowel transplants were performed. Organs transplanted per one donor (OTPD) increased to 5.5 organs after these strategies were applied.

Although 83 of 136 heart donors were ECD, no recipient died of primary graft dysfunction (PGD).

4.2 Definition

Extended donor criteria are shown in Table 4.1.

4.2.1 Heart Injury

Donor hearts are injured in great or lesser degree, by many causes, such as catecholamine storm at the completion of brain death, cardiac arrest, thoracic trauma, and maneuver of the cardiopulmonary resuscitation (CPR).

As the patients with brain injury are kept in dry condition to prevent brain edema, the heart looks hyperdynamic. To evaluate precise cardiac systolic function, central

Table 4.1 Extended criteria donor (ECD) for heart transplantation

Myocardial injury and/or underlying heart disease
Correctable valvular dysfunction or congenital heart anomaly by echocardiography (without history of open heart surgery)
Injury of the heart (history of chest trauma, open cardiac massage)
Cardiac arrest with cardiopulmonary resuscitation (>5 min)
High-dose catecholamine requirement (dopamine >15 μg/kg/min)
Left ventricular hypertrophy (wall thickness >15 mm)
Prolonged total ischemic time (>4 h)
Old age
>55 years(especially without coronary angiography)
Bypassable one- or two-vessel coronary arterial disease
Body and gender mismatch
Undersizing or oversizing by more than 20 % body weight
Female to male (especially undersized donor by more than 20 % body weight)
Infection
Local bacterial infection
Bacteremia

venous pressure at the time of evaluation should be 8–10 mmHg. It is also important to adjust hemoglobin concentration, electrolyte balance, and acid–base equilibrium.

As Swan–Ganz catheterization or coronary angiography is not performed in procurement hospitals in Japan, heart injury and underlying heart diseases are determined by evaluating hemodynamics and the dose of catecholamine and ADH injection and the wall motion and morphology by echocardiography and electrocardiogram (ECG).

As the detail was shown in the chapter "Management of Extended Criteria Donors," it is very important to evaluate donor heart function after treating diabetes insipidus, adjusting the tone of peripheral vessels and recovering the affinity of β-adrenergic receptor for adrenaline (AD) in the heart by continuously intravenous infusion of ADH [2].

As serum adrenaline reduces the density of β-adrenergic receptor [2], adrenaline should be pused as less as possible. With regard to the dose of catecholamine, less than 15 mcg/kg/min of dopamine (DOA) is acceptable.

The heart with a history of cardiac arrest with CPR can be transplanted if the cardiac function is recovered and the heart has no significant underlying disease [2, 3].

4.2.2 Underlying Heart Disease

The presence of most valvular and congenital cardiac abnormalities is a contraindication to transplantation. Therefore, the underlying heart diseases should be carefully evaluated by the echocardiogram before harvesting.

In some cases, however, "bench" repair can be performed on a donor heart with simple congenital heart disease, such as atrial septal defect, ventricular septal defect, or patent ductus arteriosus, mild or moderate mitral or tricuspid regurgitation, or other mild valvular abnormalities, such as a normally functioning bicuspid aortic valve, if the heart function is acceptable by the echocardiogram.

As the hypertrophic left ventricle (ventricular wall thickness >15 mm) is susceptible to ischemia, the use of the heart should be decided carefully. Transplantation is inadvisable if echocardiographic (>15 mm) and ECG criteria for LVH are present and TIT is longer than 4 h.

4.2.3 Total Ischemic Time

There was reported to be a significant correlation between the TIT and the early posttransplant death after HTx. The acceptable safe preservation time for HTx has been considered to be 4 h. In fact, the report of the International Society for Heart and Lung Transplantation (ISHLT) showed that the relative risk of 1 year mortality was affected by TIT longer than 6 h [4] (Fig. 4.1). However, pediatric hearts with TIT longer than 8 h were reported to be safely transplanted [3].

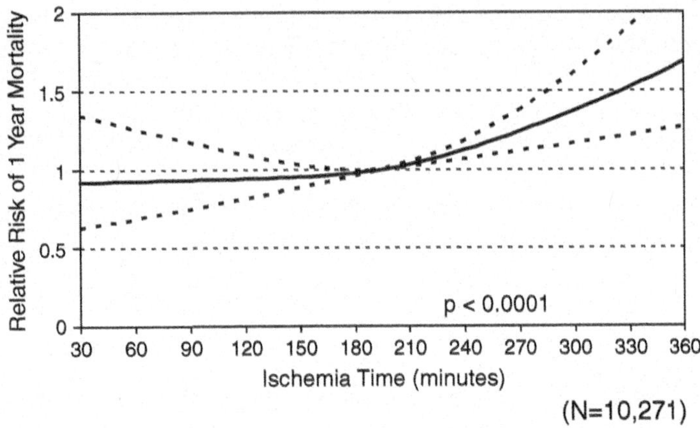

Fig. 4.1 Adult heart transplants (1/2004–6/2009). Relative risk of 1 year mortality with 95 % confidence limits with respect to ischemia time

In order to prolong safe ischemic time, many investigations were done. The author of this chapter reported that the modification of preservation solution and the application of terminal leukocyte-depleted blood cardioplegia enabled 24 h heart transplantation in large animals [5].

4.2.4 *Old Age*

As older persons have more risks of having damaged myocardium by coronary atherosclerosis, cardiac hypertrophy, and valvular disease than younger ones, older donors were generally considered to be ECD. In fact, mortalities at 1 and 5 years are affected to a great degree by donor age (Fig. 4.2) [4]. Moreover, the relative risk of developing cardiac allograft vasculopathy (CAV) within 8 years is also affected by donor age (Fig. 4.3) [4]. Therefore, in an older donor, coronary angiography and careful echocardiography are essential.

Although coronary arterial revascularization procedures can be performed in the recipient subsequently [6], little has been reported so far on the systematic use of donor hearts with significant coronary artery disease (CAD). In 59 % of those recipients [7], simultaneous bypass grafting of donor vessels was performed backtable at the time of heart transplantation using recipient conduits, mostly saphenous vein, but rarely the left anterior descending artery. Besides the reported favorable intermediate-term results with regard to survival, overall graft patency at 2 years was 82 %. One may consider brain death as a stress test such that if subsequent ECG or echocardiography is favorable, the chance of an older donor having CAD is probably low. This screening strategy without the use of coronary angiography is thought

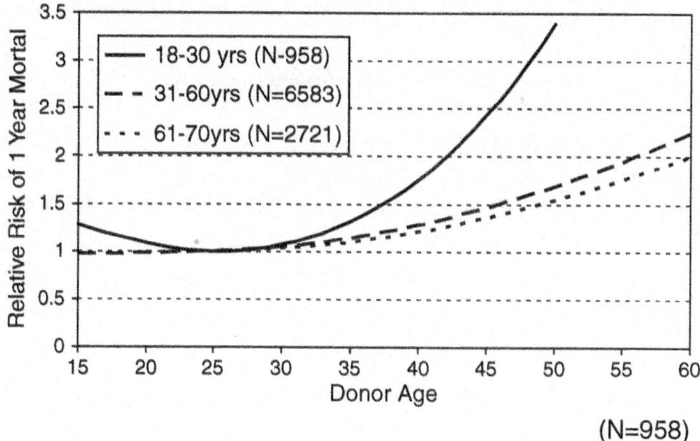

Fig. 4.2 Adult heart transplants (1/2004–6/2009). Relative risk of 1 year mortality with 95 % confidence limits with respect to donor age

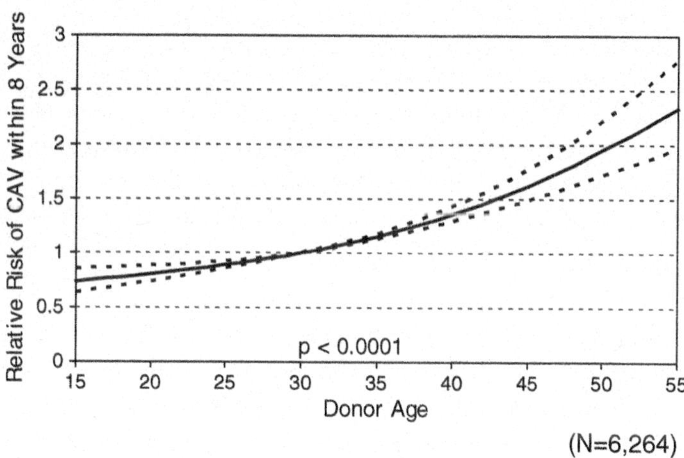

Fig. 4.3 Adult heart transplants (1/1998–6/2002). Relative risk of developing cardiac allograft vasculopathy within 8 years conditional on survival to transplant discharge with respect to donor age

to enable efficient selection of older donors for hearts [7] with the understanding that the additional presence of LVH including ECG changes generally precludes the use of such donor hearts.

4.2.5 Body Size and Gender

Despite an increased risk associated with small donor size relative to the recipient, a normal-sized adult male is considered to be suitable for most recipients. In the specific case of a small donor, size matching with body mass index or height is more accurate than weight matching, but generally undersized hearts have been used successfully with excellent long-term outcomes. Although recipient obesity is known to have an adverse effect on survival, extended donor weight above 90 kg represents also an independent risk factor for the recipient's late death. A recipient-oriented and much individualized assessment process is very important when accepting organ offers, especially from marginal donors.

Consistent with previous studies, we demonstrate that transplanting a female donor heart into a male recipient is associated with significantly higher risk of PGD [8]. On the other hand, the risk of CAV universally increased with increasing donor age (Fig. 4.3). However, recipients of male allografts had an increased risk of CAV development, regardless of the recipient's gender.

4.2.6 Infection

With regard to bacterial or yeast infection, sepsis and infectious vegetations in the heart are contraindications for the heart donor. It was reported that despite high donor organ contamination (DOC) rates, posttransplant infections due to DOC were rare under the condition of adequate preoperative antibiotic prophylaxis and aseptic organ retrievement [9]. The heart from a donor with positive blood culture without any signs of sepsis can be transplanted, if the bacteria are proved to be Gram-positive cocci and sensitive to common antibiotics.

With regard to virus infection, seropositivity against HIV, HTLV-1, and HBV surface antigen is contraindication for the heart donor. The transplantation of donor hearts with HBV core antibody is associated with a small risk of virus transmission. The use of these hearts has the potential to safely expand the current donor pool [10].

As nearly all recipients of kidney transplants from HCV-positive donors became infected with the virus, many thoracic transplant centers do not accept HCV-positive donors as seroconversion also occurs following HTx of infected organs. The transplantation of HCV-positive grafts to HCV-positive recipients is undesirable for two specific reasons: firstly, there is more than one strain of hepatitis C virus, and, secondly, the prevalence of antiviral antibody does not guarantee immediate immunity.

4.3 Viability Assay

The real goal of donor heart assessment is not to estimate the functional status of the heart just before organ harvesting but rather to predict the performance of the transplanted graft after weaning from the extracorporeal circulation and in the postoperative period. One also has to take into account the cumulative injury by "preexisting damage" of the donor heart and "brain-death-related stress."

4.3.1 Hemodynamic Assessment Before and After Brain Death

For the hemodynamic assessment as well as for the appropriate management of the donor with regard to the cause of brain death, the clinical course and pathophysiology of brain death, past history of heart disease, treatment of the patients, especially doses of inotropes [DOA, dobutamine (DOB), AD, and noradrenaline (NAD)], ADH, other pituitary hormones, and antibiotics, fluid intake and transfusion, urine output, and hemodynamic parameters, such as mean arterial pressure (MAP), preload and afterload [CVP, PCWP/LAP, pulmonary arterial pressure (PA)], cardiac output, and/or mixed-venous oxygen saturation, are required.

Multicenter analysis (1,719 consecutive primary HTx) reported that donor hearts requiring inotropic support of up to 6 μg/kg/min of DOA or DOB can be accepted as the so-called marginal grafts had acceptable outcome [11]. Even if the donor has a history of cardiopulmonary resuscitation longer than 5 min, the heart might be eligible for transplantation, if hemodynamics, cardiac function, wall motion of left ventricle, and ischemic changes in ECG are restored under optimal donor management [12].

4.3.2 Chest X-Ray

Cardiomegaly, chest trauma, or pleural effusions are checked by chest X-ray.

4.3.3 Electrocardiogram

As most BD donors have some degree of myocardial insufficiency caused by combined preexisting and brain-death-induced damage, ECG usually shows abnormality in ST segments and QRS wave. Sustained abnormalities in ST segments and QRS and multifocal ventricular ectopic beats under optimal donor management are considerably high risks.

4.3.4 Echocardiography

Echocardiography allows reliable assessment of cardiac valve function and myocardial hypertrophy as well as the verification/exclusion of congenital malformations. As global and even regional ventricular dysfunction may be brain death induced and these wall motion abnormalities may be reversible within hours, serial echocardiography is required before a graft is rejected because of myocardial dysfunction.

In the presence of LV underfilling, LV seems to be hypertrophic or to have suitable LV systolic function. Therefore, circulatory blood should be estimated by CVP, PCWP, or the size and respiratory movement of the inferior vena cava (IVC) as well as doses of inotropes prior to undergoing echocardiography to assess cardiac function.

4.3.5 Coronary Angiography

As asymptomatic coronary atherosclerosis is common even in children and young people, coronary angiography, at least in donors older than 40 years or according to the anamnesis and/or risk factors, should be performed in Western countries. However, up until now there is no evidence which kind or degree of transmitted coronary atherosclerosis really impairs the posttransplant outcome since angiography in donors younger than 60 years has been regarded as unnecessary. Of course, recent infarction and diffuse coronary sclerosis are contraindications without any doubt, but a single stenosis with good performance of the dependent myocardial area seems to be acceptable [13], especially if it is treated interventionally during donor angiography or by concomitant bypass surgery during transplantation [14].

In the future, contrast CT scan, especially cardiac CT scan, might be useful to rule out coronary arterial disease in the donor heart.

4.4 Outcome

Outcomes of HTx from ECDs in the world were already presented in each category.

Here, outcomes of HTx from all 200 consecutive brain-dead donors since the Japanese Organ Transplantation Act was issued on October 17, 1997 until November 25, 2012 were reviewed. Seventy donors were male. The mean age of the donors was 45.1 years. The cause of brain death was 119 in cerebral stroke (91 in subarachnoid hemorrhage, 7 in cerebral infarction, and 21 in cerebral bleeding), 37 in head trauma, 27 in asphyxia, and 17 in brain injury after cardiopulmonary resuscitation.

From these BD donors, 146 HTx and 1 heart–lung Tx (HLTx) were performed (heart transplanted rate was 73.5 %). One hundred and eight recipients were male. The age at HTx was 37.5 ± 12.9 years. The underlying disease of HTx was dilated cardiomyopathy in 100 patients, dilated phase hypertrophic cardiomyopathy in 14, restrictive cardiomyopathy in 3, secondary cardiomyopathy in 14, ischemic cardiomyopathy in 14, and congenital heart disease in 1 and that of HLTx was Eisenmenger syndrome with double outlet right ventricle. One hundred and thirty-one patients were implanted left ventricular assist device (LVAD) for bridge to HTx. The waiting time for HTx was 182–2,872 days (a mean of 956 days), and support days with LVAD were 29–1,607 days (a mean of 864 days). With regard to donors for HTx, age at donation was 42.3 ± 12.9 years and 86 were male. The cause of brain death was 84 in cerebral stroke (67 in subarachnoid hemorrhage, 4 in cerebral infarction, and 13 in cerebral bleeding), 31 in head trauma, 22 in asphyxia, and 10 in brain injury after cardiopulmonary resuscitation. Twenty-seven donors were older than 55 years old. Fifty-seven had a history of cardiopulmonary resuscitation longer than 5 min. Sixty-three required inotropic support of up to 10 μg/kg/min of DOA or DOB or AD/NAD.

None of the 146 heart Tx recipients died of PGD. Patient survival rate after heart Tx was 92.3 % at 10 years.

4.5 Basic Research

4.5.1 Preharvest Management of the Donor

Nilsson et al. [15] showed that glycogen stores in the hearts of brain-dead pigs could be boosted by administration of a glucose–insulin–potassium (GIK) infusion. Wheeldon et al. [16] have shown that replacement of thyroid hormone, adrenal corticosteroids, and insulin significantly improves the state and function of donor organs including the heart. The use of this aggressive treatment of marginal donors can increase the number of acceptable donor organs. A recent consensus meeting has recommended the use of a uniform and aggressive donor management procedure [17].

4.5.2 Interfering with NF-κB Signalling Pathways

Many drugs familiar to clinicians act on the NF-κB pathway. For instance, cyclosporine inhibits the enzymes involved in the early activation of NF-κB, its final cytoplasmic activation step, and its action within the nucleus. Aspirin and sulfasalazine also act at several levels to inhibit NF-κB [18]. Although these simple drugs have additional actions, they, or more selective derivatives, have a real potential to play a crucial role in future treatment of the donor and the donor organs by diminishing the inflammatory response initiated by NF-κB signalling. Sakaguchi et al. showed that gene transfection of the NF-κB decoy attenuated ischemia–reperfusion injury after prolonged heart preservation in a rat model [19].

4.5.3 Preservation Solutions

Preservation solutions are formulated to counteract the effects of perturbation of ion homeostasis. Table 4.2 shows the composition of the commonly used preservation

Table 4.2 Standard preservation solutions

Component	UW	EC	HTK	Celsior	Stanford	STHS
Ionic composition						
Na^+ (mmol/L)	30	10	10	100	25	120
K^+ (mmol/L)	120	115	10	15	30	16
Cl^- (mmol/L)	0	15	50	41.5	30	203
Mg^{2+} (mmol/L)	5	0	4	13	0	16
Ca^{2+} (mmol/L)	0	0	0.015	0.25	0	1.2
pH	7.4	7.45	7.2	7.3	8.1–8.4	7.8
Osm (mOsm/L)	320	406	310	360	440	324
Impermeants						
Lactobionate (mmol/L)	100	0	0	80	0	0
Raffinose (mmol/L)	30	0	0	0	0	0
Hydroxyethyl starch (g/L)	50	0	0	0	0	0
Mannitol (mmol/L)	0	0	30	60	12.5	0
Metabolic agents						
Glucose (mmol/L)	0	198	0	0	50	0
Adenosine (mmol/L)	5	0	0	0	0	0
Glutamate (mmol/L)	0	0	0	20	0	0
Ketoglutarate (mmol/L)	0	0	1	0	0	0
Tryptophan (mmol/L)	0	0	2	0	0	0
Buffers						
Phosphate buffer (mmol/L)	25	100	0	0	0	0
Bicarbonate buffer (mmol/L)	0	10	0	0	25	10
Histidine buffer (mmol/L)	0	0	180	30	0	0
Antioxidants						
Glutathione (mmol/L)	2	0	0	3	0	0
Allopurinol (mmol/L)	1	0	0	0	0	0

UWS University of Wisconsin solution, *EC* Eurocollins solution, *HTK* Brettschneider's histidine–tryptophan–ketoglutarate solution, *STHS* St. Thomas' Hospital solution, *Osm* osmolarity

solutions. "Extracellular" and "intracellular" solutions differ in their concentrations of Na^+ and K^+ ions. "Intracellular" solutions abolish the ionic gradients responsible for passive exchanger activity. However, several studies have shown that high potassium levels in cardioplegic solutions used during standard cardiac surgery have damaging effects on the endothelium.

Impermeants and oncotic agents play a key role in preservation solutions that include them. Molecules that are able to escape from the vascular bed but are unable to enter the cell will counteract intracellular edema and are known as impermeants. Edema places stress upon the cytoskeleton and makes the cell vulnerable to structural failure at reperfusion. Impermeants include raffinose (a trisaccharide) and lactobionate. The omission of lactobionate from University of Wisconsin solution (UWS) results in significant deterioration in stored organs and poor recovery after reperfusion. Celsior solution contains lactobionate on the basis of this observation. Mannitol is an effective oncotic agent that is a potent free radical scavenger. HTK, Celsior, and Stanford solutions contain mannitol.

The inclusion of antioxidants in preservation solutions is a useful protective strategy that can introduce free radical damage. Allopurinol is an inhibitor of the xanthine oxidase enzyme and has been incorporated into UWS. Histidine, a component of Celsior and HTK solutions, reacts with hydrogen peroxide and reduces the formation of hydroxyl radicals produced by the Fenton reaction. UWS and Celsior contain glutathione that may benefit antioxidant capacity; however, with shelf storage glutathione may become oxidized, ineffective, and potentially harmful.

4.5.4 Continuous Perfusion of the Explanted Donor Heart

Continuous perfusion has been employed in donor kidneys since the 1960s. Similar techniques have been employed in experimental heart transplantation. Experimentally, normothermic perfusion has been studied in heart as well as many organs. Normothermic perfusion enables successful transplantation of organs after ischemic damage that would be incompatible with cold preservation at 120 min warm ischemia of the canine kidney, 60 min warm ischemia of the porcine liver, and 65 min warm ischemia in porcine lung transplantation.

To date the only uses of normothermic perfusion in a clinical environment have been in the heart and lung transplantation. Approximately 80 clinical heart transplants have been carried out worldwide using the "Organ Care System" developed by the TransMedics company [20], which has been shown to be safe and effective; it also permits ex vivo donor heart assessment including identification of occult pathologic condition such as donor coronary disease.

4.5.5 Reperfusion Conditions

The ischemic conditions prevailing during the preservation phase of donor heart retrieval predispose the heart to significant injury by white blood cells when the heart receives blood during reperfusion. Therefore, the removal of the white cells responsible for causing this damage may reduce the severity of reperfusion injury. Short ischemic times seem to result in less benefit from leukocyte depletion [21]. Pearl et al. [22] have demonstrated in a clinical trial in heart transplant patients reductions in coronary sinus levels of markers of myocardial cell damage (CK-MB, lactate), mediators of reperfusion injury (thromboxane B2), and a reduction in histological signs of reperfusion injury.

Recent studies of cardiac injury have measured levels of cytokines as an index of leukocyte-induced inflammation within the heart. Several studies carried out on standard cardiac surgery patients have revealed a clinical benefit of leukocyte depletion in terminal blood cardioplegia [23]. A reduced period on ventilators in ICU and reduced length of hospital stay have been reported [23], suggesting a reduced incidence of graft injury, better performance, and reduced damage downstream from the heart, especially in the lungs. In animal experiments, leukocyte-depleted terminal blood cardioplegia (LDTC) prolonged the safe preservation period up to 24 h [5, 24]. In the clinical setting, we started HTx program using LDTC for reperfusion of the donor heart resulting in successful outcomes [25].

References

1. Matsuda H, Fukushima N, Sawa Y, Nishimura M, Matsumiya G, Shirakura R. First brain dead donor heart transplantation under new legislation in Japan. Jpn J Thorac Cardiovasc Surg. 1999;47:499–505.
2. Fukushima N, Ono M, Nakatani T, et al. Strategies for maximizing heart and lung transplantation opportunities in Japan. Transplant Proc. 2009;41(1):273–6.
3. Bailey LL, Razzouk AJ, Hasaniya NW, Chinnock RE. Pediatric transplantation using hearts refused on the basis of donor quality. Ann Thorac Surg. 2009;87(6):1902–8. discussion 1908–9.
4. Stehlik J, Edwards LB, Kucheryavaya AY, et al. The Registry of the International Society for heart and lung transplantation: twenty-eighth official adult heart transplant report–2011. J Heart Lung Transplant. 2011;30(10):1071–132.
5. Fukushima N, Shirakura R, Nakata S, et al. Study of efficacies of leukocyte-depleted terminal blood cardioplegia in 24-hour preserved hearts. Ann Thorac Surg. 1994;58(6):1651–6.
6. Laks H, Gates RN, Ardehali A, et al. Orthotopic heart transplantation and concurrent coronary bypass. J Heart Lung Transplant. 1993;12:810–5.
7. Marelli D, Laks H, Bresson S, et al. Results after transplantation using donor hearts with preexisting coronary artery disease. J Thorac Cardiovasc Surg. 2003;126:821.
8. Russo MJ, Iribarne A, Hong KN, et al. Factors associated with primary graft failure after heart transplantation. Transplantation. 2010;90(4):444–50.
9. Mattner F, Kola A, Fischer S, et al. Impact of bacterial and fungal donor organ contamination in lung, heart–lung, heart and liver transplantation. Infection. 2008;36:207–12.
10. Pinney SP, Cheema FH, Hammond K, et al. Acceptable recipient outcomes with the use of hearts from donors with hepatitis-B core antibodies. J Heart Lung Transplant. 2005;24:34–7.
11. Grauhan O. Screening and assessment of the donor heart. Cardiopulm Pathophysiol. 2011;15:191–7.
12. Young JB, Naftel DC, Bourge RC, et al. Matching the heart donor and heart transplant recipient. Clues for successful expansion of the donor pool: a multivariable, multiinstitutional report. The Cardiac Transplant Research Database Group. J Heart Lung Transplant. 1994;13:353–65.
13. Grauhan O, Siniawski H, Dandel M, et al. Coronary atherosclerosis of the donor heart: impact on early graft failure. Eur J Cardiothorac Surg. 2007;32(4):634–8.
14. Musci M, Pasic M, Grauhan O, et al. Orthotopic heart transplantation with concurrent coronary artery bypass grafting or previous stent implantation. Z Kardiol. 2004;93:971–4.
15. Nilsson B, Berggren H, Ekroth R, et al. Glucose-insulin-potassium (GIK) prevents derangement of myocardial metabolism in brain-dead pigs. Eur J Cardiothorac Surg. 1994;8(8): 442–6.
16. Wheeldon DR, Potter CD, Odura A, Wallwork J, Large SR. Transforming the "unacceptable" donor: outcomes from the adoption of a standardized donor management technique. J Heart Lung Transplant. 1995;14(4):734–42.
17. Zaroff JG, Rosengard B, Armstrong WF, et al. Maximizing use of organs recovered from the cadaver donor: cardiac recommendations. (Consensus Conference Report, March 28–29, 2001, Crystal City). J Heart Lung Transplant. 2002;21(11):1153–60.
18. Epinat JC, Gilmore TD. Diverse agents act at multiple levels to inhibit the Rel/NF-Kappa B signal transduction pathway. Oncogene. 1999;18:6896–909.

19. Sakaguchi T, Sawa Y, Fukushima N, et al. A novel strategy of decoy transfection against nuclear factor-kappaB in myocardial preservation. Ann Thorac Surg. 2001;71(2):624–9. discussion 629–30.
20. Reddy SP, Brockmann J, Friend PJ. Normothermic perfusion: a mini-review. Transplantation. 2009;87:631–2.
21. Sawa Y, Taniguchi K, Kadoba K, Nishimura M, et al. Leukocyte depletion attenuates reperfusion injury in patients with left ventricular hypertrophy. Circulation. 1996;93(9):1640–6.
22. Pearl J, Drinkwater DC, Laks H, Capouya ER, Gates RN. Leukocyte depleted reperfusion of transplanted human hearts: a randomized, double blind clinical trial. J Heart Lung Transplant. 1992;11:1082–92.
23. Sawa Y, Matsuda H, Shimazaki T, Kaneko M, Nishimura M, Amemiya A, et al. Evaluation of leukocyte depleted terminal blood cardioplegic solution in patients undergoing elective and emergency coronary artery bypass grafting. J Thorac Cardiovasc Surg. 1994;108(6):1125–31.
24. Fukushima N, Shirakura R, Nakata S, et al. Effects of terminal cardioplegia with leukocyte-depleted blood on heart grafts preserved for 24 hours. J Heart Lung Transplant. 1992;11 (4 Pt 1):676–82.
25. Fukushima N, Miyamoto Y, Ohtake S, et al. Early result of heart transplantation in Japan: Osaka University experience. Asian Cardiovasc Thorac Ann. 2004;12(2):154–8.

Part IV
Lung Transplantation

Chapter 5
How to Initiate DCD Program for Lung Transplantation

Stig Steen

5.1 Introduction

Each year more than 10,000 die in Sweden after cardiac arrest, and it has been estimated that 600,000 die yearly due to cardiac arrest in Europe and the USA, almost all out of hospital [1]. In the 1990s we began a research project to study the pathophysiology and treatment of cardiac arrest; if the best treatment cannot save a victim of cardiac arrest, would it be possible to find an ethically acceptable method to resuscitate and preserve the lungs for transplantation, under the precondition that this was the will or not against the presumed will of the victim?

5.2 Realistic Animal Experiments

An absolutely reliable way of demonstrating the efficacy of resuscitation and preservation of lung function in a DCD donor is an experimental setup in which the recipient animal is totally dependent for its survival on the function of the preserved and transplanted lung tissue. Only two models satisfy this strict criterion of testing: double-lung transplantation and single-lung transplantation followed by contralateral pneumonectomy. Of these two models, we decided to use only the latter, since that model yields the strongest evidence of excellent preservation, if the contralateral pneumonectomy can be performed without negative effects on respiratory or hemodynamic variables. We have used 60-kg pigs, which have a thorax of similar size as that of an adult human being. The size of the thorax is important when a DCD lung is studied, since big lungs take longer time to cool. Left lung transplantation is done with the donor lung to be tested, followed by right pneumonectomy.

S. Steen (✉)
Lund University, Igelösa 373, SE-225 94 Lund, Sweden
e-mail: stig.steen@med.lu.se

T. Asano et al. (eds.), *Marginal Donors: Current and Future Status*,
DOI 10.1007/978-4-431-54484-5_5,

The recipient pig is monitored for at least 24 h. Blood gases and hemodynamic parameters are compared to healthy pigs of similar size in which only right pneumonectomy has been done. Important findings with this model with relevance for lung DCD are presented in [2–4]. In the 1990s we also developed a method for evaluation of lung function ex vivo, because we thought it impossible to get an ethical permission to start a clinical uncontrolled lung DCD study without it. No medical journal agreed to publish this ex vivo lung evaluation method until it had been successfully used on a patient, but then a detailed description of the method was published in The Annals of Thoracic Surgery [5]. We also studied the endothelial function of the pulmonary artery in animal cadavers up to 6 h after death and found that the pulmonary artery can tolerate 3 h of warm ischemia in the cadaver without loss of endothelium-dependent relaxation and smooth muscle functions [6], whereas whole lungs can tolerate at least 1 h of warm ischemia after failed resuscitation [5].

5.3 Study of Human Lungs Ex Vivo After Warm and Cold Ischemia

With written consent from the patients and permission from the Ethics Committee, we studied excised human lungs or lung lobes (with small cancer tumours) using our ex vivo method, before the lungs were delivered to the pathology department. For this purpose an extra unit of erythrocyte concentrate (necessary for ex vivo evaluation) had been ordered the day before surgery. After excision of the lung and different time intervals of warm ischemia, the lung was topically cooled for up to 12 h and then evaluated ex vivo. In none of these cases had the patients been given heparin, but we did not observe any clots within the small intrapulmonary vessels, and the ventilation-perfusion relationship in these lungs as measured ex vivo was normal. The pathologists told us that they normally do not see clots in the small intrapulmonary vessels at autopsies; if they do see clots, it indicates pulmonary emboli rather than post-mortem clotting. We decided that heparin may be omitted in a clinical program if ethical or practical difficulties were to stop its use.

In 1997 we had reached the following conclusions from our experiments on animal and human lungs:

1. Topical cooling gives excellent lung preservation for 12 h.
2. Lungs tolerate a "hands off" interval of 1 h after cardiac death.
3. Intrapleural topical cooling initiated after a 1-h "hands off" interval gives excellent lung preservation for 6 h.
4. Lung function can be safely evaluated ex vivo.
5. Heparin is not essential in lung DCD, under the precondition that ex vivo evaluation is done before transplantation.

With this information in published papers or manuscripts we considered ourselves ready to initiate an ethical discussion with the aim of finding an acceptable way to perform a clinical study with uncontrolled DCD lungs.

5.4 Discussion of Ethics

In the winter of 1997 we consulted doctors, nurses, hospital chaplains, lawyers, teachers, philosophers, theologians and ordinary citizens across Sweden about how a potential uncontrolled lung DCD might be performed, if at all, with support from the general public. We learned that any type of surgery on a dead body within 1 h of unexpected death would be problematic. If the cooling of the lungs could be delayed at least 1 h and be done without surgery on the dead body, then it might be possible to get acceptance from the Ethics Committee, if the next of kin had given permission.

We returned to the laboratory after this consultation and developed an efficient technique for topical cooling of the lungs within the intact dead body by a puncture placement of intrapleural cannulae for infusion of cold preservation solution, i.e., we hoped that this technique would not be looked upon as surgery on a dead body.

In September 1997 we called for a meeting with the chief physician, the chairman of the Medical Ethics Committee, and the hospital legal and ethics experts at Lund University Hospital to discuss potential problems with the use of lungs from uncontrolled DCD donors. The discussion raised two main concerns. First, since clinical lung transplantation with uncontrolled DCD lungs had not been done before, what backup could the recipient be offered if the transplanted lungs should for unexpected reasons fail? And second, would an extra burden be added to the next of kin if the question of lung donation was raised within 1 h of an unexpected death? The first question could be satisfactorily answered since we were an ECMO center for the treatment of critical respiratory insufficiency and in the clinic we had successfully achieved 5 weeks of total extracorporeal lung assist [7]. If the transplanted lung was to fail, we could keep the patient alive, make an urgent call for new donor lungs and do re-transplantation.

However, the question about next of kin was deemed to be outside the competence of the local Ethics Committee at Lund University Hospital. No clinical study should be started before the general public in Sweden had been fully informed. Only after a favourable response from the general public would it be possible to start a clinical study.

We contacted two respected and nationally well-known TV journalists and asked for their help with this project. They made an information video and also wrote articles about the project that caught great interest. During autumn of 1997 and winter of 1998, the general public in Sweden was informed via all three national television channels, national radio, and all major newspapers (see Fig. 5.1).

The reaction was generally positive and resulted in an invitation to a hearing at the government's Medical Ethics Council where I had the opportunity to explain the project in detail. The council found the project fully acceptable, but made it clear that the formal decision to undertake a clinical study had to be taken by the Medical Ethics Committee at Lund University Hospital. I also had a meeting with the Committee for Ethical Questions of the National Board of Health and Welfare, and they found no ethical problems with the project and appreciated our information campaign to the general public.

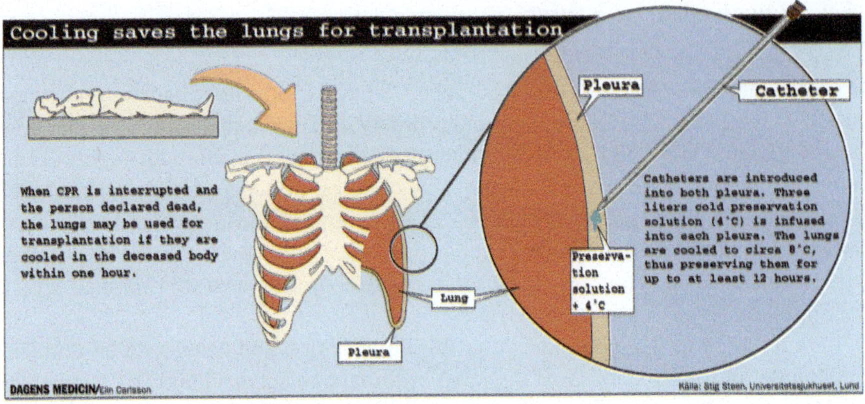

Fig. 5.1 This picture was used in the newspapers and on TV to explain to the Swedish population how lungs may be saved for transplantation after sudden cardiac death

Our application to the Medical Ethics Committee at Lund University Hospital was sent in May 1998, and the study protocol was finally approved on August 19, 1998. The committee stated that no surgery of any kind was permitted on the dead body before the next of kin had given permission, i.e., lung donation had to be discussed with the next of kin before cannulation of thorax and intrapleural cooling could be started. However, 10 min after declaration of death, intravenous heparin followed by 20 chest compressions could be given without informing the next of kin, since the law in Sweden permits some minor preparations for organ donation to be done on a dead body before the next of kin is informed.

All potential recipients had to sign a document stating that he or she had been fully informed that this type of transplantation had never been done on a patient before and that unexpected complications could therefore not be excluded.

5.5 Education of Personnel

Education of all personnel who might be involved in the procedure was started. A group of hospital chaplains accepted to be on call regarding possible needs of the next of kin and two pathologists accepted to be on call for emergency autopsy of the abdomen of the donor to rule out occult cancer. The blood bank developed a routine to deliver 2 units of crossmatched erythrocyte concentrate for the ex vivo evaluation, within 2 h after receiving blood from the donor. Key personnel in six hospitals in Southern Sweden were trained to inform the next of kin and to initiate intrapleural cooling within 1 h after declaration of death if the next of kin gave permission. Some doctors found it problematic to give heparin and do chest compressions on a dead body after a "hands off" period of only 10 min, and they were informed that heparin was not mandatory and could be omitted. All necessary equipment for intrapleural cooling was kept in a special refrigerator in each hospital, and when permission for cooling of the lungs had been obtained, the pleura puncture and infusion of the cold preservation solution was to be initiated by the surgeon or anaesthesiologist on duty (who had been given practical training on pigs and had access to an instruction video).

5.6 The First Clinical Case

The first patient was transplanted in October 2000. All the details of the case have been published in the Lancet [8]. The TV journalists who had helped us to inform the general public had been promised to film the first transplantation, which they did, and it was shown on national television the same evening and was very well received. After the Lancet article [8], the ethics behind our DCD program was analyzed in a highly influential medical ethics journal in the USA and found to be consonant with good medical practice [9].

References

1. Steen S, Liao Q, Pierre L, Paskevicius A, Sjöberg T. The critical importance of minimal delay between chest compression and subsequent defibrillation: a haemodynamic explanation. Resuscitation. 2003;58:249–58.
2. Steen S, Kimblad PO, Sjöberg T, Lindberg L, Ingemansson R, Massa G. Safe lung preservation for twenty-four hours with Perfadex. Ann Thorac Surg. 1994;57:450–7.
3. Steen S, Sjöberg T, Ingemansson R, Lindberg L. Efficacy of topical cooling in lung preservation: is a reappraisal due? Ann Thorac Surg. 1994;58:1657–63.
4. Steen S, Ingemansson R, Budrikis A, Bolys R, Roscher R, Sjöberg T. Successful transplantation of lungs topically cooled in the non-heart-beating donor for 6 hours. Ann Thorac Surg. 1997;63:345–51.
5. Steen S, Liao Q, Wierup P, Bolys R, Pierre L, Sjöberg T. Transplantation of lungs from non-heart-beating donors after functional assessment ex vivo. Ann Thorac Surg. 2003;76:244–52.
6. Bolys R, Ingemansson R, Sjöberg T, Steen S. Vascular function in the cadaver up to six hours after cardiac arrest. J Heart Lung Transplant. 1999;18:582–6.
7. Wetterberg T, Steen S. Total extracorporeal lung assist: a new clinical approach. Intensive Care Med. 1991;17:73–7.
8. Steen S, Sjöberg T, Pierre L, Liao Q, Eriksson L, Algotsson L. Transplantation of lungs from a non-heart-beating donor. Lancet. 2001;357:825–9.
9. Carlberg A. Transplanting lungs from non-heart-beating donors. Natl Cathol Bioeth Q. 2002; 2:377–80.

Chapter 6
DCD for Lung Transplantation

Takahiro Oto

6.1 Introduction

Lung transplantation has been performed as a well-accepted therapy for patients with various end-stage lung diseases [1]. Nonetheless, the wide spread of lung transplantation is limited by the donor shortage resulting in increasing number of deaths on waiting lists [2, 3].

Historically, the first attempts of most of solid organ transplants were from donation after cardiac death donor (DCD)/non-heart-beating donor (NHBD) [4, 5]. Since the introduction of brain death criteria, organs have been retrieved from brain-dead (heart-beating) donors. However, as a result of increasing donor shortage, there is now a renewed interest in DCD (NHBD) lung transplantation [6, 7]. DCD (NHBD) is expected to become the major source of organ supply in countries especially where the concept of brain death is not widely accepted by the public.

This chapter aims to describe the relevant published experimental evidences and recent clinical experiences with lung transplantation from DCD (NHBD).

6.2 Donor Criteria

6.2.1 *Maastricht Categories*

At the International Workshop on NHBDs in Maastricht, Netherlands [8], five types of DCD (NHBD) were identified. Categories I (dead on arrival), II (unsuccessful resuscitation), and V (unexpected cardiac arrest in a hospital inpatient) include

T. Oto (✉)
Department of Thoracic Surgery, Okayama University Graduate School of Medicine, Dentistry and Pharmacological Sciences, 2-5-1, Shikata-cho, Okayama, Kita-ku 700-8558, Japan
e-mail: oto@md.okayama-u.ac.jp

T. Asano et al. (eds.), *Marginal Donors: Current and Future Status*,
DOI 10.1007/978-4-431-54484-5_6, © Springer Japan 2014

uncontrolled donors and categories III (withdrawal of life-supporting therapy) and IV (cardiac arrest in brain-dead donor) comprise controlled donors.

6.2.2 *Scenarios of DCD (NHBD)*

Uncontrolled DCD (NHBD) may occur unexpectedly and may usually happen out of hospital. Emergency services may commence cardiopulmonary resuscitation as soon as possible. If the resuscitation may fail and the organs can be adequately preserved inside the cadaver, the deceased person may become a potential DCD (NHBD). In such cases, the exact length of warm ischemia is often not known and the assessment of organ function before circulatory arrest is impossible. Therefore, evaluation of viability and function of the organ by means of reliable reperfusion apparatus prior to implantation may be necessary [9, 10].

In the controlled DCD (NHBD), withdrawal of life-supporting therapy can be planned in advance in a setting of ICU or operating theater. Therefore, the moment of circulatory arrest is relatively predictable and the functional assessment before circulatory arrest is usually possible.

6.2.2.1 Inclusion Criteria for DCD (NHBD)

Detailed inclusion criteria for DCD (NHBD) have been described elsewhere [7, 11–13]. In uncontrolled DCD (NHBD), it is important to know the time of cardiac arrest and is suggested to initiate cardiopulmonary resuscitation maneuvers within 15 min after cardiac arrest. In controlled DCD (NHBD), donor inclusion criteria are generally based on the criteria for brain-dead donors set by International Society for Heart and Lung Transplantation [14]. Any DCD (NHBD) lung transplant unit guidelines may differ regarding specific lung requirements, parameters, and management principles including the timing of heparin administration and initiation of hypothermia (Fig. 6.1).

6.3 Procurement and Preservation

In principle, the warm ischemic time should be reduced as much as practical, but based on the literatures the lungs with warm ischemic time less than 60 min seem to be acceptable for transplantation [9–13]. Steen and colleagues have reintroduced “topical in situ cooling” for DCD (NHBD) lung preservation [15]. Two chest tubes are inserted and the lungs are cooled inside the body with cold Perfadex® solution for 2 h up to 18 °C. Pre-procurement interval could be safely extended by “topical in situ cooling” up to 6 h postmortem allowing distant organ procurement or next of kin to spend more time to be with the deceased relatives.

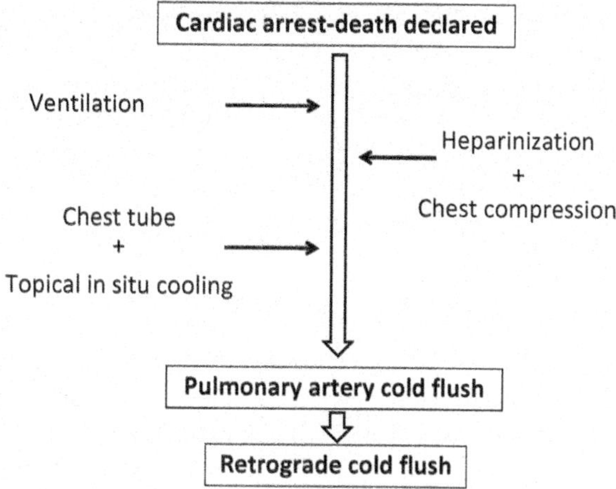

Fig. 6.1 Scheme of DCD lung procurement

6.3.1 *Timing of Heparin Administration*

Administration of heparin before cardiac arrest is a routine clinical practice in brain-dead heart-beating donor transplantation. This can be done before withdrawal of life-supporting therapy in the controlled DCD (NHBD) or before termination of resuscitative maneuver in the uncontrolled DCD (NHBD). However, an intervention aiming for organ preservation before death certification may raise ethical issues. Administration of heparin after certified death is possible with chest compressions to distribute the heparin around the circulatory system [6, 10–12]. In clinical brain-dead-donor lung transplantation, donor thromboembolism was a significant risk factor for development of post-transplant primary graft dysfunction and removal of the pulmonary emboli improved post-transplant graft function [16, 17].

6.3.2 *Definition of Warm Ischemic Time*

The definitions of warm ischemic time are relevant when attempting to cross compare different types of DCD (NHBD), for example, category I versus category III, and also compare the outcomes of varying techniques and ischemic injury therapies. Oto and colleagues described the importance of recording and defining warm ischemic time [12]. To define the start of warm ischemia, (1) oxygen saturation <85, (2) systolic arterial pressure <50 mmHg, (3) cardiac arrest, and (4) death certification were possibly all relevant [18]. Similarly, in defining the end of the warm ischemia period, (1) initiation of ventilation with 100 % oxygen, (2) topical in situ cooling, and (3) pulmonary artery flushing could be used. In the case series from Madrid and Lund, warm ischemic time was defined as a period between cardiac arrest and topical in situ cooling and the actual warm ischemia of their uncontrolled DCD (NHBD) was 65–120 min. Snell and colleagues described the association between warm ischemic time and early outcomes including post-transplant PaO_2/FiO_2 and duration of intensive care unit stay [13]. Clear definition of warm ischemic time has not been determined; therefore, we encourage individual lung transplant units to record critical time points, including the timing of systolic hypotension, cardiac arrest, ventilation reinstitution, and the onset of cold pulmonary flush perfusion.

6.4 Viability Assay

In the controlled DCD (NHBD), graft function can be assessed before withdrawal of life-supporting therapy. Chest radiograph, bronchoscopy, and arterial blood gas analysis are usually available in the same way with the brain-dead heart-beating donor setting. Postmortem functional assessment is not deemed necessary because the warm ischemic time is limited to 60 min or shorter (15 min) especially when the withdrawal of life-supporting therapy was performed in operating theater.

In the uncontrolled DCD (NHBD), graft functional assessment may be mandatory because the graft with longer warm ischemic time compared to that in the controlled setting is potentially damaged. Ex vivo lung assessment techniques have been used in clinical DCD (NHBD) lung transplantation. Ex vivo reperfusion technique has been initiated by the Lund group and further developed by the Toronto group [9, 10]. The perfusion circuit contains a reservoir, a centrifugal pump, a deoxygenator, a heater/cooler, and a leukocyte filter. The ex vivo reperfusion for assessment without additional edema formation on the graft has been achieved with a specially developed solution (Steen Solution®) [17]. The lungs are reperfused deoxygenated perfusate under controlled pulmonary arterial pressure less than 20 mmHg (Fig. 6.2). Functional assessment with measurement of perfusate gas exchange, hemodynamic parameters, and lung compliance is performed under a condition of normothermia [19]. This model also offered the possibility of ex vivo reconditioning of the lungs with marginal quality [9, 10].

6.5 Outcome

Clinical application of DCD (NHBD) lung transplantation has been intensively investigated during the last decade. The results from experimental studies are encouraging that the lung is unique among the solid organs in its tolerance of warm ischemia for up to at least 1 h. This can be endured because the lung's metabolic requirement is low, it is normally filled with well-saturated blood, and its alveoli are filled with oxygen [20–23]. This allows for the prospect of DCD (NHBD) in several scenarios, including controlled and uncontrolled situations.

The first case of successful lung transplantation from a category III DCD (NHBD) was presented in 1995 by Love and colleagues [6]. Steen and colleagues have published the first successful case of lung transplantation from a category II

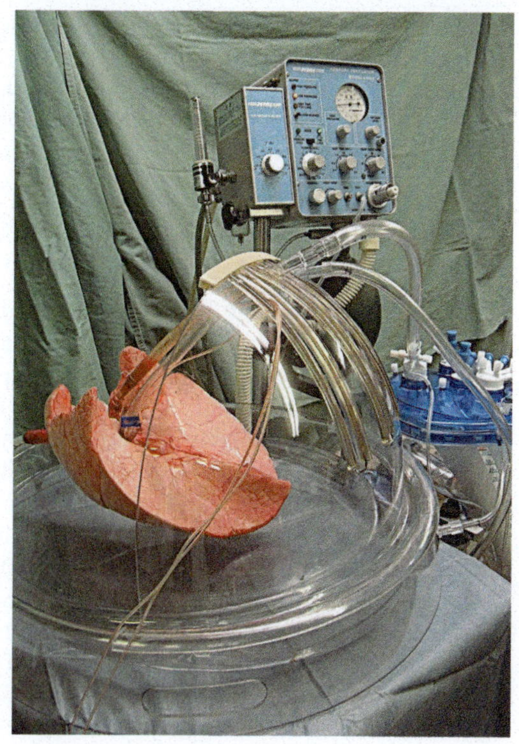

Fig. 6.2 Ex vivo lung evaluation setting at Okayama University

DCD (NHBD) in 2001 [7]. According to the US registry report, 16 DCD (NHBD) lungs in 2005 and 22 DCD (NHBD) lungs in 2006 recovered, and all 22 lungs recovered from DCD (NHBD) in 2006 were transplanted [3]. The contribution of DCD (NHBD) lungs remains low but continues to grow slowly.

Primary graft dysfunction remains a significant morbidity and mortality even after heart-beating donor lung transplantation [11]. The risk of severe primary graft dysfunction might be greater when utilizing the lungs from DCD (NHBD) that are potentially damaged by warm ischemia. From the published case series, the incidence of grade 3 primary graft dysfunction in the controlled DCD (NHBD) lung transplantation was about 13 % which was comparable to that in brain-dead-donor lung transplantation. In contrast, the incidence of grade 3 primary graft dysfunction in the uncontrolled DCD (NHBD) lung transplantation was 29 % and 1-year mortality in this group was 31 % [10, 11, 13, 19].

Bronchial healing is one of the concerns in DCD (NHBD) lung transplantation. Binns and colleagues described the risk of ischemic bronchial injury resulting in necrotic bronchial anastomosis in porcine DCD (NHBD) lung transplant after 1-h warm ischemia [24]. In the series of human DCD (NHBD) lung transplantation, no bronchial complication, except for two due to fungal and gram-negative infection, has been reported.

In the currently available case series, the low rate of acute rejection so far is noted and very reasonable lung function was seen. However, DCD (NHBD) lungs may have a potential to develop premature chronic allograft rejection or bronchiolitis obliterans syndrome (BOS). The size of the sample is too small to make any definitive conclusion; therefore, the next step for investigating DCD (NHBD) lungs relates to its long-term outcomes including the behavior of BOS.

6.6 Basic Research

Prevention of primary graft dysfunction is one of the goals in DCD (NHBD) lung transplantation. Many experimental studies have been conducted to prevent grafts from warm ischemic damage. From a practical perspective, a warm ischemic time definition starting with systolic blood pressure less than 50 mmHg and finishing with cold arterial flush provides the simplest, most universal definition that encompasses all important elements of warm ischemia [18]. In experimental condition, premortem hypoxia rather than hypotension impaired graft function [25]. To avoid graft damage during ex vivo perfusion [26], acellular perfusate has been used for ex vivo graft evaluation [10]. Therefore, ex vivo PO_2 may not be the first indication of lung injury [27]. Other physiologic parameters including graft compliance, vascular resistance, and weight may take on greater importance. Regarding intervention before and after procurement, administration of *N*-acetyl cysteine [28], protective effects of endobronchial high-flow cooled humidified air [29], partial liquid ventilation [30], aerosolized Ventavis [31] or beta-2 adrenoreceptor agonist [32], preimplantation treatment with nitroglycerin [33], and nitric oxide [34] have been described which should be considered in clinical DCD (NHBD) lung transplant practice.

6.7 Conclusion

The use of controlled DCD (NHBD) lungs for human lung transplantation is a valuable option with very acceptable early clinical outcomes. The use of uncontrolled DCD (NHBD) lungs remains to be a challenge due to its high incidence of primary graft dysfunction. The use of DCD (NHBD) has the potential to eliminate the donor shortage and to ameliorate deaths on waiting list. Establishing methods to facilitate long-term safe ex vivo reperfusion may allow DCD (NHBD) lung reconditioning and increased organ recovery rate.

References

1. Meyers BF, Lynch J, Trulock EP, Guthrie TJ, Cooper JD, Patterson GA. Lung transplantation: a decade of experience. Ann Surg. 1999;230:362–70.
2. Oto T, et al. Registry of the Japanese society of lung and heart-lung transplantation: the official Japanese lung transplantation report 2012. Gen Thorac Cardiovasc Surg. 2013;61(4):208–11.

3. Sung RS, Galloway J, Tuttle-Newhall JE, Tuttle-Newhall JE, Mone T, Laeng R, et al. Organ donation and utilization in the United States, 1997–2006. Am J Transplant. 2008;8:922–34.
4. Kootstra G, Kievit J, Nederstigt A. Organ donors: heartbeating and non-heartbeating. World J Surg. 2002;26:181–4.
5. Hardy JD, Webb WR, Dalton Jr ML, Walker Jr GR. Lung homotransplantations in man. JAMA. 1963;186:1065–74.
6. Love RB, Stringham JC, Chomiak PN. Successful lung transplantation using a non-heart-beating donor. J Heart Lung Transplant. 1995;14:S88 (abstr).
7. Steen S, Sjőberg T, Pierre L, Liao Q, Eriksson L, Algotsson L. Transplantation of lungs from a non-heart-beating donor. Lancet. 2001;357:825–9.
8. Kootstra G, Daemen JH, Oomen AP. Categories of non-heart-beating donors. Transplant Proc. 1995;27:2893–4.
9. Steen S, et al. First human transplantation of a nonacceptable donor lung after reconditioning ex vivo. Ann Thorac Surg. 2007;83:2191–4.
10. Cypel M, Yeung JC, Keshavjee S. Novel approaches to expanding the lung donor pool: donation after cardiac death and ex vivo conditioning. Clin Chest Med. 2011;32:233–44.
11. de Antonio DG, et al. Results of clinical lung transplant from uncontrolled non-heart-beating donors. J Heart Lung Transplant. 2007;26:529–34.
12. Oto T, et al. A practical approach to clinical lung transplantation from a Maastricht category III donor with cardiac death. J Heart Lung Transplant. 2007;26:196–9.
13. Snell GI, et al. Early lung transplantation success utilizing controlled donation after cardiac death donors. Am J Transplant. 2008;8:1282–9.
14. Orens JB, Boehler A, de Perrot M, Estenne M, Glanville AR, Keshavjee S, et al. A review of lung transplant donor acceptability criteria. J Heart Lung Transplant. 2003;22:1183–200.
15. Steen S, Ingemansson R, Budrikis A, Bolys R, Roscher R, Sjőberg T. Successful transplantation of lungs topically cooled in the non-heart-beating donor for 6 hours. Ann Thorac Surg. 1997;63:345–51.
16. Oto T, Excell L, Griffiths AP, Levvey BJ, Snell GI. The implications of pulmonary embolism in a multiorgan donor for subsequent pulmonary, renal, and cardiac transplantation. J Heart Lung Transplant. 2008;27:78–85.
17. Oto T, Rabinov M, Griffiths AP, et al. Unexpected donor pulmonary embolism affects early outcomes after lung transplantation: a major mechanism of primary graft failure? J Thorac Cardiovasc Surg. 2005;130:1446.
18. Levvey BJ, Westall GP, Kotsimbos T, Williams TJ, Snell GI. Definitions of warm ischemic time when using controlled donation after cardiac death lung donors. Transplantation. 2008;86:1702–6.
19. Oto T. Lung transplantation from donation after cardiac death (non-heart-beating) donors. Gen Thorac Cardiovasc Surg. 2008;56:533–8.
20. Van Raemdonck DE, Jannis NC, De Leyn PR, Flameng WJ, Lerut TE. Warm ischemic tolerance in collapsed pulmonary grafts is limited to 1 hour. Ann Surg. 1998;228:788–96.
21. Egan TM. Non-heart-beating donors in thoracic transplantation. J Heart Lung Transplant. 2004;23:3–10.
22. Rega FR, Neyrinck AP, Verleden GM, Lerut TE, Van Raemdonck DE. How long can we preserve the pulmonary graft inside the non-heart-beating donor? Ann Thorac Surg. 2004;77:438–44.
23. Rega FR, Jannis NC, Verleden GM, Flameng WJ, Lerut TE, Van Raemdonck DE. Should we ventilate or cool the pulmonary graft inside the non-heart-beating donor? J Heart Lung Transplant. 2003;22:1226–33.
24. Binns OA, DeLima NF, Buchanan SA, Mauney MC, Cope JT, Thies SD, et al. Impaired bronchial healing after lung donation from non-heart-beating donors. J Heart Lung Transplant. 1996;15:1084–92.
25. Miyoshi K, Oto T, Otani S, et al. Effect of donor pre-mortem hypoxia and hypotension on graft function and start of warm ischemia in donation after cardiac death lung transplantation. J Heart Lung Transplant. 2011;30:445–51.

26. Otani S, Oto T, Kakishita T, et al. Early effects of the ex vivo evaluation system on graft function after swine lung transplantation. Eur J Cardiothorac Surg. 2011;40:956–61.
27. Yeung JC, Cypel M, Machuca TN, et al. Physiologic assessment of the ex vivo donor lung for transplantation. J Heart Lung Transplant. 2012;31:1120–6.
28. Geudens N, Van de Wauwer C, Neyrinck AP, Timmermans L, Vanhooren HM, Vanaudenaerde BM, et al. N-acetyl cysteine pre-treatment attenuates inflammatory changes in the warm ischemic murine lung. J Heart Lung Transplant. 2007;26:1326–32.
29. Oto T, Calderone A, Pepe S, Snell G, Rosenfeldt F. High-flow endobronchial cooled humidified air protects non-heart-beating donor rat lungs against warm ischemia. J Thorac Cardiovasc Surg. 2006;132:413–9.
30. Yoshida S, Sekine Y, Shinozuka N, Satoh J, Yasufuku K, Iwata T, et al. The efficacy of partial liquid ventilation in lung protection during hypotension and cardiac arrest: preliminary study of lung transplantation using non-heart-beating donors. J Heart Lung Transplant. 2005;24:723–9.
31. Wittwer T, Franke UF, Sandhaus T, Groetzner J, Strauch JT, Wippermann J, et al. Endobronchial donor pre-treatment with ventavis: is a second administration during reperfusion beneficial to optimize post-ischemic function of non-heart-beating donor lungs? J Surg Res. 2006; 136:136–42.
32. Chen F, Nakamura T, Fujinaga T, Zhang J, Hamakawa H, Omasa M, et al. Protective effect of a nebulized beta2-adorenoreceptor agonist in warm ischemic-reperfused rat lungs. Ann Thorac Surg. 2006;82:465–71.
33. Egan TM, Hoffmann SC, Sevala M, Sadoff JD, Schlidt SA. Nitroglycerin reperfusion reduces ischemia-reperfusion injury in non-heart-beating donor lungs. J Heart Lung Transplant. 2006;25:110–9.
34. Takashima S, Koukoilis G, Inokawa H, Sevala M, Egan TM. Inhaled nitric oxide reduces ischemia-reperfusion injury in rat lungs from non-heart-beating donors. J Thorac Cardiovasc Surg. 2006;132:132–9.

Chapter 7
ECD for Lung Transplantation

Yasushi Hoshikawa, Yoshinori Okada, Tatsuaki Watanabe, and Takashi Kondo

7.1 Introduction

The short supply of donor organs has been one of the most critical problems in the area of lung transplantation (LTx), and this is especially serious in Japan. One approach to attempt to address this limitation is the use of extended criteria donor (ECD) lungs. The currently accepted criteria for suitable donor lungs (Table 7.1) were instituted in the mid-1980s during the early development of clinical LTx [1]. These criteria were chosen by early transplant physicians and surgeons based on prevailing knowledge of pulmonary physiology, but were not based upon strict scientific evidence [2]. Afterward the ever-increasing number of recipients on waiting lists compelled lung transplant doctors to consider the use of ECD lungs. Liberalization of the donor selection criteria has been gradually accepted worldwide since the mid-1990s [2]. A recent large registry study of more than ten thousand LTxs performed in the USA from 1999 to 2008 revealed that at least one variance from the criteria occurred in more than a half of transplants [3]. Although results have varied among studies, outcomes of LTx using ECD lungs have generally been acceptable [4–18]. However, proper judgment is still difficult if multiple factors are defined extended and if ECD lungs are used in high-risk recipients especially who are rapidly deteriorating on the waiting list. To properly assess and optimize ECD lungs in such circumstances, a new strategy utilizing normothermic ex vivo lung perfusion (EVLP) system has been developed, and the impact of the system on LTx has been explored in several high-flow transplant centers [19, 20].

In Japan, 124 LTxs from deceased donors have been successfully performed as of the end of 2012 [21]. These transplantations achieved a 5-year patient survival rate of 72.0 % and a 10-year survival of 57.3 % [21]. To maximize the lung

Y. Hoshikawa (✉) • Y. Okada • T. Watanabe • T. Kondo
Department of Thoracic Surgery, Institute of Development, Aging and Cancer, Tohoku University, 4-1 Seiryo-machi, Aoba-ku, Sendai 980-8575, Japan
e-mail: hoshikawa@idac.tohoku.ac.jp

T. Asano et al. (eds.), *Marginal Donors: Current and Future Status*,
DOI 10.1007/978-4-431-54484-5_7, © Springer Japan 2014

Table 7.1 Current donor lung guidelines

Age <55 years
ABO compatibility
Clear chest radiograph
PaO_2 >300 torr on $FiO_2 = 1.0$, PEEP 5 cm H_2O
Smoking history <20 pack-years
Absence of chest trauma
No evidence of aspiration/sepsis
No prior cardiothoracic surgery
No organisms on endotracheal aspirate gram stain
No purulent secretions on bronchoscopy

PaO_2 arterial difference in partial pressure of oxygen, FiO_2 fraction of inspired oxygen, *PEEP* positive end-expiratory pressure. Adapted from [23]

utilization rate in multiorgan donors, Japan Organ Transplant Network has operated a system involving the partnership of well-trained transplant consultant doctors and local doctors in assessing donor lungs and providing intensive care to donors since 2002 [22]. These consultant doctors tirelessly performed bronchial toileting for donors and provided advice on respiratory therapy, mechanical ventilation, infection controls, and circulatory management of donors. Since such sustained efforts by the consultant doctors in cooperation with local doctors have been made to effectively utilize ECD lungs, the lungs were used for transplantation in more than 60 % of brain-dead donors [22].

This chapter reviews definition and assessment methods of ECD lungs, studies showing outcomes of LTx using ECDs, and progress in recent research regarding ECD lungs.

7.2 Definition

The extended donor criteria are defined according to the standard criteria [23], which are as follows: age <55 years, ABO compatibility, clear chest radiograph, arterial difference in partial pressure of oxygen (PaO_2) >300 mmHg at 100 % fraction of inspired oxygen (FiO_2) and positive end-expiratory pressure (PEEP) of 5 cm H_2O, a cumulative smoking history of <20 pack-years, absence of chest trauma, no evidence of aspiration/sepsis, no prior cardiothoracic surgery, no organisms on endotracheal aspirate gram stain, and no purulent secretions on bronchoscopy (Table 7.1).

7.3 Viability Assay

To assess the viability of donor lungs, all donor criteria listed on Table 7.1 must be carefully evaluated. The most difficult judgment decisions pertain to the chest radiograph, the bronchoscopic findings, and the intraoperative assessment of the donor lung by means of hands-on inspection and palpation [24]. These assessments cannot be performed in quantitative form and critically depend on the experience of the retrieval surgeon. We believe that the donor bronchoscopic examination is of most importance and that the findings of copious purulent secretions, which cannot be suctioned clear, and of edematous and/or reddened bronchial mucosa coincident with chest radiograph infiltrates indicating pneumonia represent strong contraindications to the use of that lung. In Japan, a transplant consultant doctors sent from one of seven lung transplant centers assesses bronchoscopic findings and chest radiograph infiltrates at several time points to evaluate if the ECD recovers from pneumonia after suitable management.

In addition to the careful evaluation of all donor criteria, consideration must also be given to the recipient's underlying disease and the severity of illness when using an ECD lung [6]. Usually, care is taken not to place organs from truly extended donors into high-risk recipients especially with pulmonary hypertension or pulmonary fibrosis with secondary pulmonary hypertension, or into other complex cases [24].

Normothermic EVLP is currently being explored to evaluate the viability of ECD lungs. This system allows the lungs after procurement to be perfused under normothermic conditions for approximately 4 h so that the lungs can be optimized as well as continually reassessed. Steen et al. were the first to create a successful EVLP evaluation system for donating after cardiac death [19] by means of Steen solution, a hyperoncotic fluid with 15 % hematocrit [25]. Cypel et al. applied this system to the clinical trial where they evaluated early post-LTx outcomes of ECD lungs which were physiologically stable during 4 h of normothermic EVLP and compared them with those of the conventionally selected lungs [20]. ECD lungs were defined by specific criteria, including pulmonary edema and a ratio of the partial pressure of arterial oxygen to the fraction of inspired oxygen (PaO_2/FiO_2) less than 300 mmHg. Twenty out of 26 ECD lungs were transplanted after EVLP and demonstrated comparable incidence of primary graft dysfunction (PGD), 30-day mortality, bronchial complications, duration of mechanical ventilation, and length of stay in intensive care unit (ICU) and hospital, to 116 conventionally selected lungs. However, the clinical use of normothermic EVLP system for assessing ECD lungs has not yet been spread worldwide since Steen solution is not yet approved by the Food and Drug Administration (FDA) for use in the USA and also has not been approved for use based on pharmaceutical affairs law in most countries including Japan as of the end of 2012.

The use of biomarkers in bronchoalveolar lavage (BAL) fluids also has been explored to assess the viability of ECD lungs. Fisher and associates found that high IL-8 levels in the donor BAL were associated with poor outcomes after LTx, especially with development of severe PGD and with early recipient mortality [26]. Similarly, Kaneda and associates found that IL-6, IL-8, TNF-α, and IL-1β were risk factors for 30-day mortality, while IL-10 and IFN-γ were protective [27]. However, none of such biomarkers have yet been generally utilized in clinical transplantation.

7.4 Outcomes

First, several studies demonstrating the effects of the clinical use of ECDs in LTx are listed in chronological order. Kron et al. reported the efficacy of the use of 10 ECDs in LTx performed at a single center in the USA to expand the donor pool in 1993 [4]. It was the first report showing the possibility to utilize ECD lungs without an increased risk of mortality. Sundaresan et al. reported the first retrospective study comparing 44 ECDs and 89 standard donors (SDs) [5]. No differences were found between recipients of the lungs from ECDs and SDs with respect to duration of postoperative mechanical ventilation, gas exchange, and 30-day mortality. However, cardiopulmonary bypass was required more often in the ECDs than in the SDs. Gabbay et al. published their experiences in Australia with 64 ECDs and 48 SDs [2], showing no significant differences in length of ICU stay, postoperative gas exchange, 30-day mortality, and 1-, 2-, and 3-year survival between recipients of the lungs from ECDs and SDs. They found graft ischemic time was predictive of recipient gas exchange after transplantation. Bhorade et al. performed the retrospective evaluation comparing patients receiving the lungs from 52 ECDs and 61 SDs at a single center in the USA [6]. To define ECDs, the authors were the first to use following criteria: donor ventilator time >5 days and donor use of inhaled drugs (cocaine or marijuana) in addition to the previously accepted standard criteria, such as donor age, tobacco history, and abnormal chest radiograph. There were no differences in operative and early-term complications and hospital survival. Moreover, this is the first report to suggest that no alteration in lung function or 1-year survival occurs with the use of ECDs. Since the authors observed a trend toward slightly decreased pulmonary function at 1 year in single-ECD-lung recipients, they advocated to be cautious against the use of single lungs from ECDs. Pierre et al. reported the retrospective review of 128 consecutive lung or heart-lung transplants performed in Toronto comparing 63 ECDs and 65SDs [24]. This is the first to find a higher early mortality at both 30 (17.5 vs. 6.2 %, $p=0.047$) and 90 days (22.2 % vs. 7.7 %, $p=0.0391$) after transplantation using ECDs. The authors warned against using ECDs in higher-risk recipients, especially ones with pulmonary hypertension (PH), pulmonary fibrosis with PH, and cystic fibrosis with *Burkholderia cepacia* colonization. Oto et al. retrospectively reviewed 173 heart-lung and bilateral single-lung transplant recipients of whom 77 were ever smokers and 64 out of those were current smokers [7]. The authors found more than 20 pack-years was associated with impaired early oxygenation and longer ventilation time and ICU stay, but no differences in 3-year survival and incidence of death due to bronchiolitis obliterans syndrome (BOS) which is one of the major factors affecting long-term survival after LTx. Thabut et al. investigated the effect of donor characteristics on short- and long-term outcomes of a total of 785 adult patients undergoing LTx at seven centers in France [8]. The authors found donor gas exchange before harvest was significantly associated with recipient early gas exchange, duration of mechanical ventilation, and long-term survival. A nonlinear model showed a steep increase in the relative risk of death when donor PaO_2/FiO_2 before harvest was below 350 (hazard ratio 1.43; 95 % confidence interval 1.10–1.85; $p=0.01$). Lardinois et al. evaluated an impact of ECDs, especially low PaO_2 (<250 torr) before harvesting and multiple extended criteria, on early outcomes and medium-term survival of 148 consecutive recipients at a single center in Switzerland [9]. The authors did not find any difference in early and intermediate results when they analyzed survival among the number of extended criteria. Moreover, this is the first report showing that the use of ECD lungs with a PaO_2 <250 mmHg in selected cases is not associated with an unfavorable outcome. However, the authors cautioned against the use of ECD lungs with an association of PaO_2 <300 mmHg and purulent secretions. Aigner et al. retrospectively analyzed 98 consecutive lung transplantations performed at a single center in Austria during a 2-year period of time with the lungs from 26 ECDs and 72 SDs [10]. The analysis of major outcomes in the short and the medium term did not show any differences between ECDs and SDs. Kawut et al. performed a retrospective cohort study of 51 patients undergoing LTx at a single center in the USA for 2 years [11]. This study included comprehensive data reflecting the condition of the recipient at the time of transplantation. Significant differences between recipients of 27 ECD and 24 SD lungs in several primary endpoints were shown. Recipients of ECD lungs had fewer ICU-free days, a longer time to hospital discharge, and lower spirometry at 1 year than did SD lung recipients. Donor age 55 years or older and smoking were associated with fewer ICU-free days than younger donors and nonsmokers, respectively. No differences were observed in 30-day and longer-term survival between ECDs and SDs. Luckraz et al. analyzed 362 double-lung and heart-lung transplantations performed at a single center in the UK from 50 donors with low levels of PaO_2 (<300 mmHg) and 312 donors with normal PaO_2 [12]. They observed, in the low PaO_2 group, a compromised 30-day mortality rate (22 % vs. 13 %, odds ratio = 1.92) and comparable 1- and 5-year survival when compared with the normal PaO_2 group. Botha et al. retrospectively reviewed 201 patients undergoing lung or heart-lung transplantation at a single center in the UK of whom 83 received ECD lungs [13]. Recipients of ECD lungs had a higher incidence of severe PGD (43.9 % vs. 27.4 %) and 90-day organ-specific (respiratory failure or multiorgan failure with severe PGD) mortality (15.7 % vs. 5.1 %) when compared with recipients of SD lungs. They found significantly high 30-day mortality (17 %) with ECD lungs for bilateral lung transplantation with the use of cardiopulmonary bypass. Moreover, the authors advocated current heavy smoking as a risk factor for impaired oxygenation and longer ICU stay after transplantation. De Perrot et al. compared the outcome of 60 LTxs of the lungs from donors aged 60 years or more with 407 LTxs of the lungs from younger donors, all of which were performed at a single center in Toronto for 11 years [14]. The authors found the increased age is associated with borderline risk for increased 10-year mortality (39 % vs. 16 % in the younger donor group, $p=0.07$) and increased risk of BOS (65 % vs. 34 % in the younger donor group, $p=0.01$). Meers et al. analyzed 50 LTxs with the lungs from 27 ECDs and 23 SDs performed at a single center in Belgium and observed a negative impact of ECDs in terms of ICU stay and the PGD rate [15]. The study of Berman et al. [16] was based on smoking donors (n = 184) and their impact on LTx performed at a single center in the UK. Over a period of 13 years, 454 patients were included. The authors found a significant association between smoking history and lower 3-month survival (21 % vs. 13 % in the nonsmoking donor group, $n=240$, odds ratio 1.9, $p=0.04$) and also ICU stay for >2 days. No differences were observed in long-term survival and infection between recipients of the lungs from smoking and nonsmoking donors. Reyes et al. utilized multivariable survival methods to determine several donor factors, adjusted for recipient risk factors on 10,333 LTxs performed during a 10-year period of time in the USA [3]. Increasing number of variances was not associated with worse survival after LTx. Of donor guideline variables, a smoking history of greater than 20 pack-years appeared to be a small but statistically significant risk factor for mortality. Mortality did not significantly increase despite the use of donor lungs with an abnormal chest radiograph, age greater than 55 years, or a lower donor PaO_2 (as low as 230 mmHg). Recently, Zafar et al. retrospectively analyzed 12,045 LTxs performed over a 9-year period of time to assess the effect of donor PaO_2 at the time of procurement on graft survival [17]. Kaplan-Meier survival analysis on LTxs from 12,045 donors who had a PaO_2 of greater than 300 mmHg ($n=9{,}593$), of 201 to 300 ($n=582$), and of less than 200 ($n=1{,}830$) showed no difference in graft survival, irrespective of whether recipients had a single or double LTx. A Cox multivariable analysis of 21 donor characteristics also demonstrated that donor PaO_2 had no association with graft survival [17]. The study limitation is they did not look at the short-term or the acute events, such as development of PGD, sepsis, and 30-day mortality in these patients. Recently, Bonser et al. [18] retrospectively analyzed 1,295 LTxs performed during a 12-year period of time in the UK to assess the impact of donor smoking history on recipient early outcomes and survival. In this study, the authors estimated the effects of non-acceptance of the lungs from donors with positive smoking histories. This study showed increased 3-year mortality after adjustment for other independent factors such as recipient's age, cytomegalovirus mismatch, and increasing ischemic time (67.2 % vs. 55.7 %, $p=0.0002$, adjusted hazard ratio 1.36, 1.11–1.67) and an increased incidence of BOS associated with 510 smoking donors compared with 712 nonsmoking donors. Furthermore, recipients of the lungs from smoking donors were likely to spend longer in ICU and hospital and could derive less functional benefit from transplantation than recipients of the lungs from donors with negative smoking histories. The stratified Cox regression model revealed recipients receiving the lungs from donors with positive smoking histories had a significantly lower unadjusted hazard of death after registration than did those remaining on the list for a potential transplant from a donor with negative smoking history (HR 0.79, 95 % CI 0.70–0.91; $p=0.0004$).

In summary, although results have varied, outcomes of LTx using ECD lungs have generally been acceptable. Next, considerations regarding each extended criteria (age, P/F ratio, and smoking history) are listed below.

7.4.1 Age

Although the current guidelines for upper age limit suggest 55 years as maximum age, small-size studies with some dozens of donors have not shown a survival disadvantage with the use of older donors [11, 28, 29]. A larger study with hundreds of LTxs has shown that increased age (of 60 years or more) is associated with borderline risk for increased 5-year mortality, increased 10-year mortality, and increased risk of BOS [14]. A recent larger registry study with more than ten thousand LTxs has demonstrated no significant increase in mortality despite the use of donor lungs with an age greater than 55 years [3].

7.4.2 Low Ratio of Pulmonary Arterial Oxygen to Fraction of Inspired Oxygen (P/F Ratio)

Although small studies demonstrated an impact with the use of donors presenting low P/F ratio on 30-day mortality (P/F ratio <300) [12] and long-term mortality (P/F ratio <350) [8], recent larger registry studies have shown no significant increase in long-term mortality despite the use of donor lungs with a lower P/F ratio [3, 17]. In the future more and more centers will utilize EVLP to assess the viability of borderline grafts with P/F ratio of 300 mmHg or lower.

7.4.3 Smoking History

Although no study has evaluated the number of pack-years of smoking history that would preclude the lungs from being transplanted, a retrospective study by Oto et al. showed more than 20 pack-years was associated with impaired early oxygenation and longer ventilation time and ICU stay, but no differences in 3-year survival and incidence of death due to BOS [7]. The study of Berman demonstrated a significant association between smoking history and lower 3-month survival and longer ICU stay, but no differences in long-term survival and infection [16]. Recent larger studies have shown increased long-term mortality (3, 18) and an increased incidence of BOS associated with smoking donors. It is of interest that a study by Bonser revealed recipients receiving the lungs from donors with positive smoking histories had a significantly lower hazard of death after registration than did those remaining on the list for a potential transplant from a donor with negative smoking history [18].

7.5 Research

Recently, approaches for an effective reconditioning of ECD lungs by means of EVLP system have been explored. Several studies have demonstrated a high incidence of thrombi in donor lungs which cause rejection of the lungs for LTx or PGD after LTx [30–33]. Motoyama et al. reported the effect of the fibrinolytic agent plasmin administered in an EVLP model of cardiac arrest rats on pulmonary vascular resistance, dynamic compliance, and lung weight gain [34]. Plasmin administration dissolved thrombi in the rat lungs, resulting in reconditioning of the lungs as assessed by significantly decreased pulmonary vascular resistance, stable dynamic compliance, and less lung weight gain when compared with non-plasmin rats.

Although cold flush and static cold storage is the accepted standard for preservation of donor lungs in clinical transplantation, deterioration of the donated lungs still occurs. Usually, the longer the lung is kept cold and ischemic, the greater the extent of injury. To minimize this cold ischemia injury and to assess and improve ECD lungs, organ care system (OCS), a portable normothermic EVLP system, has been developed [35]. The OCS provides immediate and sustained lung recruitment starting at the donor site and substantially reduces cold ischemic time [35]. An international randomized trial is ongoing in which the impact of portable ex vivo perfusion and ventilation of donor lungs by means of the OCS on post-LTx outcomes as compared to current cold storage technique is evaluated. Interim results from this trial were presented at the International Society for Heart and Lung Transplantation (ISHLT) 33rd Annual Meeting in Montreal (http://www.transmedics.com/wt/page/pr_1366904571). The donor lungs preserved using the OCS had significantly lower incidence of severe PGD after LTx as compared to the lungs that were preserved using cold storage. In addition, other important clinical parameters like in-hospital mortality, six-month survival, rate of lung-related complications, time on mechanical ventilation, and ICU time were better in the OCS group as compared to cold storage.

References

1. Sundaresan S, Trachiotis G, Aoe M, Patterson G, Cooper J. Donor lung procurement: assessment and operative technique. Ann Thorac Surg. 1993;56:1409–13.
2. Gabbay E, Williams TJ, Griffiths AP, Macfarlane LM, Kotsimbos TC, Esmore DS, Snell GI. Maximizing the utilization of donor organs offered for lung transplantation. Am J Respir Crit Care Med. 1999;160(1):265–71.
3. Reyes KG, Mason DP, Thuita L, Nowicki ER, Murthy SC, Pettersson GB, Blackstone EH. Guidelines for donor lung selection: time for revision? Ann Thorac Surg. 2010;89(6):1756–64.
4. Kron IL, Tribble CG, Kern JA, Daniel TM, Rose CE, Truwit JD, Blackbourne LH, Bergin JD. Successful transplantation of marginally acceptable thoracic organs. Ann Surg. 1993; 217(5):518–22.
5. Sundaresan S, Semenkovich J, Ochoa L, Richardson G, Trulock EP, Cooper JD, Patterson GA. Successful outcome of lung transplantation is not compromised by the use of marginal donor lungs. J Thorac Cardiovasc Surg. 1995;109(6):1075–9.
6. Bhorade SM, Vigneswaran W, McCabe MA, Garrity ER. Liberalization of donor criteria may expand the donor pool without adverse consequence in lung transplantation. J Heart Lung Transplant. 2000;19(12):1199–204.
7. Oto T, Griffiths AP, Levvey B, Pilcher DV, Whitford H, Koshimbos TC, Rabinov M, Esmore DS, Williams TJ, Snell GI. A donor history of smoking affects early but not late outcomes in lung transplantation. Transplantation. 2004;78:599–606.
8. Thabut G, Mal H, Cerrina J, Dartevelle P, Dromer C, Velly JF, Stern M, Loirat P, Bertocchi M, Mornex JF, Haloun A, Despins P, Pison C, Blin D, Simonneau G, Reynaud-Gaubert M. Influence of donor characteristics on outcome after lung transplantation: a multicenter study. J Heart Lung Transplant. 2005;24(9):1347–53.

9. Lardinois D, Banysch M, Korom S, Hillinger S, Rousson V, Boehler A, Speich R, Weder W. Extended donor lungs: eleven years experience in a consecutive series. Eur J Cardiothorac Surg. 2005;27(5):762–7.
10. Aigner C, Winkler G, Jaksch P, Seebacher G, Lang G, Taghavi S, Wisser W, Klepetko W. Extended donor criteria for lung transplantation–a clinical reality. Eur J Cardiothorac Surg. 2005;27(5):757–61.
11. Kawut SM, Reyentovich A, Wilt JS, Anzeck R, Lederer DJ, O'Shea MK, Sonett JR, Arcasoy SM. Outcomes of extended donor lung recipients after lung transplantation. Transplantation. 2005;79(3):310–6.
12. Luckraz H, White P, Sharples LD, Hopkins P, Wallwork J. Short- and long-term outcomes of using pulmonary allograft donors with low Po2. J Heart Lung Transplant. 2005;24(4):470–3.
13. Botha P, Trivedi D, Weir CJ, Searl CP, Corris PA, Dark JH, Schueler SV. Extended donor criteria in lung transplantation: impact on organ allocation. J Thorac Cardiovasc Surg. 2006;131(5):1154–60.
14. De Perrot M, Waddell TK, Shargall Y, Pierre AF, Fadel E, Uy K, Chaparro C, Hutcheon M, Singer LG, Keshavjee S. Impact of donors aged 60 years or more on outcome after lung transplantation: results of an 11-year single-center experience. J Thorac Cardiovasc Surg. 2007;133(2):525–31.
15. Meers C, Van Raemdonck D, Verleden GM, Coosemans W, Decaluwe H, De Leyn P, Nafteux P, Lerut T. The number of lung transplants can be safely doubled using extended criteria donors; a single-center review. Transpl Int. 2010;23(6):628–35.
16. Berman M, Goldsmith K, Jenkins D, Sudarshan C, Catarino P, Sukumaran N, Dunning J, Sharples LD, Tsui S, Parmar J. Comparison of outcomes from smoking and nonsmoking donors: thirteen-year experience. Ann Thorac Surg. 2010;90(6):1786–92.
17. Zafar F, Khan MS, Heinle JS, Adachi I, McKenzie ED, Schecter MG, Mallory GB, Morales DL. Does donor arterial partial pressure of oxygen affect outcomes after lung transplantation? A review of more than 12,000 lung transplants. J Thorac Cardiovasc Surg. 2012;143(4):919–25.
18. Bonser RS, Taylor R, Collett D, Thomas HL, Dark JH, Neuberger J, Cardiothoracic Advisory Group to NHS Blood and Transplant and the Association of Lung Transplant Physicians (UK). Effect of donor smoking on survival after lung transplantation: a cohort study of a prospective registry. Lancet. 2012;380(9843):747–55.
19. Steen S, Sjoerg T, Pierre L, Liao Q, Eriksson L, Algotsson L. Transplantation of lungs from a non-heart-beating donor. Lancet. 2001;357(9259):825–9.
20. Cypel M, Yeung JC, Liu M, et al. Normothermic ex vivo lung perfusion in clinical lung transplantation. N Engl J Med. 2011;364(15):1431–40.
21. Registry Report. 2013. http://www2.idac.tohoku.ac.jp/dep/surg/shinpai/pg185.html
22. Egawa H, Tanabe K, Fukushima N, Date H, Sugitani A, Haga H. Current status of organ transplantation in Japan. Am J Transplant. 2012;12(3):523–30.
23. Orens JB, Boehler A, Perrot M, Estenne M, Glanville AR, Keshavjee S, Kotloff R, Morton J, Studer SM, Van Raemdonck D, Waddel T, Snell GI. A review of lung transplant donor acceptability criteria. J Heart Lung Transplant. 2003;22:1183–200.
24. Pierre AF, Sekine Y, Hutcheon MA, Waddell TK, Keshavjee SH. Marginal donor lungs: a reassessment. J Thorac Cardiovasc Surg. 2002;123(3):421–7.
25. Steen S, Sjoerg T, Ingemansson R, Lindberg L. Efficacy of topical cooling in lung preservation: is a reappraisal due? Ann Thorac Surg. 1994;58(6):1657–63.
26. Fisher AJ, Donnelly SC, Hirani N, Haslett C, Strieter RM, Dark JH, Corris PA. Elevated levels of interleukin-8 in donor lungs is associated with early graft failure after lung transplantation. Am J Respir Crit Care Med. 2001;163(1):259–65.
27. Kaneda H, Waddell TK, de Perrot M, Bai XH, Gutierrez C, Arenovich T, Chaparro C, Liu M, Keshavjee S. Pre-implantation multiple cytokine mRNA expression analysis of donor lung grafts predicts survival after lung transplantation in humans. Am J Transplant. 2006; 6(3):544–51.
28. Meyer DM, Bennett LE, Novick RJ, Hosenpud JD. Effect of donor age and ischemic time on intermediate survival and morbidity after lung transplantation. Chest. 2000;118(5):1255–562.

29. Pizanis N, Heckmann J, Tsagakis K, Tossios P, Massoudy P, Wendt D, Jakob H, Kamler M. Lung transplantation using donors 55 years and older: is it safe or just a way out of organ shortage? Eur J Cardiothorac Surg. 2010;38(2):192–7.
30. Stewart S, Ciulli F, Wells F, Wallwork J. Pathology of unused donor lungs. Transplant Proc. 1993;25:1167–8.
31. Ware LB, Fang X, Wang Y, Babcock WD, Jones K, Matthay MA. High prevalence of pulmonary arterial thrombi in donor lungs rejected for transplantation. J Heart Lung Transplant. 2005;24:1650–6.
32. Oto T, Rabinov M, Griffiths AP, Whitford H, Levvey BJ, Esmore DS, Williams TJ, Snell GI. Unexpected donor pulmonary embolism affects early outcomes after lung transplantation: a major mechanism of primary graft failure? J Thorac Cardiovasc Surg. 2005;130:1446–52.
33. Ware LB, Fang X, Wang Y, Sakuma T, Hall TS, Matthay MA. Selected contribution: mechanisms that may stimulate the resolution of alveolar edema in the transplanted human lung. J Appl Physiol. 2002;93:1869–74.
34. Motoyama H, Chen F, Ohsumi A, Hijiya K, Okita K, Nakajima D, Sakamoto J, Yamada T, Sato M, Aoyama A, Bando T, Date H. Protective effect of plasmin in marginal donor lungs in an ex vivo lung perfusion model. J Heart Lung Transplant. 2013;32(5):505–10.
35. Warnecke G, Moradiellos J, Tudorache I, Kühn C, Avsar M, Wiegmann B, Sommer W, Ius F, Kunze C, Gottlieb J, Varela A, Haverich A. Normothermic perfusion of donor lungs for preservation and assessment with the organ care system lung before bilateral transplantation: a pilot study of 12 patients. Lancet. 2012;380(9856):1851–8.

Chapter 8
LD for Lung Transplantation

Hiroshi Date

8.1 Criteria for Living Donation

Living-donor lobar lung transplantation (LDLLT) has been performed as a lifesaving procedure in approximately 400 patients worldwide [1]. During the past several years, LDLLT has been almost exclusively performed in Japan [1], where the average waiting time for cadaveric lungs exceeds 800 days [2]. The results of LDLLT have been reported to be equal to or better than conventional cadaveric lung transplantation [3–6]. In LDLLT, the right and left lower lobes from two healthy donors are implanted in the recipient in place of the whole right and left lungs (Fig. 8.1). Occasionally, single LDLLT can be performed for a carefully selected small recipient [7].

8.1.1 Donor Selection

Although immediate family members (relatives within the third degree or a spouse) have been the only donors in our institution, non-Japanese institutions have accepted extended family members and unrelated individuals [3]. Eligibility criteria for living lobar lung donation at Kyoto University are summarized in Table 8.1.

Preoperative workup consists of posterior-anterior and left lateral chest roentgenogram, high-resolution computed tomographic scan of the chest (at maximal inspiration and expiration), formal pulmonary function tests, measurement of room air blood gases, electrocardiogram, and Doppler echocardiogram. Three-dimensional

H. Date (✉)
The Department of Thoracic Surgery, Kyoto University Graduate School of Medicine,
54 Shogoin-Kawahara-cho, Sakyo-ku, Kyoto 606-8507, Japan
e-mail: hdate@kuhp.kyoto-u.ac.jp

T. Asano et al. (eds.), *Marginal Donors: Current and Future Status*,
DOI 10.1007/978-4-431-54484-5_8, © Springer Japan 2014

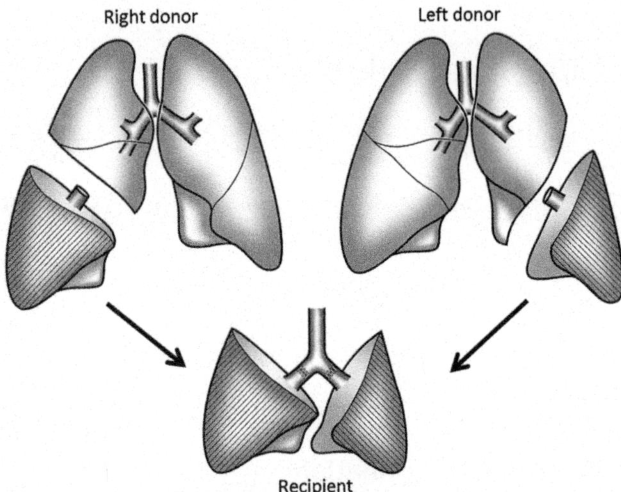

Fig. 8.1 Bilateral living-donor lobar lung transplantation. The right and left lower lobes from two healthy donors are implanted in a recipient in place of the whole right and left lungs, respectively

Table 8.1 The eligibility criteria for living lung donation (Kyoto University)

Medical criteria
Age 20–60 years
ABO blood type compatible with recipient
Relatives within the third degree or a spouse
No significant past medical history
No recent viral infection
No significant abnormalities on echocardiogram and electrocardiogram
No significant ipsilateral pulmonary pathology on computed tomography
Arterial oxygen tension ≧ 80 mmHg (room air)
Forced vital capacity, forced expiratory volume in 1 s ≧ 85 % of predicted
No previous ipsilateral thoracic surgery
No active tobacco smoking
Social and ethical criteria
No significant mental disorders proved by a psychiatrist
No ethical issues or concerns about donor motivation

multidetector computed tomography angiography is created for the confirmation of the pulmonary arterial and venous anatomy (Fig. 8.2) [8]. The completeness of pulmonary fissures is carefully evaluated by high-resolution computed tomography. Although HLA matching is not required for donor selection, a prospective cross-match to rule out the presence of anti-HLA antibodies is performed.

Potential donors should be competent, willing to donate free of coercion, medically and psychosocially suitable, fully informed of the risks and benefits as

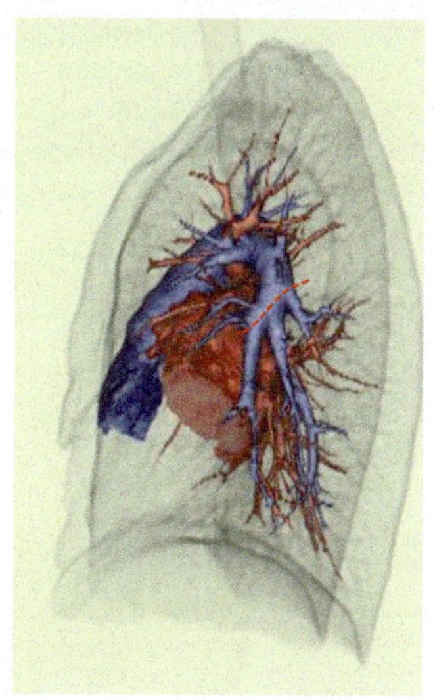

Fig. 8.2 Three-dimensional computed tomography angiography in a typical left donor. A *red dotted line* shows the planned cutting oblique line of the pulmonary artery, thus to preserve the lingular branches

a donor, and fully informed of risks, benefits, and alternative treatment available to the recipient. In our institution, potential donors are interviewed at least three times to provide them multiple opportunities to question, reconsider, or withdraw as a donor.

After a suitable donor pair is found, the larger donor with better vital capacity is selected for the donation of the right lower lobe, and the other for removal of the left lower lobe.

8.1.2 Size Matching

Appropriate size matching between the donor and recipient is important in LDLLT. It is often inevitable that small grafts are implanted in LDLLT in which only two lobes are implanted. Excessively small grafts may cause high pulmonary artery pressure, resulting in lung edema [9]. A pleural space problem may increase the risk of empyema. Overexpansion of the donor lobes may contribute obstructive physiology by early closure of small airways [10].

8.1.2.1 Functional Size Matching

For "functional size matching," we utilize graft forced vital capacity (FVC) [11]. We have previously proposed a formula to estimate the graft FVC based on the donor's measured FVC and the number of pulmonary segments implanted [5].

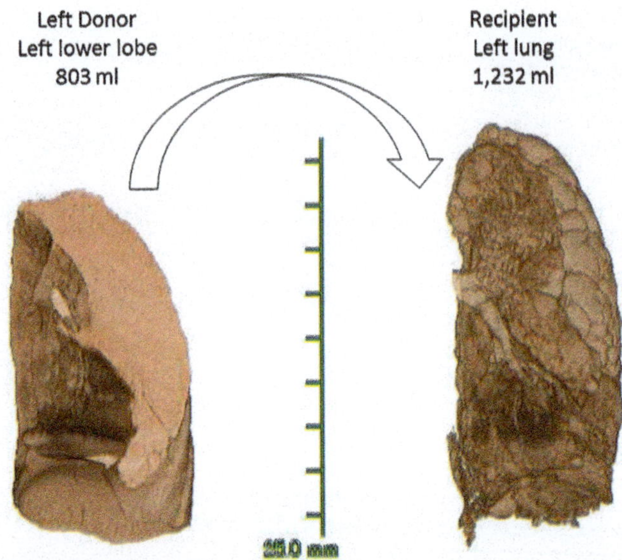

Fig. 8.3 Anatomical size matching for the left donor graft and the recipient left hemithorax, using three-dimensional volumetry. The recipient was an adult male whose left hemithorax was 1,232 mL. The left donor was his wife whose left lower lobe was 803 mL. The ratio of left donor graft to recipient left hemithorax was estimated to be 65.2 %

Given that the right lower lobe consists of 5 segments, the left lower lobe of 4, and the whole lung of 19, the total FVC of the 2 grafts is estimated by the following equation:

Total FVC of the 2 grafts = Measured FVC of the right donor × 5/19 + Measured FVC of the left donor × 4/19.

When the total FVC of the 2 grafts is more than 45 % of the predicted FVC of the recipient (calculated from a knowledge of height, age, and sex), we accept the size disparity regardless of the recipient's diagnosis:

Total FVC of the 2 grafts/Predicted FVC of the recipient > 0.45.

The recipient's mean measured FVC at 6 months after LDLLT was well correlated with the estimated graft FVC [11]. In contrast, we found no significant correlation between the recipient's predicted FVC and the recipient's measured FVC. There results indicate that the amount of lung tissue implanted, not recipient factors such as diagnosis, determines recipient FVC.

8.1.2.2 Anatomical Size Matching

For "anatomical size matching," three-dimensional computed tomography (3D CT) volumetry is performed for both the donor and the recipient (Fig. 8.3) [12, 13]. CT images are obtained using a multidetector CT scanner during a single respiratory pause at the end of maximum inspiratory effort. The upper and lower threshold of anatomical size matching has not been determined yet. We have accepted a wide range of volume ratio between the donor's lower lobe graft and the corresponding recipient's chest cavity. When the ratio was within 40–160 %, we found that recipient's adaptation ability to undersized or oversized grafts was remarkable.

8.1.3 Technique of Donor Lobectomy

The most common procedure involves a right lower lobectomy from a larger donor and a left lower lobectomy from a smaller donor. An epidural catheter for postoperative pain is placed the day before the surgery to avoid any complications related to heparinization. After induction of general anesthesia, donors are intubated with a left-sided double-lumen endotracheal tube. The donors are placed in the lateral decubitus position and a posterolateral thoracotomy is performed though the fifth intercostal space. Fissures are developed using linear stapling devices. The pericardium surrounding the inferior pulmonary vein is opened circumferentially. Dissection in the fissure is carried out to isolate the pulmonary artery to the lower lobe and to define the anatomy of the pulmonary arteries to the middle lobe in the right-side donor and to the lingular segment in the left-side donor. If the branches of middle lobe artery and lingular artery are small, they are ligated and divided. However, if such braches are large enough, arterioplasty using autopericardial patch should be performed [14].

Intravenous prostaglandin E1 is administered to decrease a systolic blood pressure by 10–20 mmHg. Five thousand units of heparin and 500 mg of methylprednisolone are administered intravenously. After placing vascular clamps in appropriate positions, the division of the pulmonary vein, the pulmonary artery, and the bronchus is carried out in this order. Vascular stamps are closed with 5-0 Prolene running suture. The bronchus is closed with 4-0 Prolene interrupted sutures. The bronchial stamp is covered with pedicled pericardial fat tissue.

On the back table, the lobes are flushed with preservation solution both antegradely and retrogradely from a bag about 50 cm above the table. The lobes are gently ventilated with room air during the flush.

8.2 Trials to Extend Living-Donor Criteria

Eligibility criteria for living lobar lung donation summarized in Table 8.1 should be strictly followed for the donor safety. Extracting more than one lobe from the donor should be prohibited. Non-Japanese institutions have accepted extended family members and unrelated individuals, which have never been accepted in Japan to exclude inappropriate motivation.

Recently, many cases of ABO-incompatible organ transplantation, especially kidney and liver transplantation, have been performed to overcome the donor organ shortage. We recently reported successful ABO-incompatible LDLLT performed in a 10-year-old boy with bronchiolitis obliterans after bone marrow transplantation for recurrent acute myeloid leukemia [15]. His blood type had changed from AB to O by the bone marrow transplantation and received type B and AB donor lobar lungs.

Finding two suitable donors with appropriate size matching is not an easy task. To overcome this problem, we have developed several surgical procedures in LDLLT from size-mismatched donors.

8.2.1 LDLLT Using Oversized Graft

For small children, the adult lower lobe might be too big. The use of oversized grafts could cause high airway resistance, atelectasis, and hemodynamic instability by the time of chest closure [16]. To overcome these problems, we have developed several techniques including single lobe transplantation with or without contralateral pneumonectomy, delayed chest closure, and downsizing the graft.

Single LDLLT from a single living donor can be performed for selected small recipients. We retrospectively investigated 14 critically ill patients who had undergone single LDLLT at three lung transplant centers in Japan [7]. Three- and five-year survival rates were 70 % and 56 %, respectively. Survival among these 14 patients was significantly worse than survival in a group of 78 patients undergoing bilateral LDLLT during the same period. Single LDLLT provides acceptable results for sick patients who would die soon otherwise. However, bilateral LDLLT appears to be a better option if two living donors are found.

We reported successful right lower lobe transplantation and simultaneous left pneumonectomy in an 8-year-old girl on a ventilator [17]. The graft donated by her mother was estimated to be 200 % larger than the right chest cavity of the recipient.

It has been reported that delayed chest closure can be safely used after cadaveric bilateral lung transplantation. This technique can be applied to LDLLT [18]. The oversized graft volume is expected to decrease during the waiting period by improvement of pulmonary edema and the dimensions of the recipient's right heart are expected to decrease because of the reduction in the afterload after LDLLT.

We reported another strategy for oversized graft by downsizing a graft on a back table. A 15-year-old boy with bronchiolitis obliterans successfully underwent bilateral LDLLT with segmentectomy of the superior segment of an oversized right lower lobe graft obtained from his father [12].

8.2.2 LDLLT Using Undersized Graft

When grafts are too small, a limited amount of vascular bed might cause high pulmonary artery pressure, resulting in lung edema [9]. Intrathoracic dead space can remain and cause complications, such as postoperative bleeding, persistent air leakage, and empyema. Moreover, hyperinflation of the grafted lungs may result in insufficient respiratory dynamics or hemodynamic collapse after LDLLT [10].

We reported a successful LDLLT in which a very large size mismatch between donor lungs and recipient chest cavity was solved by sparing the bilateral native upper lobes [19]. A recipient, 44-year-old man with bronchiolitis obliterans, was 17 cm taller than his donors, his sister, and his wife. Regarding functional size matching, the estimated graft FVC was 45.7 % of the recipient's predicted FVC. Regarding anatomical size matching, the volume ratio of the graft was only 22 % in the right side and 36 % in the left side. By sparing native upper lobes, adequate chest cavity for small grafts was provided. Candidates for this approach should have no infection in the spared lobes and minimum pleural adhesion with well-developed interlobar fissures. Considering these factors, a space-occupying, noninfectious disease, such as bronchiolitis obliterans, would be an ideal indication. Pulmonary fibrosis, pulmonary artery hypertension, emphysema, and lymphangioleiomyomatosis may also be possible indications.

8.3 Prognosis of Living Donors

Successful LDLLT largely depends on donor outcome. It is well known that the survival of recipients receiving LDLLT is similar or better than cadaveric lung transplantation. On the other hand, long-term outcomes of live donors have not been well documented. It is because the donor follow-up continues generally through 1 year and then discontinues. More studies will be needed to understand the long-term results of living lung donors.

8.3.1 Perioperative Complications in Living Donors

Relatively high morbidity after lobectomy has been described in the previous reports, but there has been no reported perioperative mortality [20, 21]. Morbidity rates varied from 20 % to 60 % depending on the definition of complications. Common complications are pleural effusion, bronchial stamp fistulas, hemorrhage, and arrhythmia. The Vancouver Forum Lung Group summarized the world experience on approximately 550 living lung donors in 2006 [22]. Approximately 5 % of them have experienced complications requiring surgical or bronchoscopic intervention.

Relatively high morbidity after living-donor lobectomy as compared to standard lobectomy may be explained by three technical differences between the two surgical procedures. First, the circumferential pericardotomy surrounding the inferior pulmonary vein may increase the risk for arrhythmias and pericarditis. Second, an oblique transection of the right lower lobe bronchus may increase the risk for bronchial fistula and stenosis. Third, administration of heparin may increase the risk of bleeding in the perioperative period.

8.3.2 Psychologic Outcome of Living Donors

The Massachusetts General Hospital (MGH) reported that living lung donors enjoyed generally satisfactory physical and emotional health [23]. Donors reported positive feelings about donation, but wished to be recognized and valued by the transplant team and the recipient. Okayama group reported that the average quality of life in the living lung donors was better than that of general population [24]. However, a fatal outcome in the recipient significantly impacted donor mental health. Interestingly, there was a significant correlation in mental health scores between the paired donors.

8.3.3 Pulmonary Function of Living Donors

The MGH group reported that mean donor FVC decreased by 16 ± 3 % [23]. Post-donation FVC value was higher than preoperatively predicted value. We prospectively evaluated pulmonary function 3, 6, and 12 months after donor lobectomy [25]. FVC and FEV1 recovered constantly up to more than 90 % of the preoperative value 1 year after donor lobectomy.

References

1. Date H. Update on living-donor lobar lung transplantation. Curr Opin Organ Transplant. 2011;16:453–7.
2. Shiraishi T, Okada Y, Sekine Y, et al. Registry of the Japanese society of lung and heart-lung transplantation: the official Japanese lung transplantation report 2008. Gen Thorac Cardiovasc Surg. 2009;57:395–401.
3. Starnes VA, Bowdish ME, Woo MS, et al. A decade of living lobar lung transplantation. Recipient outcomes. J Thorac Cardiovasc Surg. 2004;127:114–22.
4. Sweet SC. Pediatric living donor lobar lung transplantation. Pediatr Transplant. 2006; 10:861–8.

5. Date H, Aoe M, Nagahiro I, et al. Living-donor lobar lung transplantation for various lung diseases. J Thorac Cardiovasc Surg. 2003;126:476–81.
6. Date H, Aoe M, Sano Y, et al. Improved survival after living-donor lobar lung transplantation. J Thorac Cardiovasc Surg. 2004;128:933–40.
7. Date H, Shiraishi T, Sugimoto S, et al. Outcome of living-donor lobar lung transplantation using a single donor. J Thorac Cardiovasc Surg. 2012;144:710–5.
8. Chen F, Fujinaga T, Shoji T, et al. Short-term outcome in living donors for lung transplantation: the role of preoperative computer tomographic evaluations of fissures and vascular anatomy. Transpl Int. 2012;25:732–8.
9. Fujita T, Date H, Ueda K, et al. Experimental study on size matching in a canine living-donor lobar lung transplant model. J Thorac Cardiovasc Surg. 2002;123:104–9.
10. Haddy SM, Bremner RM, Moore-Jefferies EW, et al. Hyperinflation resulting in hemodynamic collapse following living donor lobar transplantation. Anesthesiology. 2002;97:1315–7.
11. Date H, Aoe M, Nagahiro I, et al. How to predict forced vital capacity after living-donor lobar-lung transplantation. J Heart Lung Transplant. 2004;23:547–51.
12. Chen F, Fujinaga T, Shoji T, et al. Perioperative assessment of oversized lobar graft downsizing in living-donor lobar lung transplantation using three-dimensional computed tomographic volumetry. Transpl Int. 2010;23:e41–4.
13. Camargo JJP, Irion KL, Marchiori E, et al. Computed tomography measurement of lung volume in preoperative assessment for living donor lung transplantation: volume calculation using 3D surface rendering in the determination of size compatibility. Pediatr Transplant. 2009;13:429–39.
14. Chen F, Miwa S, Bando T, et al. Pulmonary arterioplasty for the remaining arterial stump of the donor and the arterial cuff of the donor graft in living-donor lobar lung transplantation. Eur J Cardiothorac Surg. 2012;42:e138–9.
15. Shoji T, Bando T, Fujinaga T, et al. ABO-incompatible living-donor lobar lung transplantation. J Heart Lung Transplant. 2011;30:479–80.
16. Oto T, Date H, Ueda K, et al. Experimental study of oversized grafts in a canine living-donor lobar lung transplantation model. J Heart Lung Transplant. 2001;20:1325–30.
17. Sonobe M, Bando T, Kusuki S, et al. Living-donor single-lobe lung transplantation and simultaneous contralateral pneumonectomy in a child. J Heart Lung Transplant. 2011;30:471–4.
18. Chen F, Matsukawa S, Ishii H, et al. Delayed chest closure assessed by transesophageal echocardiogram in single-lobe lung transplantation. Ann Thorac Surg. 2011;92:2254–7.
19. Fujinaga T, Bando T, Nakajima D, et al. Living-donor lobar lung transplantation with sparing of bilateral native upper lobes: a novel strategy. J Heart Lung Transplant. 2011;30:351–3.
20. Battafarano RJ, Anderson RC, Meyers BF, et al. Perioperative complications after living donor lobectomy. J Thorac Cardiovasc Surg. 2000;120:909–15.
21. Bowdish ME, Barr ML, Schenkel FA, et al. A decade of living lobar lung transplantation. Perioperative complications after 253 donor lobectomies. Am J Transplant. 2004;4:1283–8.
22. Barr ML, Belghiti J, Villamil FG, et al. A report of the Vancouver forum on the care of the live organ donor. Lung, liver, pancreas, and intestine data and medical guidelines. Transplantation. 2006;81:1372–87.
23. Prager LM, Wain JC, Roberts DH, et al. Medical and psychologic outcome of living lobar lung transplant donors. J Heart Lung Transplant. 2006;25:1206–12.
24. Nishioka M, Yokoyama C, Iwasaki M, et al. Donor quality of life in living-donor lobar lung transplantation. J Heart Lung Transplant. 2011;30:1348–51.
25. Chen F, Fujinaga T, Shoji T, et al. Outcomes and pulmonary function in living lobar lung transplant donors. Transpl Int. 2012;25:153–7.

Part V
Liver Transplantation

Chapter 9
How to Initiate DCD Program for Liver Transplantation

Paolo Muiesan, Francesca Tinti, and Anna Paola Mitterhofer

9.1 Classification of DCD

Donation after circulatory death (DCD) can be classified using the modified Maastricht criteria [4] (Table 9.1) and, according to the setting in which cardiac death occurs, is divided into two main categories: controlled and uncontrolled. The ethics, assessment, logistics, techniques of retrieval and outcomes of transplant are very different with controlled and uncontrolled liver DCD.

Controlled donors are generally victims of a catastrophic brain injury of diverse aetiology, deemed incompatible with meaningful recovery, but whose condition does not meet formal criteria for brainstem death and whose cardiopulmonary function ceases before organs are retrieved. The procedure of withdrawal of life support therapy (WLST) is planned by the patient's medical team in agreement with the family of the injured patient. This decision is independent from, and precedes, the one to donate. In category III, circulatory arrest is induced by WLST and occurs within an intensive care unit (ICU) or in the operating room. In type IV, brain death is declared before unpredicted cardiac arrest or, to respect family wishes, donation proceeds just after cardiac arrest.

P. Muiesan (✉)
The Liver Unit, HPB Surgery and Liver Transplantation, Queen Elizabeth Hospital Birmingham, University Hospitals Birmingham NHS Trust, 3rd Floor Nuffield House, Edgbaston, Birmingham, B15 2TH, UK
e-mail: paolo.muiesan@uhb.nhs.uk

F. Tinti
The Liver Unit, HPB Surgery and Liver Transplantation, Queen Elizabeth Hospital Birmingham, University Hospitals Birmingham NHS Trust, 3rd Floor Nuffield House, Edgbaston, Birmingham, B15 2TH, UK

Department of Clinical Medicine, Sapienza University of Rome, Rome, Italy

A.P. Mitterhofer
Department of Clinical Medicine, Sapienza University of Rome, Rome, Italy

T. Asano et al. (eds.), *Marginal Donors: Current and Future Status*,
DOI 10.1007/978-4-431-54484-5_9, © Springer Japan 2014

Table 9.1 Modified Maastricht classification of DCD [4]

Category	Description	Type of DCD	Location
I	Dead on arrival (at hospital)	Uncontrolled	ED
II	Unsuccessful resuscitation	Uncontrolled	ED
III	Anticipated cardiac arrest (after withdrawal of treatment)	Controlled	ICU and ED
IV	Cardiac arrest in a brain-dead donor	Controlled	Theatre
V	Unexpected cardiac arrest in an ICU patient	Uncontrolled	ICU

Controlled forms of DCD limit ischaemic injury and are associated with the highest quality DCD organs for transplantation. Type 1 DCD yields tissue, not organs, for donation due to the ischaemic injury. *ED* emergency department; *ICU* intensive care unit

Controlled DCD occurs in the presence of organ retrieval teams and limits the ischaemic injury associated with death. The process of dying in type III DCD, however, may be associated with a prolonged agonal period of hypotension and/or hypoxia which is ultimately responsible for ischaemic injury that may prevent organ donation or be accountable for graft dysfunction or non-function of the transplanted organ. In this respect it is crucial that we recognise that long before cardio-circulatory arrest happens, there is a total lack of arterial and portal blood flow through the liver.

On the other hand, uncontrolled donation refers to donation after death that occurred suddenly and was not anticipated. In Maastricht category I, death is declared outside of hospital and the potential donor is brought to the hospital without resuscitation attempts. In type II, cardio-circulatory arrest occurs unexpectedly and resuscitation attempts are unsuccessful. Death is then declared only after failure of resuscitation attempts.

Uncontrolled DCD occurs following the unanticipated cardiac arrest of a patient; due to logistical reasons and the associated degree of ischaemic injury only deaths occurring at a centre with established organ retrieval teams and pathways are suitable for donation of liver grafts (category II). It is possible to overcome some of these logistical challenges by directing intensive medical care resources outside of the hospital. In Madrid and Barcelona a network of mobile ICU teams are tasked to patients in out-of-hospital cardiac arrest. The subsequent effect is that this also maximises rates of uncontrolled DCD.

In summary category IV can be either uncontrolled or controlled. Categories I and II are considered uncontrolled and category III is considered controlled.

9.2 DCD Liver Transplantation: The Past, a Historical Perspective

The first human liver transplant was performed in 1963 by the surgical team led by Dr. Thomas Starzl of Denver, Colorado. The initial attempts at human liver transplantation produced short-term survival. As the criteria for brain death had not yet been established, at that time organs were retrieved after the donors died of circulatory arrest after withdrawal from respiratory support.

Starzl acknowledged the role of ischaemic injury associated with DCD and described biochemical evidence of hepatocellular damage, postoperative coagulopathy and biliary necrosis in transplanted grafts at autopsy [5]. The importance of limiting ischaemic injury by hypothermic perfusion and the time from donor death to revascularisation was highlighted in these early experiments. Calne, also utilising DCD donors, recommended limiting the time from death to cold perfusion to less than 15 min [6].

Early liver transplant programs experienced many problems including peri- and postoperative care, immunosuppression and poor graft and patient survival. The recognition of brain death [7–9], legally and clinically, led to interest in recovering organs following donation after brain death (DBD). DBD limited ischaemic injury and thus became, and remains, the standard by which cadaveric liver grafts are retrieved and led to the cessation of almost all DCD programs. With the advent of cyclosporine in the 1980s, improved graft survival was observed and led to widespread acceptance of liver transplantation for patients with end-stage liver disease. Consequently the number of potential recipients increased at a rate exceeding the number of brain-dead donors. The renewed interest in DCD as a viable organ source has occurred as a result of increased demand for donor organs. In the United Kingdom there has been a tenfold increase in DCD donors between 2000 and 2010. Early experiences of DCD renal transplantation in the modern era demonstrated long-term renal function comparable to that of organs obtained following DBD [10–12]. Early liver DCD programs in the modern era suffered a high incidence of graft dysfunction and failure in addition to biliary complications [13–16]. Casavilla et al. published early experience of both uncontrolled and controlled DCD liver transplantation in a small number of subjects [14]. Only one of six uncontrolled DCD liver grafts survived longer than a month. All controlled DCD grafts functioned though two were lost due to early hepatic artery thrombosis. In a review of United Network for Organ Sharing (UNOS) data independent predictors of early DCD graft failure were prolonged cold ischaemic time (CIT) and recipient life support, highlighting the importance of recipient variables in addition to donor variables in the use of DCD liver grafts [16]. By reducing the CIT and with careful donor and recipient selection, however, graft survival and patient survival have subsequently been demonstrated equivalent between recipients of DBD and DCD livers in single-centre experiences [17, 18]. Short warm and cold ischaemic times in addition to careful donor and recipient selection appear responsible for this equivalency.

A problem almost unique to DCD liver transplantation is the association with ischaemic-type biliary lesions (ITBL), which is associated with an increased duration of donor warm ischaemia time (dWIT) (Fig. 9.1) [19–21]. The first insult contributing to biliary damage is certainly ischaemic. The resulting ischaemic injury to the microvascular endothelium leads, in the preservation phase, to cell disruption and may contribute to microvascular thrombosis, which prevents effective revascularisation and exacerbates ischaemic injury to the biliary epithelium.

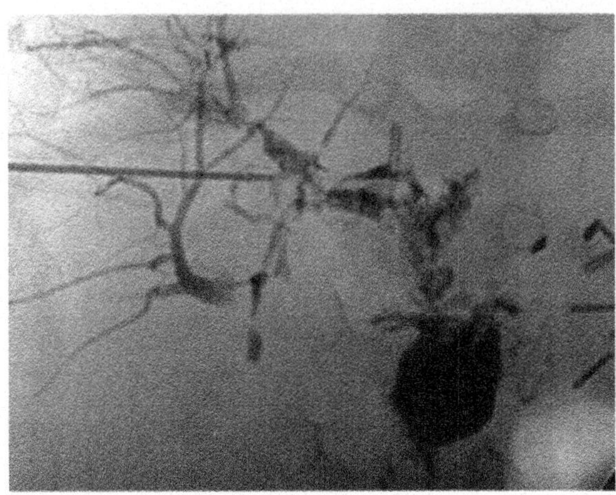

Fig. 9.1 Percutaneous cholangiogram demonstrating a DCD liver graft affected by ischaemic cholangiopathy

9.3 DCD Liver Transplantation: The Modern Era

In the present climate great emphasis is placed upon clinical outcomes; five- and ten-year graft survival and patient survival of recipients transplanted with DBD organs are well established. However, with the current rates of waiting list mortality, the use of DCD organs appears reasonable given the scarcity of DBD organs and the inherent risk of donor morbidity and mortality that is associated with living liver donation.

Ethical and legal considerations are intrinsically associated with DCD. One contemporary argument in favour of DCD is that it provides deceased patients and their families with the chance of organ donation if brain death is not the cause of death. This is essential to permit the ethical and legal justification for the process of DCD [22, 23]. It also benefits those individuals who do not recognise brain death and in whom death can only be accepted following the cessation of the heartbeat. The process associated with DCD, however, raises ethical and legal concerns [24–26]; healthcare professionals may feel a conflict of interest and be placed in particularly challenging situations when faced with patients in whom ongoing treatment is futile and who may be suitable DCD donors [27]. Further uncertainty exists on what are acceptable interventions pre- and post-mortem prior to DCD, particularly in the case of uncontrolled DCD of the liver, and what conditions must be met in order to confirm death in DCD donors.

9.4 Controlled DCD

It is essential from an ethical perspective that the decision to undertake WLST is made without consideration to the possibility of DCD. A team separate from that which is responsible for the ongoing treatment of the patient will assess the suitability of

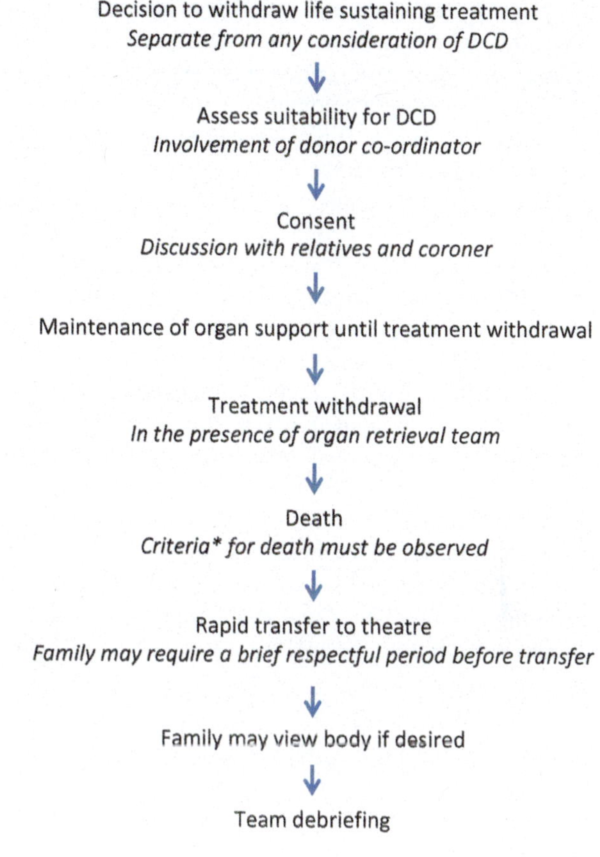

Fig. 9.2 Summary of the events and processes that occur in controlled DCD. Adapted from the Australian Guidelines on organ and tissue donation after death. The reference for this is Organ and Tissue Donation after Death, for Transplantation. Guidelines for Ethical Practice for Health Professionals. Australian Government, National Health and Medical Research Council. 2007. Available from http://www.nhmrc.gov.au/_files_nhmrc/file/publications/synopses/e75.pdf

donation. The decision to withdraw treatment precedes and must be independent from that to consider organ donation. This process is transparent to the public and no conflict of interest can be perceived. When donation is considered possible the family or next of kin are approached and consent for DCD is sought. Organ retrieval teams are dispatched to the donor hospital in a timely manner where WLST subsequently occurs. This process of events with key points is summarised in Fig. 9.2. In the United Kingdom any procedure or intervention deemed not required for that patient's ongoing medical care could be considered unethical or even unlawful. A more holistic approach to the patient recognises that an overall benefit arising from interventions may be appropriate when taking into consideration wider emotional, cultural, family and religious issues [23]. Appropriate interventions include discussing donation with family, reviewing a patient's past medical history for the purposes of donation, taking blood and serum, maintenance of life-sustaining treatment, delaying WLST until the surgical team is on site and changing a patient's location for purposes of WLST and subsequent donation. Controversial interventions are allowed in other countries and include those that can be considered as anything that places the person at risk of harm or distress and include systemic heparinisation where this might hasten death, placement of femoral catheters and cardiopulmonary resuscitation prior to the commencement of organ recovery processes [28].

Within the transplant community there is a growing concern that by promoting controlled DCD some clinicians supporting donation may avoid prolonged neurological testing that is required for DBD. Controlled DCD aims to expand the donor pool and support the already existing DBD programs that cannot meet the needs of potential recipients. A review of organ donation within European countries identified that most countries had demonstrated an increase in DBD rates between 2000 and 2009 [29]. Just 5 of 23 countries demonstrated decreased rates of DBD over the same time period. Of these, 3 were countries with expanding and outstanding controlled DCD programs (Belgium, the Netherlands and the United Kingdom).

The location of WLST is controversial. Ideally, to keep the dWIT to a minimum for the purposes of organ donation, this should occur in the theatre complex where the organ recovery procedure will occur. Treatment is withdrawn in accordance with local practice and policies and it is usually by extubation. In the United Kingdom, withdrawal commonly takes place either in the ICU or in the anaesthetic room. Withdrawal in the operating room is frequent practice in the United States and has the advantage of minimising dWIT, but it may limit the family's wishes to assist their dying relative and may not allow a complete partition of the physician declaring death from the surgeon waiting to perform the procedure.

9.4.1 Controlled DCD: Donor Selection

The increased incidence of graft dysfunction and non-function associated with DCD organs has resulted in great attention being placed upon donor selection. A very strict selection policy of the very best controlled DCD grafts has achieved excellent results so that some of these liver grafts have been also reduced to allow transplantation in children.

This process is dynamic and is influenced by events following WLST; the key component that is considered is the *functional* donor warm ischaemic time (FdWIT). FdWIT was originally defined in the United Kingdom as the duration of time from when a patient's systolic blood pressure falls below 50 mmHg or, it was later added, when the arterial oxygen saturation falls below 70 %, whichever comes first, and it ends at the commencement of cold perfusion [28]. A similar definition has been proposed in the United States and makes a distinction between the total donor warm ischaemic time (time from WLST and cold perfusion) and the true donor warm ischaemic time (from when mean blood pressure falls below 50 mmHg and cold perfusion) [30].

The tolerance of organs to warm ischaemic injury is organ dependent with the kidney being the most resistant and the heart the least so. Current practice in the United Kingdom is based upon a maximum FdWIT as follows: kidneys, 120 min; liver, 30 min; lungs, 60 min and pancreas, 30 min. These are not absolute times but

Table 9.2 British Transplantation Society guidelines on DCD

Standard criteria include
Age <50 years
BMI <30
Intensive care stay <5 days
Transaminase levels <×4 *N* values and downtrend
Withdrawal to cardiac arrest <30 min
Functional donor warm ischaemic time <20 min
Cold ischaemic time <8 h
Minimal or no steatosis <10 %

typically represent the maximum duration that an implanting surgeon would tolerate. Other factors that affect this time (to decrease it) include advanced donor age, body habitus, comorbidity and other premortem events. Despite a growing number of publications there is still paucity of high level of evidence recommendations on how to avoid early and late DCD liver graft failures.

The presence of numerous identified risk factors contributes to the complexity of a decision of acceptance or rejection of a DCD graft that needs to be made with limited time at disposal and frequently at unsocial hours. In general, adding together two or more main risk factors would suggest prudent refusal of the liver to minimise morbidity and mortality for the recipient.

From the practical viewpoint taken by the British Transplantation Society DCD livers could be divided into two subgroups: standard and extended criteria. *Standard criteria DCD* grafts achieve similar results of recipients of standard DBD livers and should be accepted for recovery and assessment (Table 9.2).

Liver grafts from donors outside the above criteria, *extended criteria* DCD, should be selected with great caution. *Extended criteria DCD* livers are at higher risk of graft loss, should be paired to suitable patients and should be used after a specific informed consent of the prospective recipient. There is no rigid rule to reject or use an extended criteria DCD liver; however, when more than one extended criterion is met, the risk of using such livers may become excessive.

9.4.2 Controlled DCD: Surgical Procedure

Casavilla originally described the super-rapid organ recovery technique for controlled DCD [14]. A midline laparotomy is followed by rapid isolation, cannulation and perfusion of the distal abdominal aorta followed by venting of the abdominal vena cava, sternotomy, clamping of the descending thoracic aorta and venting of the supradiaphragmatic inferior vena cava. In order to facilitate rapid cooling of the liver the portal system is cannulated and perfused followed by packing of the abdominal cavity with ice-cold fluid and ice. Supraduodenal portal perfusion is preferred in cases of pancreas recovery where it is usual to vent the portal vein as it appears from under the duodenum. Heparin can be added to both aortic and portal perfusion fluid in those countries where it is unlawful to administer heparin prior to certification of death. Aortic perfusion using gravity alone is insufficient to produce rapid cooling so aortic fluids are pressurised to 200 mmHg. The abdominal cavity is topically cooled using copious saline ice slush. The common bile duct is flushed profusely with saline to remove residual bile. The occurrence of left or right, accessory or replaced, hepatic arteries is more difficult to detect, given the absence of pulsation; thus, extra care is needed to avoid iatrogenic vascular injuries to the graft.

9.4.3 Choice of Preservation Solution

University of Wisconsin (UW) solution is typically preferred for perfusion as data from the UNOS database from over 17,000 liver transplants associates this solution with improved graft function compared to histidine-tryptophan-ketoglutarate (HTK) solution. This effect was particularly pronounced in cases of controlled DCD where HTK was associated with early graft loss with an odds ratio of 1.63 compared to UW solution [31]. There is no randomised evidence from which to directly influence practice in DCD liver transplantation. UW solution is not the ideal solution; however, as it is viscous, it will therefore cool more slowly than less viscous solutions and contains more potassium than other solutions.

9.4.4 Controlled DCD: Recipient Selection and Procedure

An early evaluation of the donor graft as to its suitability for transplantation is essential to limit CIT. Numerous surgeons are willing to compromise slightly on CIT in order to personally inspect the graft at its arrival before sending the recipient to the operating room. In cases where there is likely to be a protracted recipient hepatectomy, the expected duration of CIT must be known. If the hepatectomy is more difficult than anticipated, the transplant surgeon, having already performed irreversible operative procedures, may find himself/herself committed to hepatectomy but with a CIT in excess of 8 h. Furthermore, following the implantation of DCD grafts, recipients typically display more physiological stress than those of a DBD graft. This may manifest itself as cardiovascular instability, requiring escalating doses of inotropes, followed by coagulopathy during the remaining operative procedure and as postoperative organ dysfunction which may affect the liver as well as other organs. The requirement for renal support is higher following DCD liver implantation compared to DBD liver grafts. The choice of recipient should be restricted to those not requiring long difficult dissections, including retransplants or patients with previous extensive upper abdominal surgery, as this extends the CIT. High-risk patients, as those already on multi-organ support and those with severe portal hypertension, requiring robust early graft function, are not generally considered to be good candidates for DCD liver grafts. Malignancy is a good indication for

DCD liver transplantation. Patients transplanted for hepatocellular carcinoma (HCC) rather than for end-stage liver disease, given their good performance status, may better tolerate the significant reperfusion injury which follows the implantation and revascularisation of DCD livers. Patients with HCC, who are suitable for and consent to DCD grafts, experience less competition whilst waiting and are transplanted more rapidly, thus minimising the risk of dropping out for HCC progression beyond transplant criteria.

9.5 Uncontrolled DCD

Worldwide the majority of uncontrolled DCD are category I or II donors and constitute the best part of patients considered eligible for DCD in Spain, France and the Netherlands. Uncontrolled DCD are more likely to be trauma victims, younger and *healthier* individuals, yet the use of these grafts is still limited. Death often occurs after prolonged periods of resuscitation manoeuvres, leading to substantial injury from warm ischaemia, the real extent of which is difficult to assess due to the unanticipated nature of cardio-circulatory arrest that may have not occurred within the medical setting. As donation interventions need to be initiated quickly, the surrogate decision makers are unlikely to be immediately available to provide consent.

Early experience of uncontrolled DCD demonstrated very poor outcomes despite careful donor selection and relatively short periods of dWIT. Subsequent series of uncontrolled DCD predominately originate from Spain where uncontrolled DCD programs are well supported by a legal framework (Table 9.3). Contemporary uncontrolled DCD consists of advanced cardiorespiratory support, femoral cannula placement, normothermic regional perfusion (NRP) using a device similar to Extra-Corporeal Membrane Oxigenation (ECMO) and finally organ recovery (described below). Even with these processes and careful donor selection, primary non-function (PNF) still affects 10–18 % of grafts [32–36]. Graft survival and patient survival at 1 year are 49–90 % and 62–90 %, respectively. In the largest published series there is evidence of improving outcomes; 6-month graft survival was 53 % in the first half of the series compared to 88 % in the second cohort ($p=0.024$) [36]. An evolution of technical processes and a better understanding of recipient selection appear responsible for this progress. Published outcomes of liver uncontrolled DCD series are given in Table 9.3.

Despite the longer dWIT, uncontrolled donation may have theoretical advantages over controlled DCD. It has been hypothesised that brain death may lead to an upregulation of pro-inflammatory mediators and cell-surface molecules in peripheral organs to be engrafted, thus making them more susceptible to inflammatory and immune responses in the host. Due to the rapidity of events, uncontrolled donors are expected to be spared by the negative effects of severe brain injury. On the contrary, controlled DCD are likely to be affected to a degree by the *cytokine storm* given the longer duration of the central nervous system injury. Finally uncontrolled donors

Table 9.3 Published series of uncontrolled liver transplantation with outcomes

Author	LTx centre	Year	N uDCD	PNF (%)	HAT (%)	BC (%)	Re-LTx (%)	Graft survival (%)	Patient survival (%)	Follow-up (months)
Casavilla et al.	Pittsburgh	1995	6	33	17	–	50	17	67	12
Busuttil and Tanaka	UCLA	2003	16	6.25	–	–	–	75	88	12
Otero et al.	La Coruna	2003	20	25	0	5	25	55	80	24
Quintela et al.	La Coruna	2005	10	10	0	0	10	90	90	57
Fondevila et al.	Barcelona	2007	10	10	10	10	25	50	70	23
Suarez et al.	La Coruna	2008	27	18	3.6	25	–	49	62	60
Jimenez-Galanes et al.	Madrid	2009	20	10	0	5	15	80	85.5	12
Fondevila et al.[a]	Barcelona	2012	34	–	–	12	–	70	82	24

This is an update of Muiesan P: Liver transplantation using donors after cardiac death in Medical care of the liver transplant patient, Fourth Edn. 2012 Blackwell Publishing Ltd

BC biliary complications, *HAT* hepatic artery thrombosis, *LTx* liver transplant, *PNF* primary non-function

[a]Ten out of the 34 patients were previously described in the 2007 publication from the same Author

will never become controlled DCD or DBD donors and their inclusion within donor programs truly expands the donor pool.

From certain ethical perspectives uncontrolled DCD presents fewer challenges than controlled DCD. The process of dying in uncontrolled DCD is a natural spontaneous event and has not occurred following the WLST [37, 38]. In some countries where the WLST is prohibited uncontrolled DCD may be the only viable method of DCD.

9.5.1 Uncontrolled DCD: Donor Selection

Due to the established warm ischaemic injury and time required to mobilise the organ recovery teams to the donor usually kidney-only donation is possible of donors presenting to hospitals with established organ recovery pathways. Uncontrolled DCD donors of livers that are used for transplantation are typically younger, have a lower body mass index and have a more favourable biochemical profile when on ECMO [36].

Due to the risks of PNF and graft dysfunction careful selection of donors is key and resource intensive in uncontrolled liver DCD. The Barcelona experience over 8 years yielded 400 uncontrolled DCD protocol activations. One hundred and ten subjects were excluded during the process of cardiorespiratory support and then 145 further during ECMO to leave 145 organ donors from which 34 liver transplants were performed [36].

9.5.2 Uncontrolled DCD: Donor Procedure

The sequence of events that lead to liver donation in uncontrolled DCD is unique and includes (1) advanced cardiorespiratory support, (2) normothermic regional perfusion and (3) organ recovery:

1. It is important that the cardiac arrest is witnessed so that the dWIT is known with accuracy. Bystander basic life support is provided until advanced life support by medical/paramedical professionals. The duration of resuscitation that is required before death is declared varies according to local protocol; in centres with established programs this is 20 min [36]. Once this has occurred and the donor fulfils basic criteria such as age limits and mode of death a no-touch period of 5 min is required to confirm death in the absence of cardio-circulatory and respiratory functions before restarting chest compressions for the purpose of donation. This may be provided by external chest compression devices. Donor co-ordinators begin the process of organ donation; blood samples are obtained, heparin is given and the organ recovery team mobilised. Perfusion catheters are placed in the femoral artery and vein.
2. A large-bore Fogarty catheter is introduced via the contralateral femoral artery and inserted so that the balloon lies within the aorta above the origin of the coeliac axis or in the thoracic aorta to avoid warm perfusion of the cerebral circulation. NRP is commenced to maintain pump flow in excess of 1.7 L/min. Certain physiological criteria must be met during NRP including satisfactory pH and temperature. During this period an assessment of the biochemical liver function tests is performed at routine time intervals and reperfusion with warm blood allows an assessment of the liver in near-physiological conditions.
3. A full abdominal exploration is performed in the warm phase during NRP prior to cold portal and aortic perfusion and final organ recovery. This process is similar to that during DBD organ recovery.

9.6 DCD Liver Transplantation: The Future

The present use of DCD liver grafts represents the tip of the iceberg. One strategy to increase the usage of these organs is the use of NRP as an intermediate step between the donation process and implantation. This would, in theory, prevent the ischaemic/reperfusion injury and hypothermic injury associated with traditional cold storage and, in addition, allow assessment of ischaemic injury by pathological and biochemical analysis prior to implantation. In a porcine model of extreme warm ischaemic injury NRP was associated with a much improved survival over simple cold storage. Animals experienced 90 min of asystole followed by either NRP for 1 h or not and then followed by 4 h of cold storage. PNF affected 6/6 animals in the no NRP group and 1/6 in the NRP group [39]. A period of NRP permits an assessment of organ function where NRP is associated with improved bile production, haemodynamic and biochemical parameters over static cold perfusion [40]. Whether assessment during this period could discriminate between viable and non-viable human grafts remains to be established.

Ex vivo organ perfusion has shown promising results in animal models of both controlled and uncontrolled DCD. Normothermic machine perfusion (NMP) is potentially more beneficial than hypothermic machine perfusion (HMP) as it provides substrates at body temperature with which hepatocytes can ameliorate previous ischaemic injury [41, 42]. An NMP device from Oxford is about to be trialled in humans. On the other hand the group led by Guarrera used HMP for liver grafts showing a reduction in pro-inflammatory cytokine expression when compared with cold storage. In a case-controlled study HMP was associated with a lower rate of primary dysfunction compared to recipients of standard cold storage grafts (5 vs. 25 %, $p=0.08$) and significantly lower peak levels of AST, ALT, bilirubin and creatinine [43].

The introduction of uncontrolled DCD could expand the donor pool in countries/regions without an existing program without impacting upon existing controlled DCD or DBD programs. There are, however, many barriers to uncontrolled DCD programs. The provisions of trained donor co-ordinators, local pathways, organ recovery surgeons and NRP facilities are required at each site of uncontrolled DCD. This clearly presents logistical and financial challenges. Having met these a program would need to provide sufficient numbers of donors to create a genuine impact. Developing links with local prehospital teams and services is essential.

A novel technique, which aims to decrease the incidence of ITBL following DCD liver transplantation, is to reperfuse the graft with arterial blood followed by portal reperfusion. It is possible that staged portal perfusion followed by arterial perfusion prolongs the duration of warm ischaemia of the biliary tissue. In theory this strategy would limit a second warm hypoxic injury specific to the hepatic arterial circulation of the biliary tree.

9.7 Conclusions

Liver transplantation using DCD grafts increases the donor pool. However, due to concerns over graft dysfunction, non-function and ischaemic biliary injury, careful donor and recipient selection is crucial. Outcomes equivalent to DBD liver transplantation are achievable in such a setting, but many potential donor organs are not transplanted as a consequence. Uncontrolled DCD may expand the donor pool further, but it is likely that this will be at the expense of reduced graft survival.

Whether controlled DCD programs negatively impact upon rates of DBD is unclear, but recent evidence suggests this may be the case. It is essential that the transplant community works alongside allied medical professionals and lay people to maximise all forms of donation.

Strategies to decrease or limit ischaemic injury such as normothermic regional perfusion and extracorporeal machine perfusion (hypothermic or normothermic) have shown great promise in experimental models. High-quality randomised trials are required to investigate their effects in humans. Addressing ethical and legal concerns and logistical issues is a prerequisite for any group wishing to start an uncontrolled DCD liver transplant program.

References

1. Centers for Disease Control and Prevention. Vital Stat Rep. 2002;50
2. Randhawa G. Death and organ donation: meeting the needs of multiethnic and multifaith populations. Br J Anaesth. 2012;108 Suppl 1:i88–91.
3. Volk ML, Warren GJ, Anspach RR, Couper MP, Merion RM, Ubel PA. Attitudes of the American public toward organ donation after uncontrolled (sudden) cardiac death. Am J Transplant. 2010;10:675–80.
4. Kootstra G, Kievit J, Nederstigt A. Organ donors: heartbeating and non-heartbeating. World J Surg. 2002;26:181–4.
5. Starzl TE, Marchioro TL, Huntley RT, Rifkind D, Rowlands DT, Dickinson Jr TC. Experimental and clinical homotransplantation of the liver. Ann N Y Acad Sci. 1964;120:739–65.
6. Calne RY, Williams R. Liver transplantation in man. I. Observations on technique and organization in five cases. Br Med J. 1968;4:535–40.
7. A definition of irreversible coma. Report of the Ad Hoc Committee of the Harvard Medical School to Examine the Definition of Brain Death. JAMA. 1968;205:337–40.
8. Diagnosis of brain death. Statement issued by the honorary secretary of the Conference of Medical Royal Colleges and their Faculties in the United Kingdom on 11 October 1976. Br Med J. 1976;2:1187–88.
9. Diagnosis of Brain Death. Lancet. 1976;2:1069–70.
10. Weber M, Dindo D, Demartines N, Ambuhl PM, Clavien PA. Kidney transplantation from donors without a heartbeat. N Engl J Med. 2002;347:248–55.
11. Akoh JA, Denton MD, Bradshaw SB, Rana TA, Walker MB. Early results of a controlled non-heart-beating kidney donor programme. Nephrol Dial Transplant. 2009;24:1992–6.
12. Summers DM, Johnson RJ, Allen J, Fuggle SV, Collett D, Watson CJ, et al. Analysis of factors that affect outcome after transplantation of kidneys donated after cardiac death in the UK: a cohort study. Lancet. 2010;376:1303–11.
13. Foley DP, Fernandez LA, Leverson G, Chin LT, Krieger N, Cooper JT, et al. Donation after cardiac death: the University of Wisconsin experience with liver transplantation. Ann Surg. 2005;242:724–31.
14. Casavilla A, Ramirez C, Shapiro R, Nghiem D, Miracle K, Bronsther O, et al. Experience with liver and kidney allografts from non-heart-beating donors. Transplantation. 1995;59: 197–203.
15. D'Alessandro AM, Hoffmann RM, Knechtle SJ, Odorico JS, Becker YT, Musat A, et al. Liver transplantation from controlled non-heart-beating donors. Surgery. 2000;128:579–88.
16. Abt PL, Desai NM, Crawford MD, Forman LM, Markmann JW, Olthoff KM, et al. Survival following liver transplantation from non-heart-beating donors. Ann Surg. 2004;239:87–92.
17. Muiesan P, Girlanda R, Jassem W, Melendez HV, O'Grady J, Bowles M, et al. Single-center experience with liver transplantation from controlled non-heartbeating donors: a viable source of grafts. Ann Surg. 2005;242:732–8.
18. Reich DJ, Munoz SJ, Rothstein KD, Nathan HM, Edwards JM, Hasz RD, et al. Controlled non-heart-beating donor liver transplantation: a successful single center experience, with topic update. Transplantation. 2000;70:1159–66.

19. Abt P, Crawford M, Desai N, Markmann J, Olthoff K, Shaked A. Liver transplantation from controlled non-heart-beating donors: an increased incidence of biliary complications. Transplantation. 2003;75:1659–63.
20. Kaczmarek B, Manas MD, Jaques BC, Talbot D. Ischemic cholangiopathy after liver transplantation from controlled non-heart-beating donors-a single-center experience. Transplant Proc. 2007;39:2793–5.
21. Monbaliu D, Van GF, Troisi R, De HB, Lerut J, Reding R, et al. Liver transplantation using non-heart-beating donors: Belgian experience. Transplant Proc. 2007;39:1481–4.
22. Coggon J, Brazier M, Murphy P, Price D, Quigley M. Best interests and potential organ donors. BMJ. 2008;336:1346–7.
23. Richards B, Rogers WA. Organ donation after cardiac death: legal and ethical justifications for antemortem interventions. Med J Aust. 2007;187:168–70.
24. Bell MD. Non-heart beating organ donation: old procurement strategy–new ethical problems. J Med Ethics. 2003;29:176–81.
25. Bell MD. Non-heart beating organ donation: in urgent need of intensive care. Br J Anaesth. 2008;100:738–41.
26. Gardiner D, Riley B. Non-heart-beating organ donation – solution or a step too far? Anaesthesia. 2007;62:431–3.
27. Mandell MS, Zamudio S, Seem D, McGaw LJ, Wood G, Liehr P, et al. National evaluation of healthcare provider attitudes toward organ donation after cardiac death. Crit Care Med. 2006;34:2952–8.
28. Department of Health. Organ donation after circulatory death. Report of a consensus meeting. Intensive Care Society, NHS Blood and Transplant, and British Transplantation Society, 2010. Available from http://www.ics.ac.uk/intensive_care_professional/standards_and_guidelines/dcd.
29. Dominguez-Gil B, Haase-Kromwijk B, Van LH, Neuberger J, Coene L, Morel P, et al. Current situation of donation after circulatory death in European countries. Transpl Int. 2011; 24:676–86.
30. Bernat JL, D'Alessandro AM, Port FK, Bleck TP, Heard SO, Medina J, et al. Report of a national conference on donation after cardiac death. Am J Transplant. 2006;6:281–91.
31. Stewart ZA, Cameron AM, Singer AL, Montgomery RA, Segev DL. Histidine-Tryptophan-Ketoglutarate (HTK) is associated with reduced graft survival in deceased donor livers, especially those donated after cardiac death. Am J Transplant. 2009;9:286–93.
32. Fondevila C, Hessheimer AJ, Ruiz A, Calatayud D, Ferrer J, Charco R, et al. Liver transplant using donors after unexpected cardiac death: novel preservation protocol and acceptance criteria. Am J Transplant. 2007;7:1849–55.
33. Jimenez-Galanes S, Meneu-Diaz MJ, Elola-Olaso AM, Perez-Saborido B, Yiliam FS, Calvo AG, et al. Liver transplantation using uncontrolled non-heart-beating donors under normothermic extracorporeal membrane oxygenation. Liver Transpl. 2009;15:1110–8.
34. Otero A, Gomez-Gutierrez M, Suarez F, Arnal F, Fernandez-Garcia A, Aguirrezabalaga J, et al. Liver transplantation from Maastricht category 2 non-heart-beating donors. Transplantation. 2003;76:1068–73.
35. Quintela J, Gala B, Baamonde I, Fernandez C, Aguirrezabalaga J, Otero A, et al. Long-term results for liver transplantation from non-heart-beating donors maintained with chest and abdominal compression-decompression. Transplant Proc. 2005;37:3857–8.
36. Fondevila C, Hessheimer AJ, Flores E, Ruiz A, Mestres N, Calatayud D, et al. Applicability and results of Maastricht type 2 donation after cardiac death liver transplantation. Am J Transplant. 2012;12:162–70.
37. Huddle TS, Schwartz MA, Bailey FA, Bos MA. Death, organ transplantation and medical practice. Philos Ethics Humanit Med. 2008;3:5.
38. Kaufman BJ, Wall SP, Gilbert AJ, Dubler NN, Goldfrank LR. Success of organ donation after out-of-hospital cardiac death and the barriers to its acceptance. Crit Care. 2009;13:189.
39. Fondevila C, Hessheimer AJ, Maathuis MH, Munoz J, Taura P, Calatayud D, et al. Superior preservation of DCD livers with continuous normothermic perfusion. Ann Surg. 2011; 254:1000–7.

40. Gong J, Lao XJ, Wang XM, Long G, Jiang T, Chen S. Preservation of non-heart-beating donor livers in extracorporeal liver perfusion and histidine-trytophan-ketoglutarate solution. World J Gastroenterol. 2008;14:2338–42.
41. Butler AJ, Rees MA, Wight DG, Casey ND, Alexander G, White DJ, et al. Successful extracorporeal porcine liver perfusion for 72 hr. Transplantation. 2002;73:1212–8.
42. Imber CJ, St Peter SD, Lopez dC, I, Pigott D, James T, Taylor R et al. Advantages of normothermic perfusion over cold storage in liver preservation. Transplantation. 2002;73:701.
43. Guarrera JV, Henry SD, Samstein B, Odeh-Ramadan R, Kinkhabwala M, Goldstein MJ, et al. Hypothermic machine preservation in human liver transplantation: the first clinical series. Am J Transplant. 2010;10:372–81.

Chapter 10
DCD for Liver Transplantation

Naoto Matsuno and Shin Enosawa

10.1 Introduction

A critical shortage of donor liver grafts has promoted the creation of strategies to increase the donor pool. The Institute of Medicine and the Health Resources and Services Administration statement encourages using grafts from higher-risk donors in order to decrease the growing waiting list [1–3]. In March 1995, an international workshop on non-heart-beating donation was held in Maastricht. Potential donors after cardiac death (DCDs) are classified using the Maastricht classification [4]. Categories 1, 2, and 4 include uncontrolled DCDs, and Category 3 includes controlled DCDs. DCDs have come to represent the fastest growing proportion of the donor pool, thus increasing from approximately 1 % of all deceased donors in 1996 to 11 % of deceased donors in 2008. In some United Network for Organ Sharing (UNOS) regions with limited standard criteria for donors, DCDs comprise up to 16–21 % of the total donor pool [5]. Recent data regarding kidney transplants show no differences between the long-term outcomes of kidney grafts from DCDs and those from brain-dead donors (DBDs), although the incidence of delayed graft function (DGF) is higher in DCD kidneys [6–8]. Following the successful use of DCD kidney grafts for transplantation, interest has moved toward using extrarenal organs such as the liver, pancreas, and lungs [9]. Recently, a number of transplant programs have begun to use livers from DCDs. Although the use of extrarenal DCD grafts is increasing, this endeavor is still in the midst of development. In the early phase, liver

N. Matsuno (✉)
Division for Innovative Surgery and Transplantation,
National Center for Child Health and Development,
2-10-1 Okura, Setagayaku, Tokyo 157-8535, Japan
e-mail: mtnnot@yahoo.co.jp

S. Enosawa
Division for Advanced Medical Sciences, Clinical Research Center, National Center
for Child Health and Development, 2-10-1 Okura, Setagaya-ku, Tokyo 157-0074, Japan

T. Asano et al. (eds.), *Marginal Donors: Current and Future Status*,
DOI 10.1007/978-4-431-54484-5_10, © Springer Japan 2014

Table 10.1 Multiple strategies for using DCD liver graft are required

Selection criteria for donor and recipient
Development of initial flush-out solution (in situ flushing or back table)
Novel preservation system (machine perfusion is ideal) including preservation temperature
Development of preservation solution = organ recovery solution
Considering of rinse solution just before implantation
Prevention for severe reperfusion injury

transplantations from DCDs do not always show favorable post-transplant results compared to liver transplantations from DBDs. Livers from DCDs have been found to display diffuse hepatocyte necrosis, increased platelet adhesion, an absence of bile flow, and depletion of ATP. The incidence of DGF in the kidneys is high; however, it can be treated with hemodialysis until the kidneys recover. In contrast, DGF in the liver often requires retransplantation as rescue therapy. For this reason, there has been great caution in using DCD liver grafts. However, in recent years, the incidences of primary nonfunction (PNF) and severe DGF have been remarkably reduced due to the use of selected controlled DCD livers, better selection criteria, and shorter warm and cold ischemic times. Regarding preservation, the introduction of UW solution has improved the quality of cold preserved organ preservation, even for livers. However, the major principle of hypothermic liver preservation is the reduction of metabolic activity. Recently, the Barcelona group has begun to resuscitate uncontrolled DCD donors with the use of normothermic extracorporeal machine perfusion (NECMO) [10]. The use of warm perfusion may provide full metabolic support to DCD livers and establish whether a graft is viable. Again, development for clinical use of DCD liver graft is still midst. Multiple strategies will be required (Table 10.1).

10.2 Donor Criteria

The use of liver transplants from DCDs has not yet reached a majority, as with kidney transplants. Effective and rapid organ procurement, strict selection of liver grafts, and reduction of warm and cold ischemic times are important, based on the experience in some centers. There are no effective mathematical algorithms capable of differentiating livers based on transplantability. However, DCD criteria may help surgeons to create better evidence-based DCD acceptance protocols and assist in informing recipients and family members of the risks associated with specific types of DCD liver grafts.

Mateo et al. analyzed the UNOS database of 367 liver transplants from DCDs and 33,111 liver transplants from DBDs performed between 1996 and 2003 [11]. They identified the following cumulative relative risk factors for graft loss among recipients: medical conditions present at transplantation, medical history, being on life support, being hospitalized or placed in an intensive care unit, receiving dialysis, having a serum creatinine level greater than 2.0 mg/dl at the time of transplantation, and age greater than 60 years. However, low-risk recipients with low-risk DCD livers (DWIT<30 min and CIT<10 h) show graft survival rates at 1 and 3 years (81 % and 67 %) that are not statistically different from those of recipients with DBD livers. Lee et al. analyzed the data of 874 adult DCD liver transplants performed between 1996 and 2006 and found risk factors using a multivariate Cox model [12]. Five risk factors were identified based on index scores: medical history, life-support status at transplantation, DWIT, CIT, and donor age. Graft survival in recipients with low-risk DCD donors (donor age ≤45 years, DWIT ≤15 min, and CIT ≤10 h) was found to be comparable to that in recipients with DBDs. Muthur et al. analyzed data from the Scientific Registry of Transplant Recipients for DCD liver recipients who underwent transplantation between September 1, 2001 and April 30, 2009 ($n=1{,}567$) [13]. The significant predictive factors of graft failure included age ≥55 years, male sex, African-American race, HCV positivity, presence of metabolic liver disorders, transplant MELD≥35, hospitalization at transplantation, and the need for life support at transplantation ($p \leq 0.05$). The donor characteristics included age ≥50 years and weight >100 kg (both: $p \leq 0.005$). Each hour of increased cold ischemia time (CIT) was found to be associated with a 6 % higher graft failure rate ($p<0.001$). DWIT≥35 min significantly increased the graft failure rates ($p=0.002$). The recipient predictors of mortality included age ≥55 years and hospitalization at transplantation and retransplantation (all: $p \leq 0.006$). The Pittsburgh group identified the most significant parameter to be donor warm ischemic time (DWIT) (Table 10.1) [14]; this is the major factor that distinguishes DCD from DBD donors. A DWIT>20 min is associated with significantly poorer graft survival rates. Surprisingly, CIT has not been found to be significantly associated with poor outcomes in DCD patients; however, the incidence of PNF is 2.5 times higher in patients with a CIT ≤8 h than in those with a CIT >8 h. Patients who have undergone liver transplantation from DCD donors >60 years of age have a markedly high rate of biliary complications (67 %).

In conclusion, younger donors should be selected according to the length of DWIT and CIT. In general, utilizing DCD livers for transplantation requires a DWIT <30 min, donor age ≤60, and CIT <8–10 h.

10.3 Procurement and Preservation

10.3.1 Procurement

Carefully considering the risks and benefits is necessary when deciding whether to procure a DCD organ, taking into account additional extended criteria and donor or graft characteristics as older donor age, hepatic status and vital sign. Transplant team members must not be involved in decisions related to patient prognosis, withdrawal of ventilator or organ-perfusion support, or determination of death [15–19].Organs from uncontrolled DCD donors may pose different risks than those from controlled DCD donors [20, 21]. The principles of consent for donation and intervention prior to a declaration of death may be significantly different for uncontrolled and controlled DCDs [17].

10.3.1.1 Withdrawal of Ventilator and Organ-Perfusion Support

The family can be given the opportunity to spend time with the patient immediately prior to and during discontinuation of support until cessation of cardiorespiratory function. Heparin is administered prior to withdrawal of support, except in rare cases when its use might be expected to hasten death and/or is prohibited per local procurement protocol [17–19]. Phentolamine may be administered according to local procurement protocol. Specific informed consent for the administration of each of these agents is obtained from the patient's legal decision maker(s) prior to withdrawal of support. The ASTS recommends a two-minute waiting period, the Society of Critical Care Medicine recommends at least 2 min of observation [19], and the Institute of Medicine recommends 5 min of observation [15–17]. The declaration of death is the responsibility of the patient's treating care team. If withdrawal of support occurs outside of the operating room, the patient is quickly moved to the operating room after the death pronouncement.

10.3.1.2 Operative Technique

As with DBD organ procurement, there is a careful search in both the abdominal and thoracic cavities for any neoplastic or infectious processes that may present a risk of donor-related transmission. The super-rapid recovery techniques are widely used for DCD organ procurement. Most surgeons use some modification of their own procurement technique [22, 23]. The retrieval procedure developed at Kings College Hospital is a radical modification of the super-rapid technique described by Casaveilaa [24]. The procedure begins with a sternotomy and drainage of the inferior vena cava (IVC), which is divided at the level of the right atrium. The vena cava should first be vented. The importance of this procedure is to prevent organ congestion in the agonal stage. In patients with cardiac arrest, prompt sternotomy following cutting of the vena cava allows for easy and rapid perfusion. If the donor has previously undergone cardiac surgery, performing sternotomy may be time consuming, and decompression of the IVC is best achieved in the abdomen. Following the waiting period and declaration of death, the surgeons return to the operating room. Midline laparotomy is performed with rapid dissection around the inferior aorta for cannulation. The ischemic time may be reduced by starting the aortic flush and ice cooling in the abdomen immediately after cannulation. Thereafter, the thoracic or supraceliac aorta is cross-clamped. It is easier to cross-clamp the aorta in a dry field, and early sternotomy allows the descending aorta to be clamped above the diaphragm without delay after aortic perfusion. The superior mesenteric vein is identified and a second cannula is inserted into the portal vein to perfuse the liver with cold University of Wisconsin solution containing heparin. The organs may be removed en bloc or separately. Dual perfusion is also important for DCD livers due to easy formation of clots and thrombosis. The gallbladder is opened and the common bile duct is divided and flushed with UW solution to remove bile juice. In situ biliary flush is performed to minimize bile-induced epithelial damage, and the common bile duct and gallbladder are generously irrigated early after initiating the cold flush [23]. Careful dissection is performed to avoid bile duct and arterial injury. The left gastric, gastroduodenal, and splenic arteries are also divided. Particular concern is paid to the possibility for aberrant arteries because all DCD visceral dissections are performed in cold fields without blood flow (unless the ECMO technique is used) and there are no opportunities to assess the pulse. If the DCD pancreas is not going to be used, the liver is removed with the pancreatic head to avoid transecting an aberrant right hepatic artery and to minimize the extraction time. The celiac trunk is identified toward its origin from the aorta and removed with an aortic patch. The portal vein is divided at the junction with the splenic vein. The IVC is also divided above the origin of the renal vein.

10.3.1.3 Double-Balloon Triple Lumen

It is very useful when the donor has previously undergone abdominal surgery. Using a Fogarty catheter and balloon catheter, aortic perfusion is performed. The premortem annulation technique decreases the rush inherent in the super-rapid recovery technique and may decrease the warm ischemic time (WIT), particularly if withdrawal of support is performed outside of the operating room. This technique requires cannulation of the femoral artery and femoral vein prior to withdrawal of support [9, 23]. Specific informed consent is obtained if this technique is to be used [15–18]. Local anesthesia is used as appropriate. After declaration of death, a cold preservation solution is immediately infused via the femoral artery cannula, and the femoral vein cannula is opened to gravity to decompress the venous system. Thereafter, median sternotomy and midline abdominal incisions are made and the intra-abdominal organs are topically cooled with ice and then removed en bloc or separately. A few centers use premortem cannulation in conjunction with postmortem extracorporeal membrane oxygenation (ECMO) with the flow of warm oxygenated blood to the intra-abdominal organs during the interval between declaration of death and organ procurement [25]. In summary, the goals of procurement are to minimize liver congestion, improve organ perfusion, and facilitate surgical dissection to prevent extended WIT.

10.3.2 Preservation

10.3.2.1 Simple Cold Storage

There is no clear evidence regarding the optimal preservation solution for cold storage of DCD liver grafts. UW solution has been reported to produce more favorable results when compared with HTK [26]. Effectively flushing out the solution from

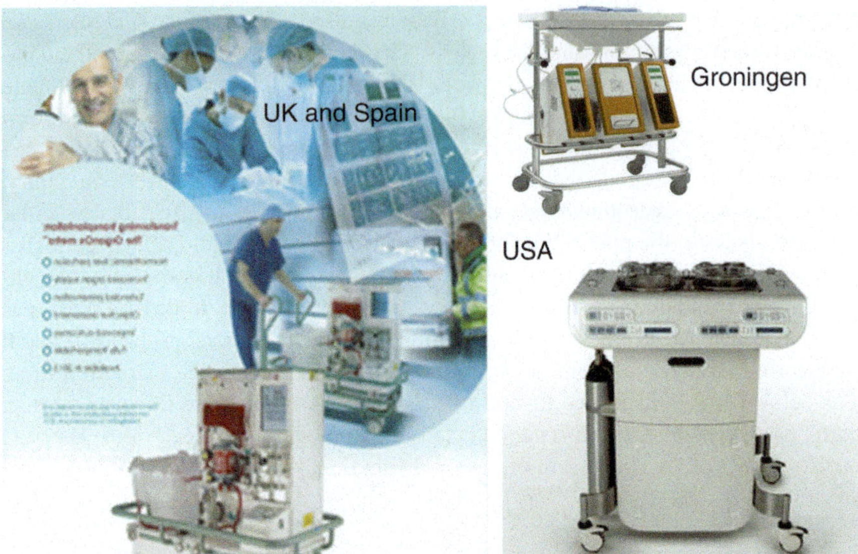

Fig. 10.1 Machine perfusion preservation systems for liver in the world. The UK group developed in both normothermic using red cells and hypothermic preservation. Organ recovery system in the USA group development hypothermic preservation machine

the DCD liver graft during retrieval is important for optimal preservation. If blood remains in the liver graft, microcirculation will cause severe injury after reperfusion at implantation and may result in PNF. Because the CIT in DCD livers is as short as possible, most of the currently available preservation solutions are suitable, including UW, HTK solution, if the preservation time is less than 8–10 h. The advantages of HTK over UW include lower cost and lower viscosity resulting in easier diffusion into the liver and faster cooling. The Kings group reported the first in situ flush-out solution with low viscosity, Marshall's solution. The use of this solution in the aorta followed by perfusion with UW solution for simple cold storage (SCS) has been proven effective [27].

10.3.2.2 Hypothermic Machine Perfusion Preservation

Although machine perfusion of the liver using hypothermia may have a theoretical advantage, its use has not become widespread in clinical practice. The Guarrera group in Colombia, New York, developed a modified Belzer machine perfusion solution, Vasosolution, containing various additives (L-arginine, *N*-acetyl cysteine, glycerol ketoglutarate, and prostaglandin E1) for successful use in human livers. The outcomes of liver transplantation were reported to be satisfactory compared with SCS (Figs. 10.1 and 10.2) [28, 29]. A new preservation solution, Polysol, was developed for machine perfusion by the Amsterdam group in 2005. Polysol

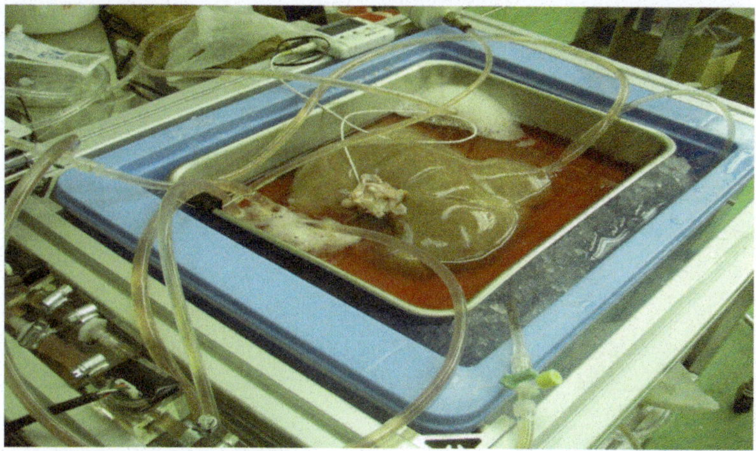

Fig. 10.2 Machine perfusion system for DCD liver graft developed in our institute demonstrated functional recovery

solution contains many vitamins and a protein-like, enriched tissue culture medium for functional recovery during preservation, which is expensive [30, 31].

10.3.2.3 Normochromic Extracorporeal Oxygenated Perfusion

Traditional methods of preservation based on static, hypothermic storage may not be best for DCD grafts because organs from DCDs have already suffered tissue damage secondary to hypoxia and hypoperfusion before the initial period of warm ischemia. Additional cold storage damage to the organ caused by hypothermic conditions may limit the ability to improve cellular function because metabolic activity is decreased in the cold. In 2002, the Hospital Clinic in Barcelona developed clinical protocol to resuscitate organs from donors and to maintain viability for transplantation (Fig. 10.3) [10]. The protocol includes cannulation of the femoral vessels to establish a normothermic extracorporeal machine oxygenation (NECMO) circuit. NECMO is used to reperfuse and deoxygenate abdominal organs after cardiac arrest while the potential DCD is evaluated and consent for organ donation is obtained. In addition, using a system of NECMO to maintain the organs offers the theoretical benefit of being able to utilize cytoprotective substances that can support recovery. In 2007, the first 10 human liver transplantations were performed with uncontrolled DCDs in which the donor was maintained with NECMO prior to organ retrieval. Ten DCD livers were transplanted, with only one graft lost to PNF and one to hepatic artery thrombosis (HAT) [10]. The great advantage of normothermic preservation, including the use of NECMO, is the ability to overcome the disadvantaged aspects of hypothermic cellular physiology [33], Additionally, any equipment failures result in unexpected warm ischemic injury. Furthermore, the use of blood-based perfusates may increase the risk of microvascular failure and sinusoidal

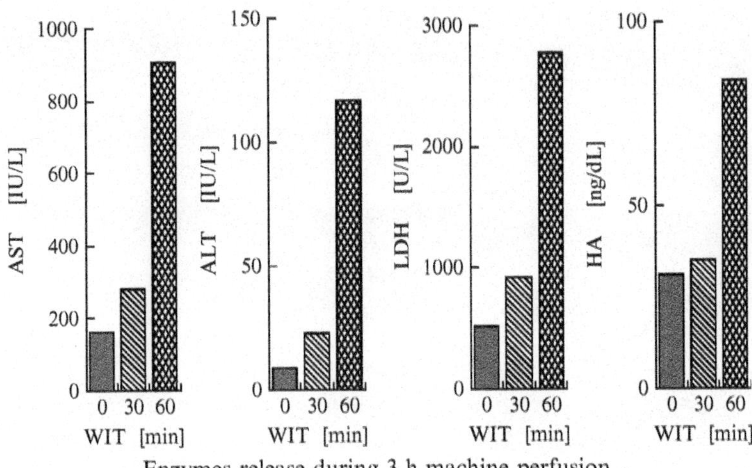

Fig. 10.3 The levels of liver enzymes (AST, LDH) in perfusate during continuous preservation and the liver function after 2 h of reperfusion

plugging and bacterial growth. Achieving normothermic organ preservation therefore remains a challenging problem. Machine perfusion preservation systems which are developing in the world were demonstrated in Fig. 10.1.

10.4 Viability Test

Making a reliable assessment of DCD liver grafts is difficult for multifactorial reasons (i.e., donor age, WIT, expected CIT, agonal stage, cause of death, etc.). Performing liver biopsies is of limited value, even in brain-dead donors. Experimentally, Ma et al. [34] investigated the histological and ultrastructural characteristics of the liver following different WITs in rats. They evaluated the degree of morphological recovery of liver grafts following rat liver transplantation and concluded that 45 min of WIT is the crucial point for liver grafts. A clinical study was conducted by Muiesan that demonstrated hepatocyte viability in DCD liver grafts for transplantation. The test is a simple assessment of graft viability using trypan blue exclusion with collagenase digestion in liver biopsies [22]. Developing a system of machine perfusion to establish viability assessments of the liver has not been easy due to the unique blood supply of liver grafts. Predicting viability by evaluating flow in the portal system is not possible because the portal flow is wide ranged and the systems used have found it difficult to generate portal pressure that demonstrates efficient portal flow in the hypothermic stage. Even tissue and vascular resistance, which provide important information in kidney preservation, are particularly low due to easy destruction in the liver. Additionally, evaluating the vascular system according to the arterial flow is difficult using rat models. The effluent aspartate aminotransferase (AST) and lactate dehydrogenase (LDH) levels collected in preservation solution have been reported to be useful and predictable biomarkers in previous reports [35–37]. Recently, Obara and Matsuno et al. developed a novel liver perfusion system (Fig. 10.1) and found that the degree of decreasing hepatic arterial pressure is correlated with the length of warm ischemic injury (up to 60 min), the levels of liver enzymes (AST, LDH) in perfusate during continuous preservation, and the liver function after 2 h of reperfusion. Pressure decreases in the hepatic artery during hypothermic preservation are significantly correlated with the length of WIT (Figs. 10.2 and 10.3) [38]. However, the liver is placed for preservation in the perfusion circuit, and the pressure on liver tissue, i.e., shear stress or gravity, differs according to how the liver is placed. This is another reason to develop a system to determine the viability of liver grafts following machine perfusion and hypothermia. On the other hand, it is not easy to establish the evaluation of viability in normothermic liver perfusion preservation, which requires blood as the perfusion solution, because the technology does not provide full metabolic support. In 2007, the first ten human liver transplantations were performed with uncontrolled DCDs, in which the donors were maintained with NECMO prior to organ retrieval. The authors also report that one method of evaluating acceptable viability is to assess whether the AST level in the perfusate is stable [11].

10.5 Outcomes

Several strategies have been developed to identify the post-transplant risk factors associated with graft failure and patient mortality following donation after cardiac death (DCD) liver transplantation.

D'Alessandro et al. from the University of Wisconsin group (UW) reported that the incidence of PNF is 10.5 % in controlled DCD donors. Graft survival is lower than that from donation after brain death (53.8 % vs. 80.9 %; $P<0.007$) [9]. In 2003, Abt et al. [39] reported that a series of controlled DCD livers had a statistically higher incidence of ischemic biliary strictures compared to DBD livers (33.3 % vs. 9.5 %; $P<0.01$), although there was no differences in patient survival between recipients with grafts from DCDs or DBDs. Muiesan at King's College Hospital reported data for 31 controlled DCD donors. The mean WIT was 14.7 min (range: 7–40 min) [22]. The overall patient and graft survival rates were 87 % and 84 %, respectively, at a median follow-up of 15 months. Both graft survival and the incidence of biliary complications were nearly identical to those of recipients of livers from DBDs. There were no graft losses due to non-anastomotic biliary stricture. The UW group reported updated outcomes of 36 recipients who received grafts from controlled DCD live donors between 1993 and 2002 [40]. The mean WIT in the DCD donors was 17.8 min. In this series, the patient and graft survival rates at 3 years were 68 % and 56 %, respectively, for DCD donations versus 84 % and 80 %, respectively, for DBD donations. The overall incidence of ischemic biliary strictures at 3 years was greater in the DCD livers (37 % vs. 12 %). The development of ischemic biliary strictures is a major source of morbidity after DCD liver transplantation. This injury is very difficult to treat, in spite of endoscopic and percutaneous biliary drainage. In addition, hepatic artery stenosis, hepatic abscesses, and bilomas are frequent in DCD livers. Fujita et al. in the University of Florida group reported the results of a comparison between 1,209 DBD donors and 24 controlled DCD donors [41]. The 1- and 3-year patient survival rates were similar (86.8 % and 81.7 % in DCD vs. 84.0 % and 76.0 % in DBD, respectively); however, the graft survival rate appeared inferior in the DCD group at both 1 year (69.1 % vs. 78.7 %) and 3 years (58.6 % vs. 70.2 %). There were no significant differences in the incidence of PNF or biliary stricture. However, all cases associated with biliary stricture in the DCD group eventually led to graft loss and the need for retransplantation. The results of these single-center studies are difficult to generalize because individualized center practices and allocation-related issues may affect donor selection. Abt et al. reported data from the UNOS database for 144 recipients of livers from DCDs. When the controlled DCD and DBD livers were compared [42], graft survival at 1 year was lower in the controlled DCDs (72.3 % vs. 80.4 %; $P=0.056$). The DCD recipients had a higher incidence of PNF (11.8 vs. 6.4 %; $P=0.008$) and retransplantation (13.9 % vs. 8.3 %; $P=0.04$) compared with the DBD recipients. Predictors of early graft failure within 60 days post-transplant include prolonged CIT (when the CIT exceeded 8 h, the incidence of graft failure within 60 days post-transplant was 30.4 %) and the use of recipient life support at the time of transplantation. Merion et al. examined a national cohort of DCD ($n=472$) and DBD ($n=23{,}598$) liver transplants performed between 2000 and 2004 using the Scientific Registry of Transplant Recipients Database. There was no categorization of DCD donation such as controlled/uncontrolled status in their analysis. Graft survival at 3 months, 1 year, and 3 years after liver transplantation was lower in the DCD recipients (83.0 %, 70.1 %, and 60.5 %) compared with that observed in the DBD recipients (89.2 %, 83.0 %, and 75.0 %; $P<0.001$) [43]. Mateo et al. analyzed the UNOS database for 367 DCD liver transplants and 33,111 DBD liver transplants performed between 1996 and 2003 [11]. The graft survival rates at 1 year and 3 years with DCD donors (71 % and 60 %; $n=367$) were significantly inferior to those with DBD donors (80 % and 72 %; $P<0.001$). However, low-risk recipients with low-risk DCD livers (DWIT<30 min and CIT <10 h) showed graft survival rates at 1 and 3 years (81 % and 67 %) that were not statistically different from those of recipients with DBD livers. Mathur et al. used a Cox regression model to analyze data derived from the Scientific Registry of Transplant Recipients for all US liver-only DCD transplants performed between September 1, 2001 and April 30, 2009 ($n=1{,}567$). Three years post-DCD liver transplant, 64.9 % of the recipients were alive with functioning grafts, 13.6 % had required retransplantation, and 21.6 % had died [13]. However, DCD and DBD grafts transplanted with MELD >30 or on organ-perfusion support (mechanical ventilation or hemodialysis) had similar graft survival, suggesting a potentially greater benefit of DCD livers in critically ill patients (Fig. 10.4) [14]. Factors associated with ischemic cholangiopathy, including older donor age, high donor weight, CIT, and DWIT, were significant predictors of graft failure. The development of ischemic biliary stricture is a major source of

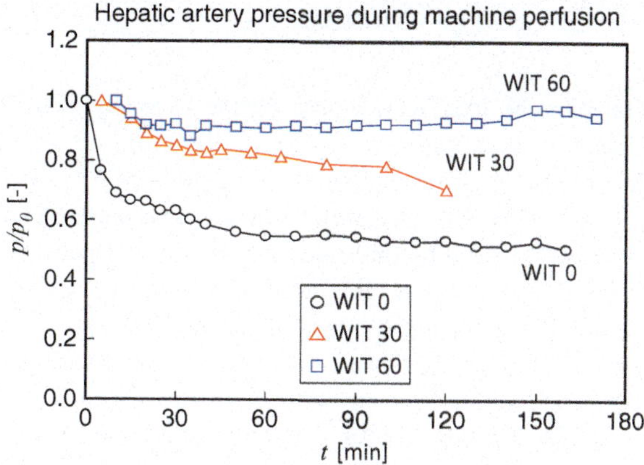

Fig. 10.4 The degree of decreasing hepatic arterial pressure is correlated with the length of warm ischemic injury (up to 60 min) during hypothermic machine preservation

morbidity after DCD liver transplant. Retransplantation is also associated with a significantly higher mortality risk. Performing retransplantation in recipients with ischemic cholangiopathy may be challenging, depending on the waiting list priority determined according to MELD. Further studies are clearly needed to identify clinical and policy strategies to reduce the incidence and improve the outcome of ischemic cholangiopathy in recipients with DCD liver grafts, such as improving organ preservation.

10.6 Basic Research

10.6.1 Small Animals

The optimal use of hypothermic machine perfusion preservation (HMP) for DCD livers has not been clearly established. Ex vivo assessment of damage showed that machine perfusion was able to reduce cellular damage induced from 30 min of warm ischemia time with 10 h of HMP compared with 10 h of SCS [44]. Dutkowski et al. [45] studied the impact of short-term hypothermic oxygenated perfusion (HOPE) at the end of cold storage. A one-hour application of HMP after 45 min of WIT and 5 h of static cold storage improved the status of the liver, with a reduction of hepatocyte necrosis, less AST release, and increased bile flow. Some studies have also investigated the perfusion temperature. For example, subnormothermic machine perfusion performed at 20 °C resulted in reduced vasoconstriction, as well as lower metabolic requirements in DCD [46] and steatotic [47] rat models. However, there are important limitations of basic research using small animals because of the difficulties associated with assessment of the animals and the impact of the hepatic artery flow. This is clearly an important factor when evaluating the clinical relevance of small animal preservation studies.

10.6.2 Large Animals

Belzer et al. tried to preserve canine livers by HMP for 8–10 h. The endothelium was damaged, and the Kupffer cells appeared swollen and disrupted after long HMP. Successful transplantation was achieved by Brettschneider et al. after 24 h of machine perfusion in a canine model [48]. Starzel et al. preserve the first 11 human livers up to 7.5 h by the same method [49]. However, the use of fresh diluted blood is inconvenient in the clinical setting. Pienaar et al. and Belzer's group reported that canine livers could be preserved successfully for 72 h by HMP by the portal vein alone [50]. However, no similar results in large animal transplant models have been published so far. Low-pressure HMP was applied via the hepatic artery in porcine livers for 2 h before transplantation and compared to similar grafts stored in cold Euro–Collins solution for the same period. Both the LDH and AST levels were consistently lower in the HMP group compared with the SCS group [35]. Guarrera et al. [51] demonstrated the outcomes of liver transplantation after 12 h of HMP or with SCS in a miniature swine model using a new preservation solution, the Vasosolution, which employs a modified Belzer-machine perfusion solution. The serum AST and total bilirubin (TBili) levels were similar in the HMP and SCS groups, indicating that HMP can be used successfully. Celsior solution was also compared with Polysol, another new preservation solution. The machine perfusion–Polysol group showed significantly less damage as demonstrated by liver function tests compared with cold storage using the Celsior solution [52]. As for DCD liver graft, most groups agree that 30 min of WIT plus 4–5 h of cold preservation results in primary loss of function in the pig liver [53, 54]; Dutkowski used a large animal model to test whether HOPE-treated DCD livers could experience the same benefits as those noted in a previous report using a rat model. The porcine DCD liver with 60 min of WIT preserved with SCS for 6 h could be rescued by a 1 h short-term HOPE [55]. When these livers were compared to those in the SCS-only group, lower values of AST and LDH after reperfusion and a higher survival rate up to 30 h in the HOPE group were demonstrated. The Pirenne group in Leuven, Belgium, designed a multifactorial biological modulation approach targeting ischemia–reperfusion injury to augment the viability of porcine liver grafts with 45 min of WIT and 4 h of SCS. In the modulation group, the DCD livers were flushed with warm Ringers containing streptokinase and a vasodilator prior to SCS. In recipients, glycine, a MAP kinase inhibitor, α-tocopherol, glutathione, and an iron chelator (apotransferrin) were administrated intravenously. This approach was effective and eliminated PNF, improving the liver function [56]. Matsuno et al. developed a new preservation machine with a temperature-controlled system. Their study showed a beneficial effect of an extracellular type solution with oxygenation in the novel continuous machine preservation, with well-preserved liver graft function. That group also reported beneficial functional recovery in the HMP group after 30 min of WIT plus 4–5 h of total ischemic time compared to the SCS-only group in a porcine liver transplantation model [57]. Furthermore, they successfully transplanted the porcine livers with 60 min. of WIT plus 4–5 h of total ischemic time by rewarming preservation from 4 to 22 °C using machine perfusion system [58]. The use of NECMO is based on experimental studies, which have shown that the recirculation of oxygenated blood at 37 °C improves the cellular energy load, reduces tissue injury, and improves the post-transplant graft function in livers damaged by the period of warm ischemia caused by cardiac arrest [58–60]. Experimental studies have demonstrated that even brief periods of cold preservation will cause injury to hepatocytes, Kupffer cells, and endothelial cells in DCD livers, even those later recirculated under normothermia. Ideally, these livers will be continuously perfused with warm, oxygenated blood during the entire ex vivo phase of preservation [61, 62]. In conclusion, machine perfusion preservation under both normothermic and hypothermic conditions is a useful way to preserve DCD liver grafts.

10.6.3 Marginal Donor Liver as a Source of Hepatocytes for Transplantation

Hepatocyte transplantation is a promising, less invasive treatment that may support liver transplantation. In addition to decreased invasiveness, the advantages of hepatocyte transplantation are [63] feasibility of partial or temporal liver support for congenital metabolic disorders or fulminant hepatic failure [64], efficient use of marginal donors or even untransplantable livers as long as intact hepatocytes are available, and [65] the possibility of a ready-to-use treatment when frozen. Regarding the last point, treating multiple patients with one liver or repeat treatment of a single patient will become a reality. However, the second point is not always correct, as hepatocytes from low-quality donors (i.e., those with steatosis, fibrosis, cirrhosis, and long-term ischemia) show low cell viability and unhealthy morphological characteristics such as swelling and budding. Moreover, damaged hepatocytes are more sensitive to cryopreservation.

10.6.3.1 Brief Summary of Clinical Hepatocyte Transplantation Focusing on Cell Donors

There are two systematic reviews of hepatocyte transplantation [63, 64]. The former described 78 cases documented up to 2006 that were categorized according to disease type, i.e., metabolic, chronic, and acute liver failure. The latter listed 24 child cases, with 12 hepatic failures and 12 metabolic disorders. Some cases overlapped between the reviews. Advanced case reports described by Fox et al. [65] and Lee et al. [66] are available from this group of cases. Fox et al. reported a case of Crigler-Najjar syndrome. They used fresh hepatocytes isolated from a 5-year-old boy whose liver was intact but unsuitable for organ transplantation, as there were no appropriate recipients compatible with this donor with respect to size and blood group. According to Fox et al., the hepatocytes were isolated at the University of Pittsburgh and transferred by air-courier service to the University of Nebraska Medical Center. Transport took approximately 5 h, and the first cell infusion was initiated 6.5 h after the cells were isolated. The cells were stored in University of Wisconsin solution at 4 °C, and this maintained good cell viability for 15 h. After hepatocyte transplantation, conjugated bilirubin was detectable in the patient's serum and the phototherapy requirement decreased. Lee et al. reported a case of glycogen storage disease type Ib. They used fresh and cryopreserved adult hepatocytes from two donor livers that were rejected for organ transplantation due to mild fibrosis and prolonged hypotension. During the first hepatocyte transplantation, 2×10^9 fresh hepatocytes were transplanted through the portal vein. Seven days later, 1×10^9 cryopreserved hepatocytes were transplanted. One month later, the same treatment was performed using the cells from the second donor. The patient received a total of 6×10^9 cells that were equivalent to 6 % of the recipient's estimated number of hepatocytes. After the hepatocyte transplantation, the patient became free of hypoglycemic symptoms despite discontinuation of cornstarch meals. Neutropenia, a serious complication of glycogen storage disease type Ib, was improved, and the patient's physical development progressed.

There are several additional case reports of hepatocyte transplantation that were not included in the reviews or cited only as conference presentations. Mitry et al. reported that hepatocytes isolated from a remnant of a split liver were transplanted into a patient with ornithine transcarbamylase deficiency [67]. They transplanted the major portions of the left and right lobes and used segment IV with or without the caudate lobe for cell isolation. Cellular viability and recovery were fairly good, and the patient was successfully bridged to transplantation. The same group reported another case treated using fresh and cryopreserved adult hepatocytes [68]. Stéphenne et al. reported the transplantation of cryopreserved hepatocytes isolated from a split liver to a 14-month-old boy who suffered from ornithine transcarbamylase deficiency [69]. After cell transplantation, the patient's condition improved, including psychomotor development, and he eventually underwent liver transplantation. Recently, hepatic progenitor cells isolated from adult livers [adult-derived human liver stem/progenitor cells (ADHLSCs)] are being used [70]. There is another report of hepatocyte transplantation into patients with urea cycle disorder [71]. Meyburg et al. used cryopreserved hepatocytes of the same lot isolated from the liver of a 9-day-old neonate that was inappropriate for whole-organ transplantation. The number of transplanted cells ranged from 0.87 to 1.89×10^9 administered by 2–6 portal vein injections. Although one patient died from norovirus and upper airway tract infections, the remaining three patients survived, and their symptoms improved. In addition to metabolic disorders, hepatocyte transplantation is performed for the treatment of acute liver failure. Schneider et al. reported a case of successful recovery from mushroom poisoning following transplantation of cryopreserved adult hepatocytes [72].

There are two reports of fetal hepatocyte transplantation; the first was performed for Crigler–Najjar syndrome type 1 treatment, and the other for biliary atresia treatment [73, 74]. Cells were procured from an aborted fetus at 18 weeks of gestation. In the former case, decreased TBili and increased conjugated bilirubin levels were observed 60 days after transplantation. In the latter case, decreased conjugated bilirubin and serum glutamic pyruvic transaminase (GPT) levels were achieved 60 days after transplantation, although there was no evidence of hepatic drainage by tracer diagnosis.

10.6.3.2 Hepatocyte Isolation from Human Liver and Elaboration from Marginal Donors

The methodology for human hepatocyte isolation is based on collagenase perfusion using a vascular system as established in experimental animals [75]. Collagenase is a type of protease that functions to decompose the triple-helical structure of collagen. Therefore, the damaging effect on cell surface proteins is minimized, unlike with other proteases. However, specific improvements have been established to address the size and intensity of the connective tissue of human liver [76, 77]. Moreover, it is critical that clinical studies perform all procedures according to good manufacturing practices (GMP). At present, most laboratories use Liberase (Roche Applied Science, Penzberg, Germany), which consists of collagenase I, collagenase II, neutral metalloproteinase, and thermolysin. Besides the available methodological descriptions, there is likely a certain amount of technical knowledge that has been unreported by each laboratory.

Because liver transplantation is approved as a treatment for end-stage hepatic failure, donor livers are preferentially allocated for organ transplantation but not hepatocyte isolation. On rare occasions, the lack of appropriate donor–recipient matching (e.g., a case of infant donor liver) provides good-quality hepatocytes [71], and fetal liver is considered to be an alternative cell source [78]. However, hepatocytes for transplantation should be obtained from marginal donors such as those with steatosis, fibrosis, cirrhosis, and long-term ischemia. Alexandrova et al. reported that no correlations were demonstrated between isolation efficiency and cold ischemia time or donor age among adult organ donors, whereas organs with severe steatosis generally did not result in successful cell isolation [79]. Two similar reports exist. Terry et al. reported that hepatocytes isolated from non-heart-beating donors and steatotic tissues were more vulnerable to the effects of cryopreservation [80]. Hughes et al. noted that although hepatocytes suitable for cell transplantation can be obtained from non-heart-beating donor livers, higher viability values may be obtained if both warm and cold ischemia times of the donor livers can be reduced prior to processing [81].

Recently, we developed a novel pretreatment for hepatocyte isolation from liver tissue that suffered from warm ischemia [82, 83]. As a solution for flushing blood from inside the tissue, the citrate-phosphate-dextrose-supplemented Euro-Collins solution allowed for high recovery and viability of hepatocytes. Citrate is well known as an anticoagulant as well as heparin, but heparin exhibits an inhibitory effect on hepatocyte isolation. Although precise mechanism remains to be resolved, citrate may have certain bio-restorative effect on liver. A beneficial effect of citrate in liver preservation was reported by Tamaki et al. [84].

To develop clinical evidence for the efficacy of hepatocyte transplantation, it is necessary to establish a stable procurement system of high-quality hepatocytes. Further research is required to improve hepatocyte isolation and cryopreservation protocols for various types of liver tissues, particularly those obtained from marginal or submarginal donors.

References

1. Sung RS, Galloway J, Tuttel-Newhall JE, et al. Organ donation and utilization in the United States 1997–2006. Am J Transplant. 2008;8(4pt 2):922–34.
2. Rotts Jr JT, Herdman R. Non-heart beating organ transplantation and ethical issues in procurement. Washington DC: National Academy Press; 1997.
3. Tuttel-Newhall JE, Krishnan SM, Levy MP, McBrude V, et al. Organ donation and utilization in the United States 1997–2007. Am J Transplant. 2009;914(Pt21):879–93.
4. Kootstra G, Daemen J, Oomen A. Categories of non-heart-beating donors. Transplant Proc. 1995;27(5):2893–4.
5. United Network for Organ Sharing. Available at: http://www.unos.org (2010). Accessed 15 Feb 2010.
6. Koffman CG, Bewick M, Chang RW, et al. Comparative study of the use of systolic and asystolic kidney donors between 1988 and 1991. Transplant Proc. 1993;25:1527–9.
7. Weber M, Dindo D, Demartines N, et al. Kidney transplantation from donors without a heartbeat. N Eng J Med. 2002;347(4):248–55.
8. Sanchez Fructuono AI, Olatz D, Torrentle J, et al. Renal transplantation from non-heart beating donors: a promising alternative to enlarge the donor pool. J Am Soc Nephrol. 2000;11(2):350–5.
9. D'Alessandro AM, Hoffman RM, Knecchtle SJ, et al. Successful extrarenal transplantation from non-heart beating donors. Transplantation. 1995;59(7):977–82.
10. Fondeviella C, Hessheimer AJ, Ruiz A, et al. Liver transplant using donors after unexpected cardiac death: novel preservation protocol and acceptance criteria. Am J Transplant. 2007;7: 1849–55.
11. Mateo R, Cho Y, Sigh G, et al. Risk factors for graft survival after cardiac death donors: an analysis of OPTN/UNOS data. Am J Transplant. 2006;6(4):791–6.
12. Lee KW, Simpkins CF, Montgomery RA, et al. Factors affecting graft survival after liver transplantation from donation after cardiac death donors. Transplantation. 2006;82(12):1683–8.
13. Mathur AK, Heimbach J, Steflick DE, et al. Donation after cardiac death liver transplantation: predictors of outcome. Am J Transplant. 2010;10:2512–9.
14. De Vera ME, Lopez-Solis R, Dvorchil I, et al. Liver transplantation using donation after cardiac death donors: long-term follow up from a single center. Am J Transplant. 2009;9:77381.
15. Institute of Medicine. Non-heart-beating organ transplantation: medical and ethical issues in procurement. Washington, DC: National Academy Press; 1997. p. 104
16. Institute of Medicine. Non-heart-beating organ transplantation: practice and protocols. Washington, DC: National Academy Press; 2000. p. 174.
17. Institute of Medicine. Organ donation: opportunities for action. Washington, DC: National Academy press; 2006. p. 358.
18. Bernat JL, D'Alessandro AM, Port FK, et al. Report of a national conference on donation after cardiac death. Am J Transplant. 2006;6:281–91.
19. Ethics Committee, American College of Critical Care Medicine, Society of Critical Care Medicine. Recommendations for non-heart-beating organ donation: a position paper by the Ethics Committee, American College of Critical Care Medicine, Society of Critical Care Medicine. Crit Care Med. 2001;29:1826–31.

20. Otero A, Co'mez-Gutie'rrez M, Sua'rez F, et al. Liver transplantation from Maastricht category 2 non-heart-beating donors. Transplantation. 2003;76:1068–73.
21. Sua'rez F, Otero A, Solla M, et al. Biliary complications after liver transplantation from Maastricht category-2 non-heart-beating donors. Transplantation. 2008;85:9–14.
22. Muiesan P, Girlanda R, Jassem W, et al. Single center experience with liver transplantation from controlled non-heart beating donors, a viable source of grafts. Ann Surg. 2005;242(5):732–8.
23. Reich DJ. Non-heart-beating donor organ procurement. In: Humar A, Matas AJ, Payne WD, editors. Atlas of organ transplantation. London: Springer; 2006.
24. Casa viella A, Ramirez C, Shapiro R, et al. Experience with liver and kidney allografts from non-heart beating donors. Transplantation. 1995;59(2):197–203.
25. Magliocca JF, Magee JC, Rowe SA, et al. Extracorporeal support for organ donation after cardiac death effectively expands the donor pool. J Trauma. 2005;58:1095–102.
26. Meine MH, Zabiteli ML, Neumann J, et al. Randomized clinical assay for hepatic grafts preservation with University of Wisconsin or histidine tryptophan-ketoglutarate solution in liver transplantation. Transplant Proc. 2006;38(6):1872–5.
27. Marshall VC, Ross H, Scot DF, et al. Preservation of cadaveric renal allografts-comparison of flushing and pumping techniques. Proc Eur Dial Transplant Asoc. 1977;14:301–9.
28. Guarrera JM, Polyak M, O'MarArrington B, et al. Pulsatile machine perfusion with Vasosol solution improves early graft function after cadaveric renal transplantation. Transplantation. 2004;77(8):1264–8.
29. Guarrera JV, Henrry SP, Samstein B, et al. Hypothermic machine preservation in human liver transplantation: the first clinical series. Am J Transplant. 2010;10:372–87.
30. Doorschodt BM, Bessems M, van Vliet AK, et al. The first disposable perfusion preservation system for kidney and liver grafts. Ann Transplant. 2004;9(2):40–1.
31. Bessems M, Doorschodt BM, van Vliet AK, et al. Improved rat liver preservation by hypothermic continuous machine perfusion using polysol, a new enriched preservation solution. Liver Transpl. 2005;11(5):539–46.
32. Vogel T, Brodkmann JG, Couissios C et al: The role of normothermic etracorporeal perfusion in minimizing ishemia reperfusion injury. Transplantation Reviews. 26 (2012)156–162.
33. Brasile L, Stubentisky BM, Booster MH, et al. Hypothermia – a limiting factor in using warm ischemically damaged kidneys. Am J Transplant. 2001;1(4):316–20.
34. Ma Y, Wang GD, Wu LW, et al. Dynamical changing patterns of histological structure and ultrastructure of liver graft undergoing warm ischemia injury from non-heart beating donor in rats. World J Gastoroenterol. 2006;12(30):1942–5.
35. Uchiyama M, Kozaki K, Matsuno N, et al. Usefulness of preservation method by machine perfusion and pentoxifylline on the liver transplantation from non-heart beating donor. J Tokyo Med Univ. 2000;58(6):743–56.
36. Bessems M, Doorschodt BM, van Marle J, et al. Improved machine perfusion preservation of the non-heart-beating donor rat liver using Polysol: a new machine perfusion preservation solution. Liver Transpl. 2005;11:1379–88.
37. van der Plaats A, Maathuis MH, T Hart NA, et al. The Groningen hypothermic liver perfusion pump: functional evaluation of a new machine perfusion system. Ann Biomed Eng. 2006;34:1924–34.
38. Obara H, Matsuno N, Enosawa S, et al. Pre-transplant screening and viability evaluation of a liver graft using a machine perfusion. Transplant Proc. 2012;44(4):959–61.
39. Abt P, Crawford M, Desai N, et al. Liver transplantation from controlled non-heart-beating donors: an increased incidence of biliary complications. Transplantation. 2003;75:1659–63.
40. Foley DP, Fernandez LA, Leverson G, Chin LT, et al. Donation after cardiac death: the University of Wisconsin experience with liver transplantation. Ann Surg. 2005;242:724–31.
41. Fujita S, Mizuno S, Fujikawa T, et al. Liver transplantation from donation after cardiac death: a single center experience. Transplantation. 2007;84:46–9.
42. Abt PL, Desai NM, Crawford MD, et al. Survival following liver transplantation from non-heart beating donors. Ann Surg. 2004;239:87–92.

43. Merion RM, Pelletier SJ, Goodrich N, et al. Donation after cardiac death as a strategy to increase deceased donor liver availability. Ann Surg. 2006;244:555–62.
44. Lee CY, et al. Functional recovery of preserved livers following warm ischemia: improvement by machine perfusion preservation. Transplantation. 2002;74:944–51.
45. Dutkowski P, Furtner K, Tian Y, et al. Novel short-term hypohermic oxygenated perfusion (HPE) system prevents injury in rat liver graft from nonheart beating donor. Ann Surg. 2006;24:968–76.
46. Olschewski P. The influence of storage temperature during machine perfusion on preservation quality of marginal donor livers. Cryobiology. 2010;60:343–7.
47. Vanteui M. Correlation between the liver temperature employed during machine perfusion and reperfusion damage: role of Ca^{2+}. Liver Transpl. 2008;14:494–503.
48. Brettschneider L, Dalonze P, Huget C, et al. Successful orthotopic transplantation of liver homografts after 8–25 hours preservation. Surg Forum. 1967;18:376.
49. Starzl TE. Experience in hepatic transplantation. Philadelphia: Saunders; 1969.
50. Pinaar BH, Lindel SL, van Gulik T, et al. Seventy-two-hour preservation of the canine liver by machine perfusion. Transplantation. 1990;49(2):258–60.
51. Guarrera JV, Esterves J, Boykin J, et al. Hypothermic machine perfusion of liver grafts for transplantation; technical development in human discard and miniature swine models. Transplantation Proc. 2005;37(1):323–5.
52. Bessems M, Doorscodt BM, van Vliet PS, et al. Improved rat liver preservation by hypothermic continuous machine preservation of the pig liver using a new preservation solution. Polusol Transplant Proc. 2006;28:1238–42.
53. Monbaliu D, Crabbé T, Roskams T, et al. Livers from non-heart-beating donors tolerate short periods of warm ischemia. Transplantation. 2005;79:1226–30.
54. Takada Y, Taniguchi H, Fukunaga K, et al. Hepatic allograft procurement from non-heart-beating donors: limits of warm ischemia in porcine liver transplantation. Transplantation. 1997;63(3):369–73.
55. de Rougemont O, Breilenstein S, Leskosek B, et al. One hour hypothermic oxygenated perfusion (HOPE) protects nonviable liver allografts donated after cardiac death. Ann Surg. 2009;250:674–83.
56. Monbaliu A, Vekemans K, Hoektra H, et al. Multifactorial biological modulation of warm ischemia reperfusion injury in liver transplantation from non-heart-beating donors eliminates primary nonfunction and reduces bile salt toxicity. Ann Surg. 2009;250(5):808–17.
57. Shigeta T, Matsuno N, Obara H, et al. Functional recovery of donation after cardiac death liver graft by continuous machine perfusion preservation in pigs. Transpl Proc. 2012;44:946–7.
58. Shigeta T, Matsuno N, Obara, H. et al: Impact of Rewarming Preservation by Continuous Machine Perfusion: Improved Post-Transplant Recovery in Pigs Transpl Proc. (2103) 45, 1684–1689.
59. Galcia-Valdecasas JC, Tabet J, Valern R, et al. Liver conditioning after cardiac arrest: the use of normothermic recirculation in an experimental animal model. Transpl Int. 1998;11: 424–32.
60. Net M, Valero R, Almenara R, et al. The effect of normothermic recirculation is mediated by ischemic preconditioning in NHBD liver transplantation. Am J Transplant. 2005;5:2385–93.
61. Readdy P, Bhattacharinjya S, Maniaku N, et al. Preservation of porcine non-heart-beating donor livers by sequential cold storage and warm perfusion. Transplantation. 2004;17:1328–32.
62. Readdy P, Greenwood J, Maniaka N, et al. Non-heart beating donor porcine livers: the adverse effect of cooling. Liver transplant. 2005;16:35–8.
63. Fisher RA, Strom SC. Human hepatocyte transplantation: worldwide results. Transplantation. 2006;82(4):441–9.
64. Meyburg J, Schmidt J, Hoffmann GF. Liver cell transplantation in children. Clin Transplant. 2009;23 Suppl 21:75–82.
65. Fox IJ, Chowdhury JR, Kaufman SS, Goertzen TC, Chowdhury NR, Warkentin PI, Dorko K, Sauter BV, Strom SC. Treatment of the Crigler-Najjar syndrome type I with hepatocyte transplantation. N Engl J Med. 1998;338(20):1422–6.

66. Lee KW, Lee JH, Shin SW, Kim SJ, Joh JW, Lee DH, Kim JW, Park HY, Lee SY, Lee HH, Park JW, Kim SY, Yoon HH, Jung DH, Choe YH, Lee SK. Hepatocyte transplantation for glycogen storage disease type Ib. Cell Transplant. 2007;16(6):629–37.
67. Mitry RR, Dhawan A, Hughes RD, Bansal S, Lehec S, Terry C, Heaton ND, Karani JB, Mieli-Vergani G, Rela M. One liver, three recipients: segment IV from split-liver procedures as a source of hepatocytes for cell transplantation. Transplantation. 2004;77(10):1614–6.
68. Puppi J, Tan N, Mitry RR, Hughes RD, Lehec S, Mieli-Vergani G, Karani J, Champion MP, Heaton N, Mohamed R, Dhawan A. Hepatocyte transplantation followed by auxiliary liver transplantation–a novel treatment for ornithine transcarbamylase deficiency. Am J Transplant. 2008;8(2):427–52.
69. Stéphenne X, Najimi M, Smets F, Reding R, de Ville de Goyet J, Sokal EM. Cryopreserved liver cell transplantation controls ornithine transcarbamylase deficient patient while awaiting liver transplantation. Am J Transplant. 2005;5(8):2058–61.
70. Sokal EM. From hepatocytes to stem and progenitor cells for liver regenerative medicine: advances and clinical perspectives. Cell Prolif. 2011;44 Suppl 1:39–43.
71. Meyburg J, Das AM, Hoerster F, Lindner M, Kriegbaum H, Engelmann G, Schmidt J, Ott M, Pettenazzo A, Luecke T, Bertram H, Hoffmann GF, Burlina A. One liver for four children: first clinical series of liver cell transplantation for severe neonatal urea cycle defects. Transplantation. 2009;87(5):636–41.
72. Schneider A, Attaran M, Meier PN, Strassburg C, Manns MP, Ott M, Barthold M, Arseniev L, Becker T, Panning B. Hepatocyte transplantation in an acute liver failure due to mushroom poisoning. Transplantation. 2006;82(8):1115–6.
73. Khan AA, Parveen N, Mahaboob VS, Rajendraprasad A, Ravindraprakash HR, Venkateswarlu J, Rao P, Pande G, Narusu ML, Khaja MN, Pramila R, Habeeb A, Habibullah CM. Treatment of Crigler-Najjar Syndrome type 1 by hepatic progenitor cell transplantation: a simple procedure for management of hyperbilirubinemia. Transplant Proc. 2008;40(4):1148–50.
74. Khan AA, Parveen N, Mahaboob VS, Rajendraprasad A, Ravindraprakash HR, Venkateswarlu J, Rao P, Pande G, Narusu ML, Khaja MN, Pramila R, Habeeb A, Habibullah CM. Management of hyperbilirubinemia in biliary atresia by hepatic progenitor cell transplantation through hepatic artery: a case report. Transplant Proc. 2008;40(4):1153–5.
75. Seglen PO. Preparation of isolated rat liver cells. Methods Cell Biol. 1976;13:29–83.
76. Guguen Guillouzo C, Campion JP, Brissot P, Glaise D, Launois B, Bourel M, Guillouzo A. High yield of preparation of isolated human adult hepatocytes by enzymatic perfusion of the liver. Cell Biol Int Rep. 1982;6:625–8.
77. Dorko K, Freeswick PD, Bartoli F, Cicalese L, Bardsley BA, Tzakis A, Nussler AK. A new technique for isolating and culturing human hepatocytes from whole or split livers not used for transplantation. Cell Transplant. 1994;3(5):387–95.
78. Gridelli B, Vizzini G, Pietrosi G, Luca A, Spada M, Gruttadauria S, Cintorino D, Amico G, Chinnici C, Miki T, Schmelzer E, Conaldi PG, Triolo F, Gerlach JC. Efficient human fetal liver cell isolation protocol based on vascular perfusion for liver cell-based therapy and case report on cell transplantation. Liver Transpl. 2012;18(2):226–37.
79. Alexandrova K, Griesel C, Barthold M, Heuft HG, Ott M, Winkler M, Schrem H, Manns MP, Bredehorn T, Net M, Vidal MM, Kafert-Kasting S, Arseniev L. Large-scale isolation of human hepatocytes for therapeutic application. Cell Transplant. 2005;14(10):845–53.
80. Terry C, Mitry RR, Lehec SC, Muiesan P, Rela M, Heaton ND, Hughes RD, Dhawan A. The effects of cryopreservation on human hepatocytes obtained from different sources of liver tissue. Cell Transplant. 2005;14(8):585–94.
81. Hughes RD, Mitry RR, Dhawan A, Lehec SC, Girlanda R, Rela M, Heaton ND, Muiesan P. Isolation of hepatocytes from livers from non-heart-beating donors for cell transplantation. Liver Transpl. 2006;2(5):713–7.
82. Hsu H-C, Matsuno N, Machida N, Enosawa S. Improved recovery of hepatocytes isolated from warm ischemic rat liver by citrate phosphate dextrose (CPD)-supplemented Euro-Collins solution. Cell Med. 2013 http://dx.doi.org/10.3727/215517913X666521

83. Hsu H-C, Matsuno N, Tanaka R, Enosawa S. Improvement of hepatocyte recovery in rat liver tissue subject to one hour warm ischaemic injury by using citrate phosphate dextrose added to Euro-Collins perfusion solution. Transplant Proc. Transpl (2013). Proc, 45, 1700–1703.
84. Tamaki T, Kamada N, Wight DG, Pegg DE. Successful 48-hour preservation of the rat liver by continuous hypothermic perfusion with haemaccel-isotonic citrate solution. Transplantation. 1987;43(4):468–71.

Chapter 11
ECD for Adult Liver Transplantation

Masahiko Taniguchi and Hiroyuki Furukawa

11.1 Introduction

Since Starzl [1] performed the world's first deceased-donor liver transplant in 1963, more than 6,000 deceased-donor liver transplants have been performed annually in the USA. There, as in other parts of the world, the biggest problem with liver transplants is the unequivocal shortage of donors. In response, countries mostly in Europe and the USA have explored extended criteria donors (ECD), which include elderly donors and donors with a fatty liver. This paper describes the current state of and problems with these ECD.

11.2 Definition

11.2.1 Donor Criteria for Deceased-Donor Liver Transplants

Selection of appropriate donors is essential to the success of a deceased-donor liver transplant. Aspects that must be considered when selecting a donor include age, body mass index (BMI), medication being taken, a history of drinking, the presence or lack of liver disease, a history of infection, and a history of malignancy. Moreover, causes of death and changes in hemodynamics and liver function must also be considered. Criteria for selection of an ideal donor include a donor age of 50 or younger, normal liver function and a lack of liver disease, stable hemodynamics, a lack of severe abdominal trauma, no systemic infection, a lack of malignancy, and normal kidney function [2].

M. Taniguchi (✉) • H. Furukawa
Division of Gastroenterologic and General Surgery, Department of Surgery,
Asahikawa Medical University, Asahikawa, Hokkaido, Japan
e-mail: m-tani@asahikawa-med.ac.jp

T. Asano et al. (eds.), *Marginal Donors: Current and Future Status*,
DOI 10.1007/978-4-431-54484-5_11, © Springer Japan 2014

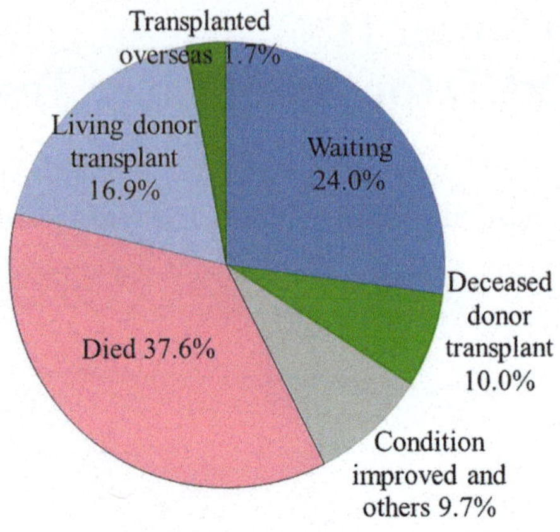

Fig. 11.1 Removal reasons (total 1,677 cases)

11.2.2 Definition of ECD

Procedures such as living-donor liver transplantation and split transplantation have been performed to cope with the shortage of donors, but these procedures have reached their limit. The reality is that surgeons must rely on liver transplants from marginal donors, i.e., liver transplants from ECD. Although there are no set criteria for ECD, there are tentative criteria. These include elderly donors, donors with a fatty liver, donors infected with HBV, donors infected with HCV, donors with hypernatremia, donors receiving prolonged respiratory care in the ICU, a liver that has been ischemic for some time as a result of cardiac arrest or low blood pressure, a donor with a high BMI, a donor using vasoactive drugs, and a liver that has been stored (both warm and cold) for a prolonged period [3, 4].

11.2.3 Outcome

In Japan, 402 individuals were registered with the Japan Organ Transport Network (http://www.jotnw.or.jp/) as candidates for a deceased-donor liver transplant as of December 2012. Since candidates for a deceased-donor liver transplant were first registered in October 1997, a total of 1,677 candidates registered prior to the end of December 2012 (Fig. 11.1). Of these patients, 168 (10.0 %) received a deceased-donor liver transplant and 284 (16.9 %) received a living-donor liver transplant in Japan, 29 (1.7 %) received a deceased-donor liver transplant overseas, and 631 (37.6 %) died. Changes in the number of liver transplant recipients since 1999 are shown in Fig. 11.2. More than 2 years has passed since the revision of the Organ Transplant Act. The number of candidates who received a deceased-donor liver transplant in Japan increased about 5 times a year compared to the number who

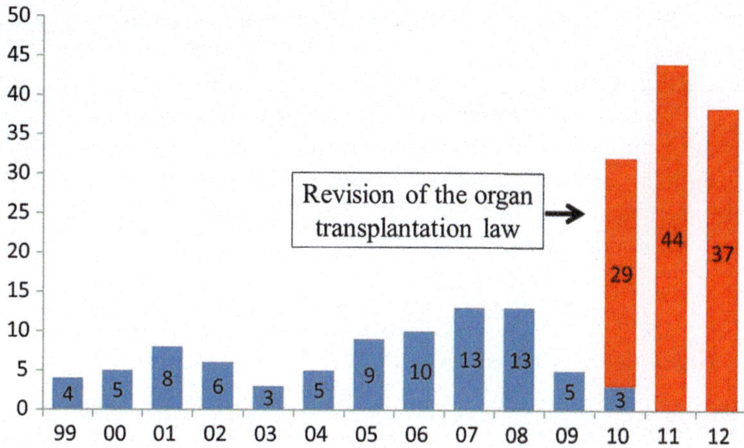

Fig. 11.2 Changes in the number of liver transplants in Japan

Table 11.1 Multivariate analysis for the 3-month patient survival

	Coefficient (SE)	Odds ratio (95 % CI)	*P*-value
MELD score ≥25	4.213 (1.387)	12.3 (1.7–90.3)	0.0133
Donor age ≥55 years	2.514 (1.015)	14.0 (1.6–119.5)	0.0159
CIT ≥600 min	2.639 (1.094)	67.6 (4.5–1024.9)	0.0024

(Quote from [5])

received a transplant before the act was revised. However, one in three individuals still die without receiving a liver transplant; so the stark reality is that there is an unequivocal shortage of donors in Japan as well.

Although the revision of the Organ Transplantation Law in July 2010 allowing organ procurement with family consent has increased the number of deceased donors, it remains insufficient. In this situation of a serious organ shortage, the use of ECD is inevitable. We analyzed ECD and recipient factors to determine which ones impacted early recipient outcomes [5]. From February 1999 to January 2011, 100 deceased-donor liver transplantations were performed in Japan, including 85 consecutive adult cases that were studied to evaluate whether 6 recipient and 16 donor factors affected the 3-month recipient survival. Upon univariate analysis, model for end-stage liver disease (MELD) score ≥25, donor age ≥55 years, and cold ischemia time (CIT) ≥10 h significantly reduced the 3-month survival. Multivariate analysis confirmed the independent contributions of three adverse factors including MELD score ≥25, donor age ≥55 years, and CIT ≥10 h (Table 11.1). Three-month recipient survivals with 0, 1, 2, and 3 positive factors were 100 %, 94.4 %, 53.8 %, and 0 %, respectively.

The importance of analyzing both donor and recipient factors simultaneously has been emphasized to match donors and recipients to compensate for their risks.

From this study, MELD score, CIT, and donor age were observed to independently impact the 3-month recipient survival rates. Subgroup analysis showed recipients with more RFs to have inferior 3-month survival; however, it was more than 66.7 % when CIT was maintained within 10 h. To minimize CIT, further efforts to reduce transportation time and to adjust donor and recipient operative times are mandatory. In the long term, we must promote deceased donation to reduce recipient MELD scores by shortening the waiting time and revise the allocation system to minimize CIT by giving priority to the local area.

11.3 Basic and Clinical Research

11.3.1 Elderly Donors

Problems with grafts from elderly donors are the presence of severe arteriosclerosis and problems with the liver parenchyma, e.g., fatty liver [6, 7]. These two conditions have a profound negative impact on the graft survival rate soon after transplantation [7]. Typically, a donor age of over 60 has a massive impact on the outcome of a transplant. However, the number of transplants of grafts from elderly donors has increased over the past few years as a way to cope with the shortage of donors. Surgeons in Spain in particular are actively performing transplants of grafts from elderly donors. Fewer than 15 % of potential donors in the USA are of age 60 or over, but in Spain more than 30 % of these potential donors are of age 60 or over. As a result, the number of donors in Spain increased 136 % compared with 33 % increase in the USA [8]. Nevertheless, there is no question that considering grafts from elderly donors increases the number of available grafts, thus reducing the number of patients who die while awaiting a transplant.

But what are the outcomes of transplant grafts from elderly donors? According to the Spanish Registry for Liver Transplantation, the 1-year survival rate is 76 % for a recipient of a graft from a donor ageing 60–69, while that for a recipient of a graft from a donor ageing 80–89 is 72 %. These figures differ a little from the 1-year survival rate of 80 % for a recipient of a graft from a donor ageing 15–60. Nevertheless, the 5-year survival rate for a recipient of a graft from a donor ageing 60–69 is 56 % and that for a recipient of a graft from a donor ageing 80–89 is 51 %, but that for a recipient of a graft from a donor ageing 15–60 is 66 %, so the difference in survival rates has increased. This is because elderly donors are obviously more susceptible to liver cancer, recurrence of hepatitis C, and recurrence of an underlying illness [9]. Currently, liver transplants from elderly donors have outcomes on par with liver transplants from younger donors, provided there are no other risks besides the donor's age [10]. This is because recipients are chosen in light of the condition of the graft and risk factors on the part of the recipient. A liver transplant from an elderly donor to a low-risk recipient will not affect the transplant's outcome. Thus, having an elderly donor is becoming less of a factor for a less satisfactory transplant outcome.

11.3.2 Fatty Liver

Thirteen to twenty-six percent of brain-dead donors have a fatty liver [11]. Fatty infiltration of the liver is classified as either macrovesicular or microvesicular steatosis. Microsteatosis is reversible, so it is not associated with the incidence of primary graft nonfunction or the recipient's survival rate [12, 13]. In contrast, the extent of macrovesicular steatosis is associated with the recipient's prognosis. Normally, severe macrovesicular steatosis of more than 60 % often leads to primary nonfunction, thus precluding the use of the liver [14]. A liver transplant from a donor with moderate (30–60 %) macrovesicular steatosis involves a high incidence of primary nonfunction compared to transplantation of a normal liver (13 % vs. 3 %) [15]. If the donor and recipient have no other risk factors, then a transplant from a donor with moderate macrovesicular steatosis results in a post-transplant outcome equivalent to a transplant from a normal donor [16]. Given the ever-increasing number of deaths of patients awaiting a transplant, efforts must be made to improve the outcomes of transplants from donors with moderate macrovesicular steatosis.

11.3.3 Donors After Cardiac Death

The particulars have taken up other section (DCD Liver).

11.3.4 HBV-Positive Donors

Liver transplantation from an HBcAb-positive donor to a recipient who is HBsAb-positive or HBcAb-positive results in few problems. However, hepatitis B often recurs when such a liver is transplanted to other recipients [17]. Thus, hepatitis B immunoglobulin and antivirals must be used after liver transplantation from an HBcAb-positive donor [18].

11.3.5 HCV-Positive Donors

There are few significant differences in the post-transplant survival rate when a liver from an HCV-positive donor is transplanted to a patient with HCV-related cirrhosis compared to a liver from an HCV-negative donor [19, 20]. However, a liver transplant from an elderly and HCV-positive donor exacerbates fibrosis more than a transplant from an elderly and HCV-negative donor and is more susceptible to graft failure [21]. Recipients in whom the donor strain of HCV became predominant after transplantation are known to have a longer relapse-free survival than recipients who retained their own HCV strain [22]. A graft from an HCV-positive donor with fibrosis or inflammation is not suitable for transplantation, so a liver biopsy prior to transplantation is crucial.

11.3.6 Matching of ECD Grafts and Recipients

Use of ECD grafts has reduced the deaths of transplant candidates [23]. From 2000 to 2007, the number of liver transplants performed in the USA increased from 4,595 to 6,228 (a 26.2 % increase). Presumably this is the result of introducing a system of organ allocation based on the MELD score and encouraging the use of marginal donors.

Which patients should receive an ECD graft? A large-scale retrospective study of over 1,000 patients at UCLA [24] scored extended criteria based on a donor age of 55 and over, donor hospitalization for longer than 5 days, a cold ischemia time of more than 10 h, and a warm ischemia time of more than 40 min. According to the study, a higher ECD score (donor score, or DS) resulted in a higher post-transplantation mortality rate. In other words, a higher DS results in greater risk, so recipients in poor condition prior to transplantation (a high MELD score) are more likely to have a poorer outcome after transplantation. A DS of 2 or less means that a transplant is possible with little risk in many cases, but a DS of more than 2 means that a transplant should be avoided in risky cases, e.g., urgent cases. Similarly, a study of 650 patients in Spain found that an elderly donor, a fatty liver with 30 % of more steatosis, and cold ischemia time were extended criteria associated with primary graft dysfunction [25]. Matching a donor with a high ECD score and a recipient with a MELD score of 29 or higher is most likely to lead to graft failure.

According to data from the Organ Procurement and Transplantation Network (OPTN) and current conditions in the USA, 12,056 liver transplants were performed from June 2002 to June 2005. Of these, 2,873 (23.8 %) were transplants of a graft from an ECD. An ECD graft is most often (33 %) transplanted to a recipient with a MELD score of <15 [4]. Based on an analysis of data covering 20,023 liver transplants in the US Scientific Registry of Transplant Recipients, Feng et al. [26] calculated the donor risk index (DRI). ECD grafts from a donor age of 40 or older or a DCD donor or grafts that were a split/partial graft closely correlated graft failure. Feng et al. reported that grafts with an increased DRI have been preferentially transplanted into older candidates with moderate disease severity (nonstatus 1 with lower MELD scores) and without hepatitis C. Although the use of an ECD graft is a significant risk factor for graft failure, there is no correlation between the use of an ECD graft and the recipient's MELD score. The same group later conducted a follow-up of 28,165 recipients in the USA, and they found that patients with a low MELD score had a higher mortality rate from receipt of a high DRI graft than from waiting for a transplant. That said, patients with a MELD score of 20 or higher did receive some survival benefit even when they received a DRI graft. Based on these findings, recipients with a high MELD score benefit more from a high DRI graft than recipients with a low MELD score. Matching a high DRI graft and a recipient with a low MELD score results in less of a survival benefit for the recipient and reduces the chances for a recipient with a high MELD score to receive a transplant, so such matches should be avoided [27].

11.4 Conclusion

This paper has described the use of ECD in liver transplants. As mentioned earlier, the unequivocal shortage of donors is a global problem. This is particularly true for Japan, where far fewer deceased-donor liver transplants are performed in comparison to Europe and the USA. Because there are so few deceased-donor liver transplants, organs must not be wasted and transplants should be successful so that the wishes of their donors can be satisfied. To that end, liver transplant surgeons must strive more than their counterparts in Europe and the USA to perform transplants from ECD and reduce the risk of ECD grafts.

References

1. Starzl TE, Marchioro TL, Vonkaulla KN, Hermann G, Brittain RS, Waddell WR. Homotransplantation of the liver in humans. Surg Gynecol Obstet. 1963;117:659–76. PubMed PMID: 14100514. Pubmed Central PMCID: 2634660. Epub 1963/12/01. eng.
2. Mehrabi A, Fonouni H, Muller SA, Schmidt J. Current concepts in transplant surgery: liver transplantation today. Langenbecks Arch Surg. 2008;393(3):245–60. PubMed PMID: 18309513. Epub 2008/03/01. eng.
3. Silberhumer GR, Pokorny H, Hetz H, Herkner H, Rasoul-Rockenschaub S, Soliman T, et al. Combination of extended donor criteria and changes in the model for end-stage liver disease score predict patient survival and primary dysfunction in liver transplantation: a retrospective analysis. Transplantation. 2007;83(5):588–92. PubMed PMID: 17353779. Epub 2007/03/14. eng.
4. Maluf DG, Edwards EB, Kauffman HM. Utilization of extended donor criteria liver allograft: Is the elevated risk of failure independent of the model for end-stage liver disease score of the recipient? Transplantation. 2006;82(12):1653–7. PubMed PMID: 17198254. Epub 2007/01/02. eng.
5. Furukawa H, Taniguchi M, Fujiyoshi M, Oota M, Japanese Study Group of Liver T. Experience using extended criteria donors in first 100 cases of deceased donor liver transplantation in Japan. Transplant Proc. 2012;44(2):373–5.
6. Grazi GL, Cescon M, Ravaioli M, Ercolani G, Pierangeli F, D'Errico A, et al. A revised consideration on the use of very aged donors for liver transplantation. Am J Transplant. 2001;1(1):61–8. PubMed PMID: 12095041. Epub 2002/07/04. eng.
7. Verran D, Kusyk T, Painter D, Fisher J, Koorey D, Strasser S, et al. Clinical experience gained from the use of 120 steatotic donor livers for orthotopic liver transplantation. Liver Transpl. 2003;9(5):500–5. PubMed PMID: 12740794. Epub 2003/05/13. eng.
8. Chang GJ, Mahanty HD, Ascher NL, Roberts JP. Expanding the donor pool: can the Spanish model work in the United States? Am J Transplant. 2003;3(10):1259–63. PubMed PMID: 14510699. Epub 2003/09/27. eng.

9. Cuende N, Grande L, Sanjuan F, Cuervas-Mons V. Liver transplant with organs from elderly donors: Spanish experience with more than 300 liver donors over 70 years of age. Transplantation. 2002;73(8):1360. PubMed PMID: 11981439. Epub 2002/05/01. eng.
10. Grande L, Rull A, Rimola A, Garcia-Valdecasas JC, Manyalic M, Cabrer C, et al. Outcome of patients undergoing orthotopic liver transplantation with elderly donors (over 60 years). Transplant Proc. 1997;29(8):3289–90. PubMed PMID: 9414718. Epub 1998/01/01. eng.
11. Imber CJ, St Peter SD, Handa A, Friend PJ. Hepatic steatosis and its relationship to transplantation. Liver Transpl. 2002;8(5):415–23. PubMed PMID: 12004340. Epub 2002/05/11. eng.
12. Urena MA, Moreno Gonzalez E, Romero CJ, Ruiz-Delgado FC, Moreno SC. An approach to the rational use of steatotic donor livers in liver transplantation. Hepatogastroenterology. 1999;46(26):1164–73. PubMed PMID: 10370686. Epub 1999/06/17. eng.
13. Fishbein TM, Fiel MI, Emre S, Cubukcu O, Guy SR, Schwartz ME, et al. Use of livers with microvesicular fat safely expands the donor pool. Transplantation. 1997;64(2):248–51. PubMed PMID: 9256182. Epub 1997/07/27. eng.
14. Selzner M, Clavien PA. Fatty liver in liver transplantation and surgery. Semin Liver Dis. 2001;21(1):105–13. PubMed PMID: 11296690. Epub 2001/04/12. eng.
15. Strasberg SM, Howard TK, Molmenti EP, Hertl M. Selecting the donor liver: risk factors for poor function after orthotopic liver transplantation. Hepatology. 1994;20(4 Pt 1):829–38. PubMed PMID: 7927223. Epub 1994/10/01. eng.
16. Burke A, Lucey MR. Non-alcoholic fatty liver disease, non-alcoholic steatohepatitis and orthotopic liver transplantation. Am J Transplant. 2004;4(5):686–93. PubMed PMID: 15084161. Epub 2004/04/16. eng.
17. Prieto M, Gomez MD, Berenguer M, Cordoba J, Rayon JM, Pastor M, et al. De novo hepatitis B after liver transplantation from hepatitis B core antibody-positive donors in an area with high prevalence of anti-HBc positivity in the donor population. Liver Transpl. 2001;7(1):51–8. PubMed PMID: 11150423. Epub 2001/01/11. eng.
18. Nery JR, Nery-Avila C, Reddy KR, Cirocco R, Weppler D, Levi DM, et al. Use of liver grafts from donors positive for antihepatitis B-core antibody (anti-HBc) in the era of prophylaxis with hepatitis-B immunoglobulin and lamivudine. Transplantation. 2003;75(8):1179–86. PubMed PMID: 12717200. Epub 2003/04/30. eng.
19. Ghobrial RM, Steadman R, Gornbein J, Lassman C, Holt CD, Chen P, et al. A 10-year experience of liver transplantation for hepatitis C: analysis of factors determining outcome in over 500 patients. Ann Surg. 2001;234(3):384–93. discussion 93–4. PubMed PMID: 11524591. Pubmed Central PMCID: 1422029. Epub 2001/08/29. eng.
20. Marroquin CE, Marino G, Kuo PC, Plotkin JS, Rustgi VK, Lu AD, et al. Transplantation of hepatitis C-positive livers in hepatitis C-positive patients is equivalent to transplanting hepatitis C-negative livers. Liver Transpl. 2001;7(9):762–8. PubMed PMID: 11552208. Epub 2001/09/12. eng.
21. Khapra AP, Agarwal K, Fiel MI, Kontorinis N, Hossain S, Emre S, et al. Impact of donor age on survival and fibrosis progression in patients with hepatitis C undergoing liver transplantation using HCV+ allografts. Liver Transpl. 2006;12(10):1496–503. PubMed PMID: 16964597. Epub 2006/09/12. eng.
22. Vargas HE, Laskus T, Wang LF, Lee R, Radkowski M, Dodson F, et al. Outcome of liver transplantation in hepatitis C virus-infected patients who received hepatitis C virus-infected grafts. Gastroenterology. 1999;117(1):149–53. PubMed PMID: 10381921. Epub 1999/06/26. eng.
23. Barshes NR, Horwitz IB, Franzini L, Vierling JM, Goss JA. Waitlist mortality decreases with increased use of extended criteria donor liver grafts at adult liver transplant centers. Am J Transplant. 2007;7(5):1265–70. PubMed PMID: 17359503. Epub 2007/03/16. eng.
24. Cameron AM, Ghobrial RM, Yersiz H, Farmer DG, Lipshutz GS, Gordon SA, et al. Optimal utilization of donor grafts with extended criteria: a single-center experience in over 1000 liver transplants. Ann Surg. 2006;243(6):748–53. discussion 53–5. PubMed PMID: 16772778. Pubmed Central PMCID: 1570573. Epub 2006/06/15. eng.

25. Briceno J, Ciria R, de la Mata M, Rufian S, Lopez-Cillero P. Prediction of graft dysfunction based on extended criteria donors in the model for end-stage liver disease score era. Transplantation. 2010;90(5):530–9. PubMed PMID: 20581766. Epub 2010/06/29. eng.
26. Feng S, Goodrich NP, Bragg-Gresham JL, Dykstra DM, Punch JD, DebRoy MA, et al. Characteristics associated with liver graft failure: the concept of a donor risk index. Am J Transplant. 2006;6(4):783–90. PubMed PMID: 16539636. Epub 2006/03/17. eng.
27. Schaubel DE, Sima CS, Goodrich NP, Feng S, Merion RM. The survival benefit of deceased donor liver transplantation as a function of candidate disease severity and donor quality. Am J Transplant. 2008;8(2):419–25. PubMed PMID: 18190658. Epub 2008/01/15. eng.

Chapter 12
LD for Liver Transplantation

Hiroto Egawa

12.1 Criteria for Living Donation

12.1.1 Principles

First of all, donation should be based on voluntary will and the donor should be healthy. A donor candidate should be fully informed about benefits and adverse effects to the donor and recipient after transplantation and the expected prognosis of the recipient. Japanese transplant law requires confirmation of voluntary will, fully consented form, and full understanding of the risks and benefits to the donor, and a psychologist should confirm it. A donor is chosen from relatives including spouses. Emotional relatives should be strictly assessed by ethical committees to avoid organ trade.

12.1.2 Practice

When a recipient has an appropriate indication for liver transplantation, the donor candidates consent initially. The informed consent for donor candidates should be obtained separately from the recipient. The donor candidates should be interviewed by a psychologist as well as his or her family. During these procedures, voluntary will should be confirmed.

For donor safety, extrahepatic diseases as well as hepatic diseases are assessed. Histories of alcohol, tobacco, and other supplement use are important. Height and weight are important for size matching and body mass index is also mandatory to

H. Egawa (✉)
Institute of Gastroenterology, Tokyo Women's Medical University,
8-1, Kawada-cho, Shinjuku-ku, Tokyo 162-8666, Japan
e-mail: egawa@kuhp.kyoto-u.ac.jp

T. Asano et al. (eds.), *Marginal Donors: Current and Future Status*,
DOI 10.1007/978-4-431-54484-5_12, © Springer Japan 2014

preclude steatosis. Varices of the lower extremities should be checked to assess risks for deep vein thrombosis.

Laboratory tests consisted, at least, of blood type, blood cell counts, renal and hepatic function tests, and screening of infectious diseases. The serology of hepatitis B, hepatitis C, treponema, adult T cell leukemia, human immunodeficiency virus, Epstein-Barr virus, and cytomegalovirus is standard. Positivity of HCV, treponema, ATL, and HIV is basically a contraindication, although there were literatures of challenging HCV, treponema, and ATL. Positivity of HB antigens is a contraindication. On the other hand, a person with positive HB antibody can donate his or her liver when the recipient is treated with HB immune globulin or vaccination, because HB virus stays in the hepatocytes.

HbA1c is important to assess diabetes as well as blood glucose levels. When at least one of them is abnormal, 75 g glucose tolerance test is indicated. The homeostasis model assessment (HOMA) (fasting plasma glucose level × fasting plasma insulin level ÷ 405) is important to estimate steady-state beta cell function and insulin sensitivity [1]. The high value indicates insulin resistance, which is a risk for nonalcoholic steatohepatitis. To assess risks for deep vein thrombosis, proteins C and S should be measured.

Human leukocyte antigens (HLA) are analyzed not to search suitable donors but to avoid graft-versus-host diseases (GVHD) in LDLT [2]. When a parent donates the liver to his or her child, homozygous HLA should be neglected. The importance of cross-match test has been a controversy in the field of liver transplantation. However, recent development of single bead method to analyze individual antibody to HLA enabled us to assess risks of positive anti-HLA antibodies in liver transplantation [3]. Strategies for positive donor HLA-specific antibody are not established in liver transplantation.

Radiological examinations are important not only to analyze anatomy for liver resection but also to assess adequate graft volume for a recipient and adequate reserved volume for a donor. The remnant liver volume exceeds 30 % in the right lobe without the middle hepatic vein and 35 % in the right lobe with the middle hepatic vein (MHV+). The remnant liver has normal quality and complete perfusion, for MHV+ donor as well as MHV− donor. To obtain complete perfusion of the remnant liver without MHV, it is necessary to make sure that the significant hepatic vein that drains segment 4 is present after the MHV is removed from the remnant liver. However, it is wise to avoid MHV+ with remnant liver volume <35 % in an elderly donor [4]. For favorable outcomes of recipients, the graft volume should be guaranteed. The reported indicators are graft-recipient weight ratio (GRWR) and standard liver volume ratio (SLR) [5, 6]. Although the minimal requirement to avoid small-for-size syndrome (SFS) is not fixed, GRWR >0.8 and SLR>30 % are desirable. On the other hand, a too large graft does not match to a small baby, but this problem can be solved surgically [7, 8]. CT scan is a powerful device to assess steatosis. The ratio of CT density between the liver and the spleen indicates the degree of fatty infiltration well [9]. The value >1.2 is desirable and that >1.0 is the minimal requirement.

HLA-related donor-specific antibody (DSA) used to be controversial in liver transplantation, because sensitivity and specificity of lymphocyte cross-match test did not satisfy clinical requirements. Recently, single bead technique enables us to identify sensitized HLA and to quantify the amount of DSA. It offers virtual cross-match test beside a conventional one. Strongly positive DSA is an important risk that should be avoided by changing a donor or aggressive desensitization.

Neglect of malignant diseases is important. Common gastrointestinal cancers and breast and gynecological cancers are checked regularly.

12.2 Background: Historical Trials to Extend Living Donor Criteria

There are two ways to expand donor criteria: choose marginal donors and expand social regulation. In marginal donors, there are healthy donors whose grafts do not match to recipients and donors with sick background. The former reasons are old age, blood type incompatibility, SFS, and positive HLA-DSA. Generally the upper limit of age of living donors is 65 years and an application of older donors is strictly assessed by institutional committees. Strategies for ABO blood type-incompatible LDLT were established and the 1-year patient survival is 10 % lower than the identical LDLT [10–12]. SFS is aggressively challenged. To obtain larger grafts, donor hepatectomy was innovated for a left lobe graft with the caudate lobe, a right lobe graft, and a right lobe graft with the middle vein. Further, to treat SFS, surgical innovations were made and the safe minimal limit of GRWR is decreased from 1.0 to 0.7 [13–16]. The situations between 0.6 and 0.7 of GRWR are still experimental. Positive HLA-DSA is a future issue.

It is a principle that the donor is healthy. But, as long as donors and recipients do not suffer any problems relating to background diseases of donors, such donors are acceptable. In liver diseases, steatosis is the most common. The laboratory data should be normal. Donor candidates with positive findings of CT scan and US require treatments by dietary treatment and exercise. Liver biopsies are performed, if necessary, to confirm the degree of fatty infiltration and to neglect steatohepatitis. Although positive HBs Ab is not a sign of ongoing hepatitis, recipients transplanted with the livers should be administrated with hepatitis B immunoglobulin (HBIG) to avoid reactivation of hepatitis [17]. Diabetes mellitus and hypertension requiring medications are contraindications. When dietary and physical treatments successfully discontinue medications, those candidates are acceptable. Domino liver transplantation using a liver graft of a recipient of familial amyloid polyneuropathy (FAP) is not frequent but regularly performed worldwide [18, 19]. This transplantation is lifesaving but the chance of onset of FAP in the long term after transplantation is not low [18].

Social limitation should be explored carefully. To avoid organ trade, living donors are chosen in relatives or spouses according to principle. In western countries, there are LDLT from emotional relatives. In Japan, living donor transplantation from nonrelatives is approved by institutional ethical committees and also assessed by the ethical committee of Japan Society of Transplantation.

12.3 Prognosis for Living Donors in Japan

One-year patient survival of LDLT was 83 % in 2010 registry by the Japanese Liver Transplantation Society including 5,653 LDLT until 2009 [20]. Hashikura et al. reported donor complications in a multicenter study including 3,565 donors until 2006 [21]. In total, 299 donors (8.4 %) suffered complications related to liver donation. Postoperative complications included biliary complications in 3.0 %, reoperation in 1.3 %, severe aftereffects in two (0.06 %), and death (apparently related to donor surgery) in one donor (0.03 %). The incidence of postoperative complications in left and right lobe donors was 8.7 % and 9.4 %, respectively.

References

1. Matthews DR, Hosker JP, Rudenski AS, Naylor BA, Treacher DF, Turner RC. Homeostasis model assessment: insulin resistance and beta-cell function from fasting plasma glucose and insulin concentrations in man. Diabetologia. 1985;28(7):412–9.
2. Kiuchi T, Harada H, Matsukawa H, Kasahara M, Inomata Y, Uemoto S, Asonuma K, Egawa H, Maruya E, Saji H, Tanaka K. One-way donor-recipient HLA-matching as a risk factor for graft-versus-host disease in living-related liver transplantation. Transpl Int. 1998;11 Suppl 1:S383–4.
3. Miyagawa-Hayashino A, Yoshizawa A, Uchida Y, Egawa H, Yurugi K, Masuda S, Minamiguchi S, Maekawa T, Uemoto S, Haga H. Progressive graft fibrosis and donor-specific HLA antibodies in pediatric late liver allografts. Liver Transpl. 2012;18(11):1333–42.
4. Egawa H. Minimizing the risks for living donors of right lobe liver grafts. Nat Rev Gastroenterol Hepatol. 2011;8(5):251–2.
5. Kiuchi T, Kasahara M, Uryuhara K, Inomata Y, Uemoto S, Asonuma K, Egawa H, Fujita S, Hayashi M, Tanaka K. Impact of graft size mismatching on graft prognosis in liver transplantation from living donors. Transplantation. 1999;67(2):321–7.
6. Kawasaki S, Makuuchi M, Ishizone S, Matsunami H, Terada M, Kawarazaki H. Liver regeneration in recipients and donors after transplantation. Lancet. 1992;339(8793):580–1.
7. Kasahara M, Fukuda A, Yokoyama S, Sato S, Tanaka H, Kuroda T, et al. Living donor liver transplantation with hyperreduced left lateral segments. J Pediatr Surg. 2008;43:1575–8.
8. Mizuta K, Yasuda Y, Egami S, Sanada Y, Wakiya T, Urahashi T, et al. Living donor liver transplantation for neonates using segment 2 monosegment graft. Am J Transplant. 2010; 10:2547–52.
9. Iwasaki M, Takada Y, Hayashi M, Minamiguchi S, Haga H, Maetani Y, Fujii K, Kiuchi T, Tanaka K. Noninvasive evaluation of graft steatosis in living donor liver transplantation. Transplantation. 2004;78(10):1501–5.
10. Egawa H, Teramukai S, Haga H, Tanabe M, Fukushima M, Shimazu M. Present status of ABO-incompatible living donor liver transplantation in Japan. Hepatology. 2008;47(1): 143–52.
11. Egawa H, Ohmori K, Haga H, Tsuji H, Yurugi K, Miyagawa-Hayashino A, et al. B-cell surface marker analysis for improvement of rituximab prophylaxis in ABO-incompatible adult living donor liver transplantation. Liver Transplant. 2007;13(4):579–88.
12. Ikegami T, Taketomi A, Yoshizumi H, Harada N, Iguchi T, Hashimoto N, et al. Rituximab, IVIG, and plasma exchange without graft local infusion treatment; a new protocol in ABO incompatible living donor liver transplantation. Transplantation. 2009;88:303–7.
13. Takayama T, Makuuchi M, Kubota K, Sano K, Harihara Y, Kawarasaki H. Living-related transplantation of left liver plus caudate lobe. J Am Coll Surg. 2000;190(5):635–8.

14. Sugawara Y, Makuuchi M, Imamura H, Kaneko J, Kokudo N. Outflow reconstruction in extended right liver grafts from living donors. Liver Transplant. 2003;9(3):306–9.
15. Ito T, Kiuchi T, Yamamoto H, Oike F, Ogura Y, Fujimoto Y, et al. Changes in portal venous pressure in the early phase after living donor liver transplantation: pathogenesis and clinical implications. Transplantation. 2003;75(8):1313–7.
16. Ogura Y, Hori T, El Moghazy WM, Yoshizawa A, Oike F, Mori A, et al. Portal pressure <15 mm Hg is a key for successful adult living donor liver transplantation utilizing smaller grafts than before. Liver Transplant. 2010;16(6):718–28.
17. Uemoto S, Sugiyama K, Marusawa H, Inomata Y, Asonuma K, Egawa H, Kiuchi T, Miyake Y, Tanaka K, Chiba T. Transmission of hepatitis B virus from hepatitis B core antibody-positive donors in living related liver transplants. Transplantation. 1998;65(4):494–9.
18. Asonuma K, Ohya Y, Isono K, Takeichi T, Yamamoto H, Lee KJ, Okumura K, Ando Y, Inomata Y. Current state of domino transplantation in Japan in terms of surgical procedures and de novo amyloid neuropathy. Amyloid. 2012;19 Suppl 1:75–7.
19. Tincani G, Hoti E, Andreani P, Ricca L, Pittau G, Vitale V, Blandin F, Adam R, Castaing D, Azoulay D. Operative risks of domino liver transplantation for the familial amyloid polyneuropathy liver donor and recipient: a double analysis. Am J Transplant. 2011;11(4):759–66.
20. The Japanese Liver Transplantation Society. Liver transplantation in Japan: registry by the japanese liver transplantation society. Ishoku. 2010;46:624–36.
21. Hashikura Y, Ichida T, Umeshita K, Kawasaki S, Mizokami M, Mochida S, Yanaga K, Monden M, Kiyosawa K, Japanese Liver Transplantation Society. Donor complications associated with living donor liver transplantation in Japan. Transplantation. 2009;88:110–4.

Part VI
Kidney Transplantation

Chapter 13
How to Initiate a DCD Programme for Kidney Transplantation

Srikanth Reddy and Rutger Ploeg

13.1 Introduction

Organ donation after circulatory death (DCD) has become an important source of organs for transplantation. The number of DCD donors is increasing in contrast to donation after brain death (DBD). This decline in DBD donors has been attributed to better road safety and improved care of patients with major trauma and cerebrovascular haemorrhage. There has been a considerable experience with DCD donor kidney transplantation. DCD kidneys have a higher incidence of delayed graft function but similar long-term function compared to DBD donors. Maastricht Category 1 and 2 donors are also termed "uncontrolled" and there is little experience with this type of donation. Most of these donors are patients presenting to the emergency department after a cardiac arrest out of the hospital or in the hospital with unsuccessful resuscitation. After declaration of death, organ donation is considered. Hence, these organs sustain a prolonged warm ischaemia. Category 3 donors are term "controlled". These patients are usually in the intensive care unit where a decision is made to withdraw support due to poor prognosis. Family consent for donation is obtained and the retrieval team mobilised prior to withdrawal of support. Hence warm ischaemia can be minimised. Controlled donation is being very successfully implemented in countries such as the UK.

S. Reddy (✉) • R. Ploeg
Nuffield Department of Surgical Sciences, Churchill Hospital, Oxford Transplant Centre, The University of Oxford, Oxford OX3 7LJ, UK
e-mail: srikanth.reddy@ouh.nhs.uk; rutger.ploeg@nds.ox.ac.uk

T. Asano et al. (eds.), *Marginal Donors: Current and Future Status*,
DOI 10.1007/978-4-431-54484-5_13, © Springer Japan 2014

13.2 Guidance for Clinical Protocols

There is a potential conflict of interest between caring for a potential donor and recipient. Hence, the Institute of Medicine in the United States and NHS Blood and Transplant in the UK provide clinical and ethical guidance. The clinical and moral requirements governing DCD organ procurement policy are summarised below.

13.2.1 Potential Donors

Organ donation should not influence the management of any patient. The team in charge of the patient should have decided to withdraw support due to poor prognosis and futility of treatment. Only then should donation be considered.

13.2.2 Consent

Informed consent must be obtained from the next of kin prior to starting the donation process in controlled donation and prior to retrieval in all the donors.

13.2.2.1 Interventions Prior to Death

Life-sustaining care of controlled donors is allowed until provision is made for organ retrieval. Blood tests including blood grouping and tissue typing are allowed. As regards any other intervention, there are clear differences between countries. Practice in the UK prevents administration of drugs or inserting additional cannulas to facilitate donation. In some countries, cannula can be placed and drugs including heparin and phentolamine administered with the consent of the family, unless contraindicated for medical reasons.

13.2.2.2 Management of Donor After Withdrawal of Support

Consensus is required about the management of the airway including extubation and sedation if the donor is in obvious distress after withdrawal of support. A senior medical professional needs to be in attendance at the time of withdrawal of support. This will allow care of donor after withdrawal of support and also prompt certification of death following cardiopulmonary arrest.

13.2.3 *Organs Can Only Be Taken from Donors After Death*

Until the moment of cessation of circulation and cardiac arrest, the donor is "alive". The first international workshop on DCD recommended a 10 min period after cardiopulmonary arrest prior to retrieval. In the USA and the UK, this period was changed to 5 min. This hands-off period is to ensure no auto-resuscitation and perfusion to the brain.

13.3 Necessity of a National and Institutional Framework

A national framework is required to provide legal and ethical guidance to establish and run a DCD programme. The responsibility of initiating and operating the programme remains at the local level in the hospitals. There needs to be a clear written policy and the following issues should also be considered.

13.3.1 *Recognition of DCD Donation*

DCD donation including controlled and uncontrolled should be legally recognised to safeguard the personnel facilitating donation.

13.3.2 *Education*

Education of public and healthcare personnel will increase donation. Sufficient trained organ donor procurement coordinators need to be based in hospitals throughout the country. Education will increase the public support and identification of suitable donors by healthcare personnel. In the UK and other countries, there is still a high rate of refusal of consent up to 40 %. Improved training of professionals will decrease this refusal rate.

13.3.3 *Donor Selection*

All potential donors are considered, but in the UK, chronic renal failure with GFR <30 mL/h and cortical necrosis on biopsy are considered specific contraindications for kidney donation.

13.3.4 Approaching the Family

The family is taken through the process by the donor coordinators. Structured electronic forms for assessment of the donor including past medical history and appropriate investigations need to be developed and should be accessible to the donation, retrieval and transplant teams.

13.3.5 Organ Allocation

HLA typing is performed early during the workup of donors and organs allocated to suitable recipients. A balance has to be established between HLA and age matching and cold ischaemia time. National sharing will improve HLA matching but could increase the cold ischaemia.

13.3.6 Organ Retrieval

Dedicated multi-organ retrieval teams should undertake retrieval and warm ischaemia should be minimised. Retrieval is performed by rapid laparotomy and thoracotomy and organs are cold flushed. Heparin should be added to the flush solution. Many donors do not arrest immediately after withdrawal of support. With controlled donation, for both outcome based and logistic reasons, the UK has a policy of not retrieving kidneys if cardiac arrest does not occur within 3 h of withdrawal of support. At the time of obtaining consent the family should be informed that donation would not proceed in such an event.

Strategies have been designed to recirculate oxygenated blood following cardiac arrest. Closed external cardiac massage has been used manually or mechanically with simultaneous mechanical ventilation. Donors have been placed on cardiopulmonary bypass at either normothermic or hypothermic temperatures in order to recirculate oxygenated blood. Results in Spain, the USA and France have demonstrated good function and survival of kidneys obtained from these donors. In most countries restoration of cerebral circulation after death is prohibited and therefore arteries supplying the head have to be occluded prior to the recirculation of blood.

13.3.7 Warm Ischaemia Time

The first international DCD workshop recommended that it be counted from the moment of cessation of circulation arrest until the start of hypothermic flush. However, after withdrawal of support, some donors have a long agonal phase prior to cardiac arrest with severe hypoxia and hypotension. Therefore in the UK, the concept of functional warm ischaemia is used. This is the time between hypotension (BP < 50 mmHg) or low saturation (<70 %) and start of cold flushing of the organs. A functional warm ischaemia of 90 min appears to be acceptable for kidneys but age and other co-morbidities have to be taken into consideration as well.

13.4 Organ Preservation

UW solution has been shown to be superior to other solutions such as hyperosmolar citrate. Hypothermic machine preservation has been shown to reduce the risk of delayed graft function but adds to the logistics though the machines are easily portable. The increased cost of machine perfusion is offset by the decreased need for dialysis following transplantation. Viability testing during preservation has been investigated. Low resistance during perfusion and glutathione-S-transferase has been shown to be useful in predicting outcome by some authors.

13.5 Recipient

Emphasis should be based on appropriate early recipient selection and minimising cold ischaemia. A national and local allocation scheme needs to be in place to identify appropriate recipients. HLA typing of the donor needs to be performed early in the workup. Recipients should be chosen early. Where feasible, a virtual X match should be used. If not, blood samples should be obtained from the donor well in advance and tissue typing performed. There needs to be good access to operating theatres.

13.6 Uncontrolled Donation

Setting up an uncontrolled DCD programme is more challenging but could yield additional organs. The donor pathway for the uncontrolled donors is different to controlled donors. Donation is considered only after declaration of death. It is possible that the next of kin will not be available at the moment of death. Interventions may have to be performed on the donors prior to obtaining consent from the donors, but retrieval surgery is performed only after consent has been obtained. Practice and regulations also vary in different countries. In those countries that practise “presumed consent” the initiation of donation in the absence of the family is possible unless the patient is registered as having opted out. Most countries, however, practise a system of “opting in”, and consent must be sought from the family of the donor. Delays in obtaining consent are likely to cause irreparable damage to the organs.

In countries such as Spain, cannulation of femoral vessels and in situ cooling using a double-balloon triple-lumen catheter in the femoral artery to selectively perfuse visceral organs are allowed prior to obtaining consent, but retrieval surgery is performed only after consent. Some centres have started to use in situ oxygenated normothermic reperfusion techniques prior to retrieval of the organs. Pilot studies have demonstrated good results.

Centres undertaking uncontrolled donation need to have staff in the emergency department with appropriate expertise to perform interventions on the donor immediately after certification of death. A separate room with all the resources needs to be made available for this in the emergency department. Consent is then obtained from the families. The donor is then moved to the operating theatre where organs are rapidly retrieved. Donation is feasible only in the patients who are on the donor register or in countries with opting-out system. The duration of warm ischaemia is often unpredictable and the yield of the organs is much lower compared to controlled donation.

Chapter 14
DCD for Kidney Transplantation

Takashi Kenmochi, Takehide Asano, Naotake Akutsu, Taihei Ito, Mamoru Kusaka, and Kiyotaka Hoshinaga

14.1 Introduction

The concept of brain death was introduced with the Harvard criteria in 1968 [1]. However, brain dead (DBD) donors were not used for organ transplantation in Japan until the enforcement of the Japanese Organ Transplant Law in 1997. Therefore, prior to this, all cadaveric kidney transplantations were performed using DCD donors according to the law regarding DCD for cornea and kidney transplantation. Due to a severe shortage of deceased donors, kidney transplantation is mainly performed using living donors in Japan. Changes in the number of kidney transplantation (Fig. 14.1) showed 212 patients underwent kidney transplantation from deceased donor in 2011, while 1,389 patients underwent living donor kidney transplantation [2]. Even after the enforcement of the Japanese Organ Transplant Law in 1997, the number of DBD donors remained low, such were only several donors per year. Although the number of DBD donors has been increased since the enforcement of the revised Japanese Organ Transplant Law in July 2010, deceased donor kidney transplantation is still mainly performed from DCD donors. Therefore, a history of deceased donor kidney transplantation is almost equal to the history of kidney transplantation using DCD donors.

T. Kenmochi (✉) • T. Ito
Department of Organ Transplant Surgery, Fujita Health University,
1-98 Dengakugakubo, Kutsukake-cho, Toyoake, Aichi 470-1192, Japan
e-mail: kenmochi@fujita-hu.ac.jp

T. Asano • N. Akutsu
Department of Surgery and Clinical Research Center, Chiba-East National Hospital,
673 Nitonacho, Chuo-ku, Chiba, Chiba 260-8712, Japan
e-mail: asano@cehpnet.com

M. Kusaka • K. Hoshinaga
Department of Urology, School of Medicine, Fujita Health University,
1-98 Dengakugakubo, Kutsukake-cho, Toyoake, Aichi 470-1192, Japan

T. Asano et al. (eds.), *Marginal Donors: Current and Future Status*,
DOI 10.1007/978-4-431-54484-5_14, © Springer Japan 2014

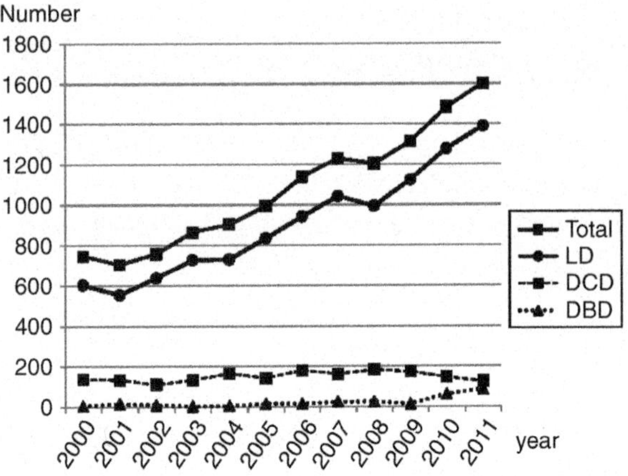

Fig. 14.1 Changes in the number of kidney transplantation in Japan (Data from The Japanese Society for Clinical Renal Transplantation [2])

Table 14.1 Maastricht criteria for DCD donors

Category	Status of the donor	Hospital department	Status of procurement
Category I	DOA	Accident or ER	Uncontrolled
Category II	Resuscitation without success	Accident or ER	Uncontrolled
Category III	Awaiting cardiac arrest (withdrawal of life-sustaining therapy)	ICU	Controlled
Category IV	Cardiac arrest while brain dead	ICU	Uncontrolled

In March 1995, Koostra et al. have introduced the classification of DCD donors into four categories (Table 14.1) [3]. Category III, in which donors were on awaiting cardiac arrest after withdrawal of life-sustaining therapy, is considered to be suitable for organ donation for transplantation because of a short period of warm ischemia. The condition of DCD donors in Japan is, however, different from those in other countries like the United States and Europe. The withdrawal of life-sustaining therapy (respirator) is rarely performed even though the donor is diagnosed to be a brain death except for an approval of donor families for the donation as DBD donors. Therefore, the DCD donors in Japan are difficult to be classified to any Maastricht categories. The condition of procurement is uncontrolled because of no withdrawal of respirator and long-lasting hypotension and oliguria (anuria) are frequently observed until cardiac arrest.

In Japan, early kidney transplantation from DCD donors was performed by regional sharing rules. Several transplantation centers in each region, in which the devoted transplant surgeons were working, conducted the registration of the recipients, procurement, organ sharing, and transplantation. Since Japan Organ Transplant Network (JOTNW) was established in 1995, the regulation of registration of the patients, procurement, organ sharing, and transplantation in all organs including the heart, lung, liver, pancreas, small intestine, and kidney have been conducted by JOTNW.

In this chapter, we describe the current status of kidney transplantation using DCD donors in Japan.

14.2 Donor Criteria

In reference to the data book edited by JOTNW in 2008, the number of DCDs from 1995 to 2006 was only 80 ± 13.1 (59–102) per year [4] (Fig. 14.2). Although mean age of DCD donors was 46.7 ± 16.8 years, ages of 292 donors were from 50 to 59 years and 187 donors were from 60 to 69 years. Thirty-nine donors showed the age of more than 70 years (Fig. 14.3). High age donor was, thus, common in Japan. Gender of DCD donors was 613 males (63.9 %) and 347 females (36.1 %). Furthermore, cerebrovascular disease (CVD) was the most frequent cause of death (56.3 %) in DCD donors in Japan (Fig. 14.4). The condition of the DCD donors in Japan is significantly poor as in comparison with other countries.

Exclusion criteria of the DCD donors for kidney transplantation were confirmed as shown in Table 14.2, which was determined by the Japan Society for Transplantation and JOTNW [5]. Once the donor candidate was considered to fulfill the indication for

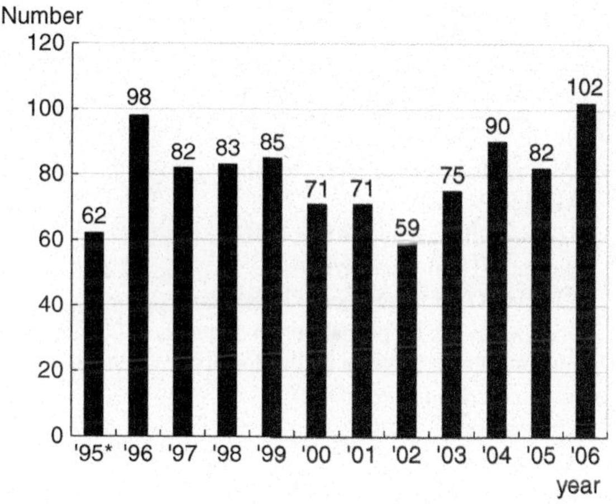

Fig. 14.2 Changes in the number of DCD donors in Japan (JOTNW, 1995–2006)

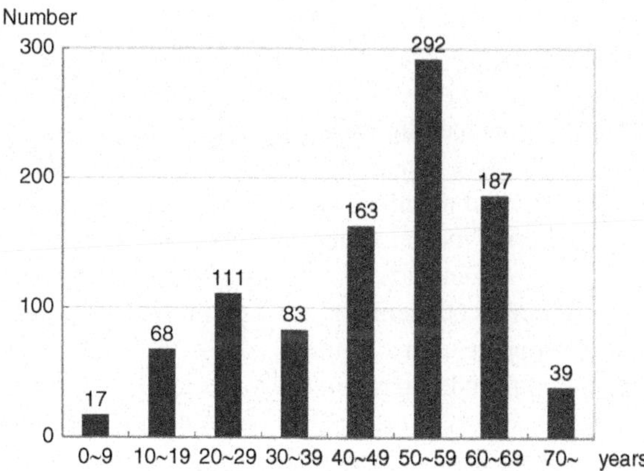

Fig. 14.3 Ages of DCD donors in Japan (JOTNW, 1995–2006)

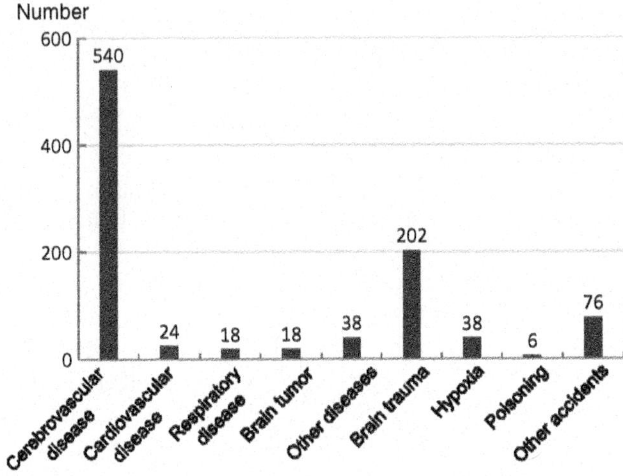

Fig. 14.4 Cause of death in DCD donors in Japan (JOTNW, 1995–2006)

Table 14.2 Exclusion criteria of the DCD donors for kidney transplantation (Japan Organ Transplant Network Website) [5]

Contraindications
Documented cases of sepsis or other systemic infectious diseases
AIDS (HIV positive)
Adult T-cell leukemia (ATL), HTLV-1 positive
Hepatitis (HBsAg positive)
CJD (vCJD) or its suspect of infection
Malignancy (as for primary brain tumors or solid tumors treated and diagnosed to be cured, judgment may be given by the doctors to see the patient)
Relative contraindications
Kidney disease
HCV positive
Age: >70 years old

DCD donors, donation was not necessarily achieved because of long-lasting hypotension and anuria until cardiac arrest. Since the clear criteria have not been determined concerning with age and duration of hypotension and anuria, final judgment of donation depends on each procurement team and transplantation team. In our institution, final judgment of capability of donation for kidney transplantation is done by considering the following donor factors: age (>70 years old), cause of death (CVD), episode of cardiac arrest (>30 min), use and amount of catecholamine, duration of hypotension (<60 mmHg), and anuria (>24 h). In addition to the donor factors, a power Doppler ultrasonography is useful for the examination of blood flow in the kidney graft and determination to progress to donation. In case of marginal donor candidate, that is considered to be borderline for donation, JOTNW consults to the medical consultant doctors in each organ transplantation followed by the final decision whether donation is possible or not, using medical consultant system.

Age is the most important risk factor of DCD donors for organ transplantation as well as DBD donors. The extended criteria donor (ECD) of kidney transplantation, which were defined by United Network for Organ Sharing (UNOS), includes (1) >60 years or (2) >50 years plus at least the two following factors: CVD as the cause of death, hypertension, and >1.5 mg/dl of serum creatinine [6]. As for the age of DCD donor, donor criteria in Japan recommend less than 70 years. According to the analysis of kidney transplantation from DCD donors [7], kidney graft survival was significantly lower in the donor of which age was over 40 years as compared to the donor with less than 40 years. Odds ratio of multivariate analysis is 1.67. However, no significant difference was observed between the donors with 40–59 years and those with ≥60 years. Since aging of the donor must provide the risks which influence on both short-term and long-term graft survival, age matching between donor and recipient should be recommended at the recipient selection for kidney transplantation.

Unlike in other countries, long-lasting hypotension and anuria before cardiac arrest in the agony are the major risk factors of DCD donors in Japan, because a withdrawal of life-sustaining therapy (respirator) is rarely performed even though the donor is diagnosed to be brain dead. Accurate evaluation of these risks is difficult and, therefore, the duration of hypotension and anuria is not included in the criteria (Table 14.2). In our experiences, in case of young donor without a use of catecholamine, the donor tolerates long-lasting hypotension and anuria up to 48 h or longer and might provide the viable kidneys for transplantation. However, high age donor with a use of a high amount of catecholamine tolerates shorter duration (within 24 h) (Kenmochi T, Asano T Unpublished data). We use power Doppler ultrasonography as the evaluation of the blood flow in the kidneys. If the blood flow is poorly detected or resistance of arterial flow (PI, RI) is extremely high, we usually give up the donation of the kidneys whether the duration of hypotension and anuria is long or short.

One of the recent major issues is concerning with the HCV-positive donors. HCV infection may occur by the transplantation of the kidney from the HCV-positive donors [8]. Therefore, a use of HCV-positive donors for kidney transplantation is still controversial. Previously or even currently in some institutions, the kidneys of HCV-positive donors were transplanted into the HCV-positive recipient as recommended in the international guideline [9]. However, superinfection may occur in the recipient when the genotype of HCV differs from that in the donor [10]. Currently, we recognize the HCV donor is indicated for kidney transplantation when the copies of HCV (RT-PCR) show low number, the genotype is the same as that in the recipient, and furthermore informed consent including the explanation of risks of development of HCV is obtained with a document.

14.3 Procurement and Preservation of the Kidneys from DCD Donors

The principles of kidney procurement from DCD donors have been considered to be a rapid cooling of the kidneys and rapid wash out of the blood from the kidneys. We consider that in situ cooling technique with a roller pump and surface cooling with

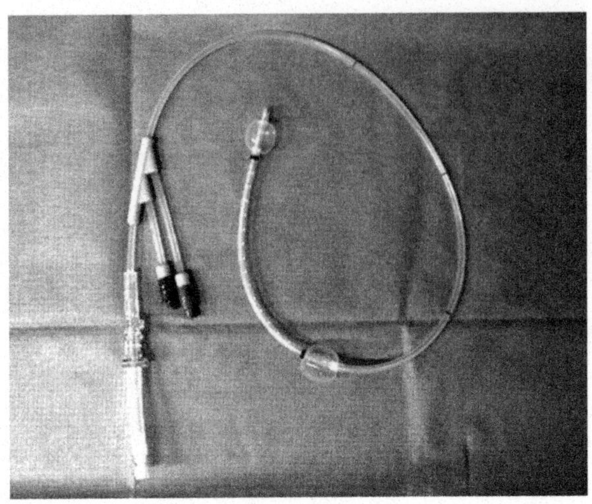

Fig. 14.5 A double-balloon silicon catheter with triple lumens (Dept. of Transplant Surgery, Fujita Health University Hospital)

crushed ice insertion into the abdomen before the procurement of kidneys are essential for the purpose of maintaining the viability of the kidney [11]. There are two techniques for the procurement of kidneys from DCD donors depending on the status of the donor. When the donor was clinically diagnosed to be brain dead, we perform a cannulation into an abdominal aorta with a double-balloon catheter via a femoral artery, cannulation into a vena cava with a catheter, and subsequent systemic heparinization in intensive care unit (ICU) before cardiac arrest, while, in case of no diagnosis of brain death, heparinization is done immediately after cardiac arrest and we have to move the donor immediately from the ICU to the operating room with a lasting of cardiac massage.

The double-balloon catheter, which was first introduced in 1975 [12], is inserted into an abdominal aorta via femoral artery at the bedside in ICU (Fig. 14.5). Also, a large (28 to 30 Fr) silicon tube was inserted into via femoral vein. From venous cannulation tube or central (or peripheral) venous line, 400 units/kg of heparin is injected for systemic heparinization at the time of cannulations. The injection of heparin is added every 6–8 h until cardiac arrest. As for the timing of cannulation, we perform both arterial and venous cannulations when the blood pressure of the donor continuously declined to less than 60 mmHg.

Historically in 1980s, we used Ringer's lactate as an initial machine wash out solution for the procurement of kidneys from DCD donors. Thereafter, we used originally modified Euro-Collins' solution, of which glucose was placed by D-mannitol. Belzer developed the University of Wisconsin solution for organ preservation in 1988 [13] and achieved prolonged preservation of the kidney [14]. Belzer demonstrated that the cell edema was prevented with a colloid pressure and maintained the viability of organs during cold storage (especially liver and pancreas), and, therefore, UW solution may be of use for initial wash out solution for in situ perfusion. Based on the excellent outcome of Belzer's paper, we investigated the efficacy of UW solution as an initial wash out solution for the procurement of kidneys and pancreas with 30 min warm ischemia using a large animal model (Beagle dos) [15]. Although UW solution was significantly effective for the procurement of the pancreas in comparison with Ringer's lactate and modified Collins' solution, no significant difference was obtained between UW solution and modified Collins' solution for the procurement of the kidneys. We have clinically introduced UW solution for perfusate of in situ machine wash out for the procurement of kidneys since October 1990 [16]. Although the edema of the small intestine and the pancreas was decreased, the outcome of kidney transplantation provided no advantage of UW solution as compared to modified Collins' solution. In addition, high cost was a major problem because 10 liters of solution were totally needed for in situ machine wash out. Therefore, we developed newly designed initial wash out solution, named CMH solution, for the procurement of liver and pancreas in addition to kidneys from DCD donors. In CMH solution, D-mannitol was added to keep crystalloid pressure and hydroxyethyl starch (HES) was added to keep colloid pressure. After the confirmation of the utility of this solution in a large animal model [17], we have introduced it to clinical application. Immediate graft function and duration of withdrawal from hemodialysis were significantly improved using CMH solution for the procurement of kidneys from DCD donors as compared to UW solution [16]. However, the production of CMH solution was unfortunately suspended and we currently use Euro-Collins' solution.

Also, other major teams of kidney transplantation using DCD donor have introduced in situ cooling technique [18–26]. The choice of the solution for in situ cooling as initial wash out is controversial. Euro-Collins' solution, HTK, and even Ringer's lactate are used in Japan based on the efficacy and economic reasons. Recently, extracorporeal membrane oxygenation (ECMO) was introduced for the normothermic perfusion technique in organ donation from the controlled donor [27] in place of hypothermic perfusion with a cold electrolyte preservation solution. This attempt is attractive and may become a breakthrough of organ procurement from DCD donors.

The technique of kidney procurement from DCD donors has previously reported and described in detail. The outline of our technique is described as follows. When the donor was not diagnosed to be brain dead, the cannulation into the abdominal aorta was firstly performed after laparotomy. Usually, we used from 24 to 28 Fr. silicon tube for cannulation. Immediately after the cannulation, the vena cava was cut in the thoracic cavity by the division of right diaphragm, and in situ machine wash out was started. Enough amount of crushed ice was inserted into the abdominal cavity. Infusion rate is initially 300–600 mL/min for 10 min and then reduced to 100 or 50 mL/min depending on the effective flush out of the blood and cooling. Since the double-balloon catheter was previously inserted in the donors with diagnosis of brain death, we confirm the condition of in situ cooling such as flushing of the blood and effective cooling of organs and insert enough amount of crushed ice. The infusion rate is regulated according to the condition of in situ wash out.

After the confirmation of effective flush out and cooling of small intestine and kidneys, the operation is started. Firstly, both kidneys were mobilized from retroperitoneal space and both ureters are dissected from the surrounding tissue.

The division (ligation and cut) of superior mesenteric artery and the division of mesocolon and mesenterium provide the good view for kidney procurement. Abdominal aorta is divided above both renal arteries and vena cava is also divided above both renal veins followed by en bloc excision of the both kidneys with ureters, aorta, and vena cava. The grafts are moved into the back table and the kidneys are divided into two grafts each. Usually, aorta is divided at the center of anterior and posterior wall and vena cava is preferable to be attached to the right kidney graft because the renal vein is shorter in the right graft than that in the left.

UW solution is a standard cold storage solution for simple cold storage of all organs from both DBD and DCD donors in Japan. Especially UW solution has an advantageous efficacy in cold storage of ischemically damaged kidneys [28]. After procurement, the kidney grafts are divided to each kidney and flushed out with UW solution at the back table and preserved in UW solution in a sterile plastic container or plastic bag on ice in the special cooler box which JOTNW designated.

Another option of preservation of the kidney is machine perfusion technique. Machine perfusion has the advantages including capability of recovery of microcirculation of the organs resulting in long-term preservation period and viability assay [29–36]. Matsuno et al. demonstrated that machine perfusion was utilized for preconditioning of the highly damaged kidney graft from poor condition DCD donors and for the viability assay indicating whether it was able to be transplanted or not [37–41]. Major disadvantage of machine perfusion is difficulty of transportation of the kidney grafts because of a big perfusion machine. Recently, Organ Recovery Systems™ developed a portable hypothermic perfusion machine "LifePort," which has a compact size and capability of battery operation for up to 24 h. This machine is easily transportable. Using this machine, early graft function was improved [42], thus resulting in the expansion of donor pool [43]. In our experimental and clinical studies, machine perfusion with KPS-1 solution was significantly useful for the preservation of ischemically damaged kidneys as compared to a cold storage with UW solution [44].

14.4 Viability Assay

Viability assay for the kidney graft which predicts the function after transplantation is essential for kidney transplantation from DCD donors. Viability assay for the kidney graft should be able to predict the development of primary nonfunction (PNF) after transplantation.

First consideration of viability assay is the evaluation of the donor conditions: age, cause of death, past history, episode of cardiac arrest, use and amount of catecholamine, and duration of hypotension (anuria). From these conditions, highly experienced transplant professionals (surgeons or coordinators) decide to advance to the procurement. In addition, the procurement technique of the kidneys influences the viability. High-leveled trained procurement team should perform cannulation correctly and start in situ cooling immediately after cardiac arrest to shorten the warm ischemic time (WIT). Final determination of the kidney procurement is usually performed by visual appearance of uniform perfusion of the graft after in situ perfusion. If the kidney graft was not uniformly perfused, we decide by microscopic findings at 0 h biopsy. In case of vessels' thrombosis dominant in the specimen, we have to give up the transplantation.

In contrast, a viability assay is possible when a machine perfusion technique is used for the preservation of the kidney grafts. Matsuno et al. demonstrated that perfusion flow rate can predict the function of the kidney after transplantation using a machine perfusion technique [38]. Also, Belzer et al. demonstrated that if the resistance to flow drops and flow rate increases in continuous perfusion, this indicates that there is no intravascular thrombosis such that the kidney would be suitable for transplantation [45]. Using continuous machine perfusion technique, we also achieved experimentally the viability assay of procured canine pancreas and liver [46, 47].

14.5 Outcome of Kidney Transplantation from DCD Donors in Japan

14.5.1 Current Status of Kidney Transplantation from DCD Donors in Japan

In Japan, 297,126 patients were undergoing hemodialysis at 2010 and only 12,388 patients (4.2 %) were registered to JOT and waiting for deceased donor kidney transplantation. Mean waiting time of the recipients who underwent deceased donor kidney transplantation in 2010 was 5,616 days (15.4 years), while the mean waiting time of the recipients whose ages were less than 16 years old was 525 days (1.4 years) due to the selection rule which had the priority of young aged (<16 years) recipients. Two thousand seven hundred and eighty-eight patients on waiting list died before transplantation from 1995 to 2010 and a shortage of deceased donors was ultimately severe issue in organ transplantation in Japan. Patient survival of the recipients who underwent deceased donor kidney transplantation was shown in Fig. 14.6. Patient survival was highly maintained for 10 years after transplantation in spite of long waiting period of the recipients. Graft survival as shown in Fig. 14.7 showed its improvement year by year. Three-year graft survival was improved to 86.6 % in 2005–2009. However, three-year graft survival was 95.2 % in living donor kidney transplantation in 2005–2009, which was significantly higher than that in deceased donor kidney transplantation. The lower graft survival of deceased donor kidney transplantation as compared to living donor kidney transplantation includes several reasons. First reason is that more than 95 % of all deceased donors were DCD donors with poor conditions such as old age, episode of cardiac arrest, and CVD as a cause of death. Secondly, the recipients tended to be old age and had several complications such as arteriosclerosis and cardiovascular diseases due to a long-term history of hemodialysis.

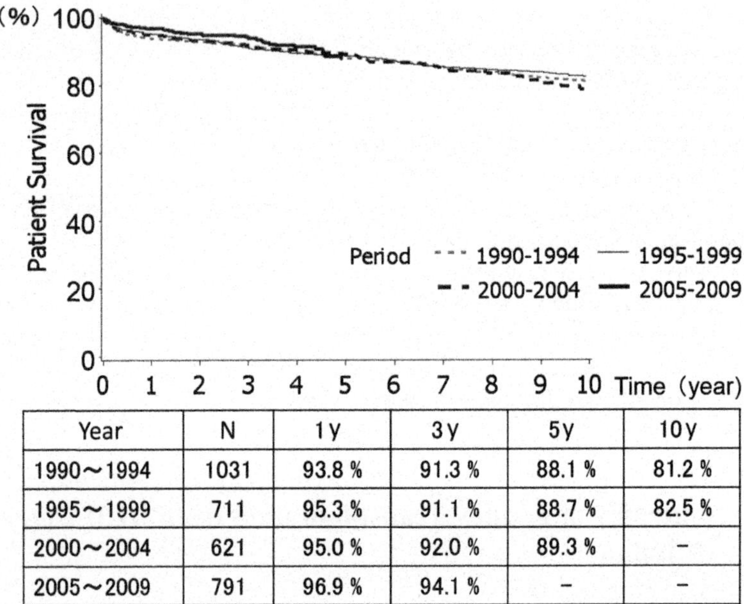

Year	N	1y	3y	5y	10y
1990～1994	1031	93.8 %	91.3 %	88.1 %	81.2 %
1995～1999	711	95.3 %	91.1 %	88.7 %	82.5 %
2000～2004	621	95.0 %	92.0 %	89.3 %	–
2005～2009	791	96.9 %	94.1 %	–	–

Fig. 14.6 Patient survival after kidney transplantation from deceased donors in Japan (JOTNW, 1995–2010)

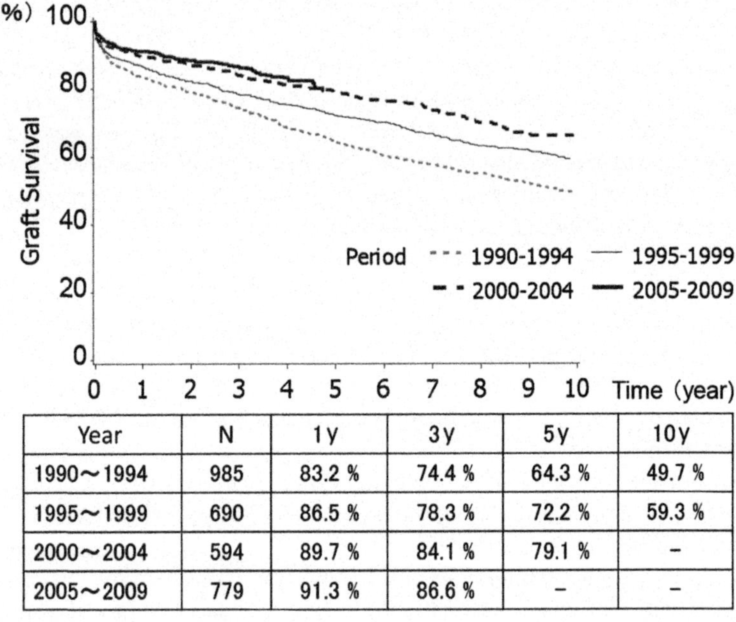

Year	N	1y	3y	5y	10y
1990～1994	985	83.2 %	74.4 %	64.3 %	49.7 %
1995～1999	690	86.5 %	78.3 %	72.2 %	59.3 %
2000～2004	594	89.7 %	84.1 %	79.1 %	–
2005～2009	779	91.3 %	86.6 %	–	–

Fig. 14.7 Graft survival after kidney transplantation from deceased donors in Japan (JOTNW, 1995–2010)

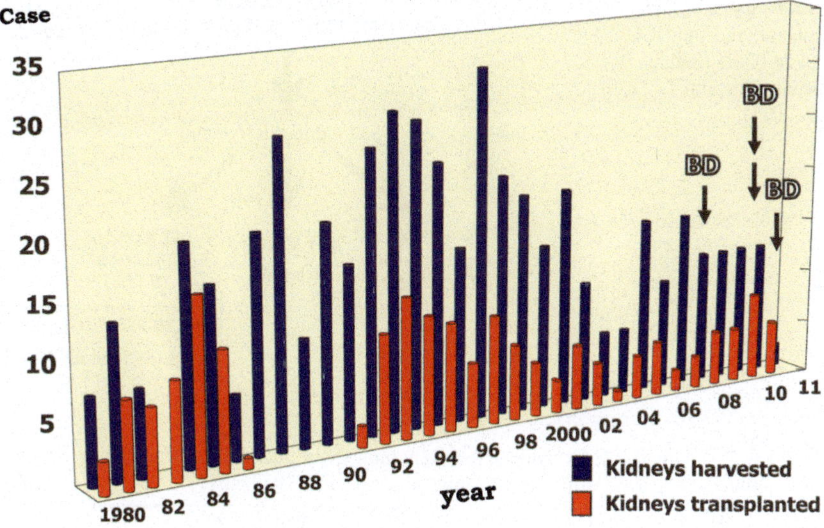

Fig. 14.8 Number of the DCD donors in Fujita Health University Hospital (1979–2011)

14.5.2 Outcome of the Kidney Transplantation from DCD Donors in a Single Institution

Fujita Health University Hospital is a representative institution of organ donation and kidney transplantation from DCD donors in Japan. Professor Hoshinaga has started and conducted the project of organ donation and kidney transplantation from DCD donors in this institution. The present author of this chapter is currently a member of transplant team in this institution. We introduce, herein, the outcome of organ donation and transplantation in our institution. The outcome of kidney transplantation using DCD donors was investigated and the risk factors affecting the prognosis of the kidney were analyzed. Since April 1979, 527 kidneys were procured from 266 DCD donors in our institution, using in situ regional cooling technique (Fig. 14.8). An excellent graft survival was noted in our series and only 47 (8.9 %) grafts had been discarded (Fig. 14.9). Four hundred and forty-three grafts transplanted since 1983 through 2011 were enrolled in this study. The age of the donors and recipients ranged from 0.7 to 75 (mean 47.6) and from 7 to 72 (mean 41.7). The WIT ranged from 1 to 71 min (mean 11.7). The serum creatinine level before cardiac arrest ranged from 0.4 to 5.4 mg/dL (mean 1.49). All the patients were treated with immunotherapy consisting of calcineurin inhibitors, steroid, and other immunosuppressants. Following kidney transplantations, PNF was noted in 27 patients (6.5 %), immediate function (IF) was 58 (13.1 %), and DGF was 358 (80.9 %). Factors which influenced the development of PNF were compared between IF and DGF group and PNF group and WIT showed the significant

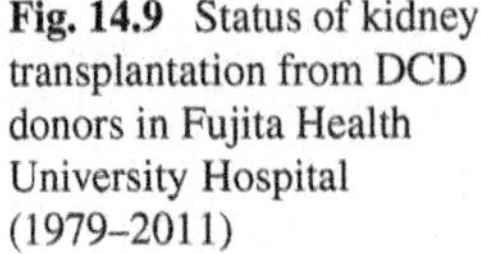

Fig. 14.9 Status of kidney transplantation from DCD donors in Fujita Health University Hospital (1979–2011)

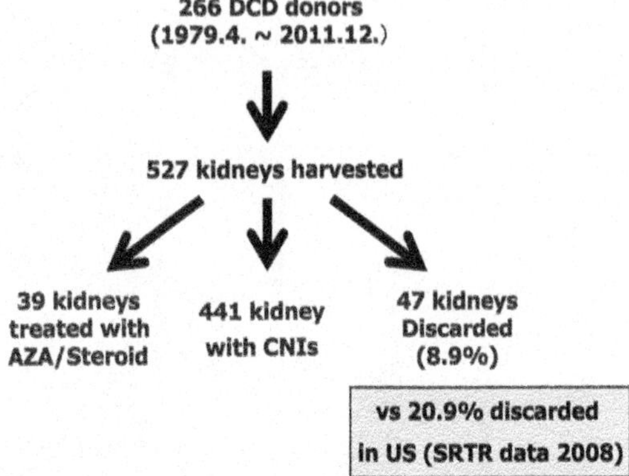

Table 14.3 Comparison of the factors between immediate and delayed function group and primary nonfunction group (Fujita Health University Hospital (1979–2011)

	IF and DGF (n=386)	PNF (n=27)	p-value
Donor age (y/o)	46.2 (0.8–75)	47.4 (6–73)	NS
Recipient age (y/o)	41.2 (7–65)	42.0 (8–65)	NS
WIT (min)	12.0 (1–71)	22.1 (1–71)	p=0.01
TIT (min)	804 (244–2,603)	834 (252–1,875)	NS

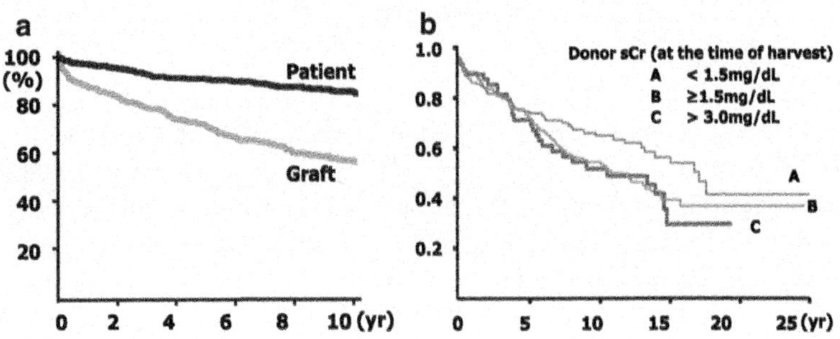

Fig. 14.10 Overall patients and graft survival after kidney transplantation from DCD donors (a) and the graft survival depending on the serum creatinine levels (b) at harvesting in Fujita Health University Hospital (1979–2011)

difference (Table 14.3). The 1-, 3-, 5-, 10-, and 15-year patient survival rates were 97.0 %, 92.1 %, 90.0 %, 82.9 %, and 78.4 %, respectively. The 1-, 3-, 5-, 10-, and 15-year graft survival rates were 86.1 %, 75.6 %, 68.5 %, 52.8 %, and 40.8 %, respectively (Fig. 14.10a). The significant risk factors for graft failure were donor age, cause of death (CVA), donor hypertension, and WIT, while serum creatinine levels at harvest did not significantly influence to the graft survivals (Fig. 14.10b). From these outcomes, kidney grafts recovered from DCD donors had a good renal function as well as an excellent long-term graft survival, when in situ regional cooling technique was applied. DCD donors should be the excellent resources of deceased donor kidneys and they can increase the donor pool for kidney transplantation, especially in our country.

References

1. Beecher H. A definition of irreversible coma. Report of the Ad Hoc Committee of the Harvard Medical School to examine the definition of brain death. JAMA. 1968;205:337–40.
2. The Japanese Society for Clinical Renal Transplantation. Annual progress report from the Japanese renal transplant registry: number of renal transplantation in 2011. Jpn J Transplant. 2012;47(6):400–15. Japanese.
3. Kootstra G, Daemen JH, Oomen AP. Categories of non-heart-beating donors. Transplant Proc. 1995;27(5):2893–4.
4. JOTNW Data Book 2007. Japan Organ Transplant Network Ed. Tokyo, 2008.
5. Japan Organ Transplant Network Website (in Japanese). http://www.jotnw.or.jp/studying/15_2.html.
6. Metzger RA, Delmonico FL, Feng S, Port FK, Wynn JJ, Merion RM. Expanded criteria donors for kidney transplantation. Am J Transplant. 2003;3 Suppl 4:114–25.
7. The Japanese Society for Clinical Renal Transplantation. Annual progress report from the Japanese renal transplant registry: number of renal transplantation in 2009, part 2. Jpn J Transplant (in Japanese). 2010;45(6):595–620.
8. Pereira BJ, Milford EL, Kirkman RL, Levey AS. Transmission of hepatitis C virus by organ transplantation. N Engl J Med. 1991;325(7):454–60.
9. Natov SN, Pereira BJ. Management of hepatitis C infection in renal transplant recipients. Am J Transplant. 2002;2(6):483–90.
10. Widell A, Månsson S, Persson NH, Thysell H, Hermodsson S, Blohme I. Hepatitis C superinfection in hepatitis C virus (HCV)-infected patients transplanted with an HCV-infected kidney. Transplantation. 1995;60(7):642–7.
11. Asano T, Kenmochi T, Isono K. Organ preservation. Nihon Geka Gakkai Zasshi (Japanese). 1996;97(11):958–63.
12. Garcia-Rinaldi R, Lefrak EA, Defore WW, Feldman L, Noon GP, Jachimczyk JA, DeBakey ME. In situ preservation of cadaver kidneys for transplantation: laboratory observations and clinical application. Ann Surg. 1975;182(5):576–84.
13. Belzer FO, Southard JH. Principles of solid-organ preservation by cold storage. Transplantation. 1988;45(4):673–6.
14. Ploeg RJ, Goossens D, Vreugdenhil P, McAnulty JF, Southard JH, Belzer FO. Successful 72-hour cold storage kidney preservation with UW solution. Transplant Proc. 1988;20(1 Suppl 1):935–8.
15. Kenmochi T, Fukuoka T, Hayashi R, Suzuki S, Amemiya H, Asano T. Experimental study on the effect of UW solution as the in situ machine wash out solution. Jpn J Transplant (Japanese). 1991;26(2):127–32.
16. Kenmochi T, Asano T, Isono K. Current status in the preservation of the kidneys. Law Temp Med. 1997;23(4):242–7.
17. Arita S, Asano T, Kenmochi T, Enomoto K, Isono K. An initial wash-out solution for "in situ machine wash-out". Transplant Proc. 1991;23(5):2589–91.
18. Shiroki R, Hoshinaga K, Horiba M, Izumitani M, Tsukiashi Y, Yanaoka M, Naide Y, Kanno T. Favorable prognosis of kidney allografts from unconditioned cadaveric donors whose procurement was initiated after cardiac arrest. Transplant Proc. 1997;29(1–2):1388–9.
19. Hoshinaga K, Shiroki R, Fujita T, Kanno T, Naide Y. The fate of 359 renal allografts harvested from non-heart beating cadaver donors at a single center. Clin Transpl. 1998;12:213–20.

20. Kato M, Mizutani K, Hattori R, Kinukawa T, Uchida K, Hoshinaga K, Ono Y, Ohshima S. In situ renal cooling for kidney transplantation from non-heart-beating donors. Transplant Proc. 2000;32(7):1608–10.
21. Kusaka M, Kubota Y, Sasaki H, Maruyama T, Hayakawa K, Shiroki R, Hoshinaga K. Is pulsatile perfusion necessary for renal transplantation engrafting kidneys from cardiac death donors? Transplant Proc. 2006;38(10):3388–9.
22. Hoshinaga K, Fujita T, Naide Y, Akutsu H, Sasaki H, Tsukiashi Y, Nishiyama N, Yanaoka M, Shinoda M, Kanno T. Early prognosis of 263 ren al allografts harvested from non-heart-beating cadavers using an in situ cooling technique. Transplant Proc. 1995;27(1):703–6.
23. Matsuno N, Sakurai E, Uchiyama M, Kozaki K, Tamaki I, Kozaki M. Use of in situ cooling and machine perfusion preservation for non-heart-beating donors. Transplant Proc. 1993; 25(6):3095–6.
24. Kinukawa T, Ohshima S, Fujita T, Ono Y. Exploration of the system for cadaver kidney transplantation with the non-heart-beating donor: efficacy of in situ cooling and low-dose cyclosporine. Transplant Proc. 1993;25(1 Pt 2):1524–6.
25. Matsuno N, Kozaki M, Sakurai E, Uchiyama M, Iwahori T, Kozaki K, Kono K, Tanaka M, Tamaki T, Tamaki I. Effect of combination in situ cooling and machine perfusion preservation on non-heart-beating donor kidney procurement. Transplant Proc. 1993;25(1 Pt 2):1516–7.
26. Fujita T, Matsui M, Yanaoka M, Shinoda M, Naide Y. Clinical application of in situ renal cooling: experience with 61 cardiac-arrest donors. Transplant Proc. 1989;21(1 Pt 2):1215–7.
27. Magliocca JF, Magee JC, Rowe SA, Gravel MT, Chenault 2nd RH, Merion RM, Punch JD, Bartlett RH, Hemmila MR. Extracorporeal support for organ donation after cardiac death effectively expands the donor pool. J Trauma. 2005;58(6):1095–101. discussion 1101–2.
28. Booster MH, van der Vusse GJ, Wijnen RM, Yin M, Stubenitsky BM, Kootstra G. University of Wisconsin solution is superior to histidine tryptophan ketoglutarate for preservation of ischemically damaged kidneys. Transplantation. 1994;58(9):979–84.
29. Belzer FO, Ashby BS, Dunphy JE. 24-hour and 72-hour preservation of canine kidneys. Lancet. 1967;2(7515):536–8.
30. Belzer FO, Ashby BS, Huang JS, Dunphy JE. Etiology of rising perfusion pressure in isolated organ perfusion. Ann Surg. 1968;168(3):382–91.
31. Toledo-Pereyra LH, Condie RM, Malmberg R, Simmons RL, Najarian JS. A fibrinogen-free plasma perfusate for preservation of kidneys for one hundred and twenty hours. Surg Gynecol Obstet. 1974;138(6):901–5.
32. Johnson RW, Anderson M, Flear CT, Murray SG, Taylor RM, Swinney J. Evaluation of new perfusion solution for kidney preservation. Transplantation. 1972;13(3):270–5.
33. Garvin PJ, Codd JE, Newton WT, Willman VL. Perfusate composition in renal preservation. Arch Surg. 1977;112(1):67–8.
34. McAnulty JF, Ploeg RJ, Southard JH, Belzer FO. Successful five-day perfusion preservation of the canine kidney. Transplantation. 1989;47(1):37–41.
35. Hoffmann RM, Stratta RJ, D'Alessandro AM, Sollinger HW, Kalayoglu M, Pirsch JD, Southard JH, Belzer FO. Combined cold storage-perfusion preservation with a new synthetic perfusate. Transplantation. 1989;47(1):32–7.
36. Ozaki A, Asano T, Amemiya H, Ochiai T, Sato H. Kidney transplantation. Successful 96-hour preservation of canine kidneys using a new machine. Transplant Proc. 1977;9(1):247–9.
37. Matsuno N, Sakurai E, Tamaki I, Uchiyama M, Kozaki K, Kozaki M. The effect of machine perfusion preservation versus cold storage on the function of kidneys from non-heart-beating donors. Transplantation. 1994;57(2):293–4.
38. Matsuno N, Sakurai E, Tamaki I, Furuhashi K, Saito A, Zhang S, Kozaki K, Shimada A, Miyamoto K, Kozaki M. Effectiveness of machine perfusion preservation as a viability determination method for kidneys procured from non-heart-beating donors. Transplant Proc. 1994;26(4):2421–2.
39. Kozaki K, Sakurai E, Tamaki I, Matsuno N, Saito A, Furuhashi K, Uchiyama M, Zhang S, Kozaki M. Usefulness of continuous hypothermic perfusion preservation for cadaveric renal grafts in poor condition. Transplant Proc. 1995;27(1):757–8.

40. Matsuno N, Sakurai E, Uchiyama M, Kozaki K, Miyamoto K, Kozaki M. Usefulness of machine perfusion preservation for non-heart-beating donors in kidney transplantation. Transplant Proc. 1996;28(3):1551–2.
41. Matsuno N, Sakurai E, Uchiyama M, Kozaki K, Miyamoto K, Kozaki M, Nagao T. Role of machine perfusion preservation in kidney transplantation from non-heartbeating donors. Clin Transplant. 1998;12(1):1–4.
42. Guarrera JV, Polyak M, O'Mar Arrington B, Kapur S, Stubenbord WT, Kinkhabwala M. Pulsatile machine perfusion with Vasosol solution improves early graft function after cadaveric renal transplantation. Transplantation. 2004;77(8):1264–8.
43. Reznik ON, Bagnenko SF, Loginov IV, Moisiuk YG. Increasing kidneys donor's pool by machine perfusion with the LifePort–pilot Russian study. Ann Transplant. 2006;11(3):46–8.
44. Akutsu N, Kenmochi T, Saito T, Saigo K, Maruyama M, Iwashita C, Otsuki K, Ito T, Asano T. Efficacy of hypothermic machine perfusion for preservation of canine kidney and pancreas with warm ischemia. Organ Biol (Japanese). 2011;18(1):81–6.
45. Belzer FO, Ashby BS, Gulyassy PF, Powell M. Successful seventeen-hour preservation and transplantation of human-cadaver kidney. N Engl J Med. 1968;278(11):608–10.
46. Kenmochi T, Asano T, Nakagouri T, Enomoto K, Isono K, Horie H. Prediction of viability of ischemically damaged canine pancreatic grafts by tissue flow rate with machine perfusion. Transplantation. 1992;53(4):745–50.
47. Uematsu T, Asano T, Enomoto K, Goto T, Suzuki T, Nakajima K, Ochiai T, Isono K. Predictable viability assay of isolated canine liver using hypothermic continuous machine perfusion. Transplant Proc. 1987;19(1 Pt 2):1321–3.

Chapter 15
Machine Perfusion Preservation for Kidney Transplantation

Naoto Matsuno

15.1 Introduction

The large gap between organ supply and demand emphasizes the importance of using all available donor sources. The shortage of donors for kidney transplantation is a universal problem. The waiting list has continued to grow, and the discrepancy between demand and supply is still increasing. The use of marginal donors is a promising way to increase the supply. In particular, the use of organs from non-heart-beating donors (NHBD) or donation after cardiac death (DCD) is acquiring increasing importance as a potential source of vital organs for clinical transplantation. However, with these expanded donor criteria (ECD), difficulties have been experienced because of preexisting organ damage from hypotension, which is associated with poor perfusion of kidney grafts. Unlike the recipients with heart beating donor kidneys, recipients of NHBD organs experience a higher incidence of primary nonfunction (PNF) and delayed graft function requiring postoperative hemodialysis (HD), prolonged hospitalization, and difficulties in the diagnosis of acute rejection. Long-term graft function and survival might be adversely affected by a delayed function of the kidneys after transplantation [1, 2]. The two approaches to preservation prior to transplantation are simple cold storage (SCS) and machine perfusion (MP). The simplicity, lower cost, and need for transport make cold storage the method of choice for the majority of renal transplant centers. However, continuous machine perfusion supplies or helps regenerate metabolic substances lost during warm ischemia and maintain near physiological conditions. It also maintains the intracellular pH and discharges waste, dilutes or neutralizes catabolic substances, and reduces sodium-dependent tissue edema (Fig. 15.1) [3, 4]. The histological integrity may be related to improved perfusion of the renal cortex microcirculation

N. Matsuno (✉)
Division for Innovative Surgery and Transplantation, National Center for Child Health and Development, 2-10-1 Okura, Setagayaku, Tokyo 157-8535, Japan
e-mail: mtnnot@yahoo.co.jp

T. Asano et al. (eds.), *Marginal Donors: Current and Future Status*,
DOI 10.1007/978-4-431-54484-5_15, © Springer Japan 2014

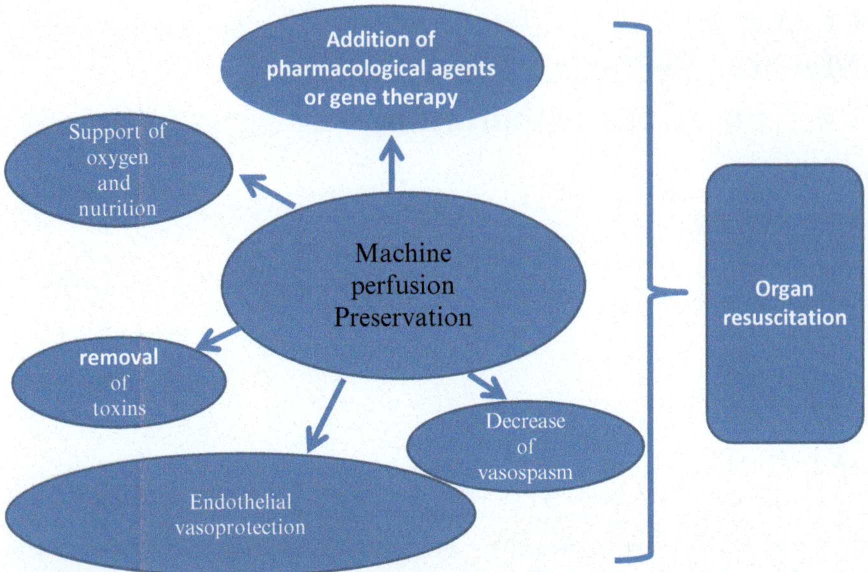

Fig. 15.1 The multiple role of machine perfusion preservation

Table 15.1 The advantages and disadvantages of machine perfusion compared to cold storage

Advantages	Disadvantages
Lower incidence of DGF	Higher cost in the short term
Continuous monitoring of parameters during perfusion	Endothelial injury is possible
Decreased vasospasm	Logistically more complex
Ability to provide metabolic support	Possible equipment failure
Potential for pharmacological manipulation	

with the removal of red cells. These metabolic and physiological benefits lead to a reduction in the need for post-transplant dialysis by lowering the incidence of post-transplant acute tubular necrosis, resulting in a shorter hospital stay and better long-term survival. Another advantage of MP is the ability to perform viability testing. The perfusate chemistry, changes in the flow, and resistance during machine perfusion can be synchronously measured as a pretransplant viability test (Table 15.1). Within the marginal kidney donor pools, hypothermic machine perfusion (HMP) may be of major importance, because it can expand the utilization of ECD and DCD kidneys.

15.2 Preservation Using Machine Perfusion: A Brief History

The introduction of kidney perfusion in clinical practice started in the late 1960s by Belzer. Belzer had already been working on the continuous hypothermic isolated perfusion and auto-kidney transplantation with blood [5, 6] and cryoprecipitated plasma. Dextrose insulin, hydrocortisone, penicillin, magnesium sulfate, and phenolsulfonthalein were added to the plasma. One of the most noteworthy achievements followed in 1967. Canine kidneys were transplanted successfully following 72 h of pulsatile hypothermic machine perfusion preservation [7]. The HMP of the first human kidney became a clinical reality soon thereafter: a patient received a kidney preserved for 17 h using this preservation circuit and had acceptable function post-transplant [8]. In the 1970s, HMP was used by transplant centers mainly in the United States and Europe to preserve and transport kidneys. Concerning the machine perfusion solutions, several groups improved the existing perfusion solution by adding or omitting various components [9]. Silica gel-filtered plasma was developed at the University of Minnesota. An advantage of this solution over the cryoprecipitated plasma was the achievements of better stability [10]. Consequently, different perfusion machines were developed and used clinically for kidney preservation. In 1980, however, the development of the UW solution produced by the same UW group allowed surgeons to preserve kidneys for much longer, up to 72 h, by SCS [11]. The development of the UW solution provided an alternative to machine preservation, and as such, most centers abandoned the clinical use of MP.

Over the last few decades, the success of kidney transplantation as the treatment of choice for end-stage renal failure has led to an increasing shortage of suitable organs. This shortage has forced the transplantation community to (re-) consider the transplantation of organs from marginal donors, such as older donors, hemodynamically unstable donors, as well as non-heart-beating donation. Thereafter, the machine perfusion of kidneys from these marginal donors regained worldwide interest. Thus, static cold preservation using the UW solution has reached the end of its development, and machine perfusion preservation methods which provide an optimized physiological environment to evaluate organ viability, resuscitation, and modulation before transplantation are now the focus of research and clinical use.

As for the machines used for perfusion, the Koostra group's machine was used in the early days, then a modified Gambro machine [12]. The solution used was their modified University of Wisconsin solution, which omitted starch. The Newcastle DCD kidney team also used a locally manufactured UW solution without starch [13]. Currently, there are two commercially available renal perfusion devices: the LifePort, from Organ Recovery Systems, and the RM3, from Waters Medical Systems (Figs. 15.2 and 15.3). The technology and utilization have increased exponentially with time, with approximately 25 % to 35 % of all transplanted kidneys in the United States now being preserved before transportation via hypothermic machine perfusion [14].

15.3 Outcomes: Clinical Use of SCS Versus MP

Both in animal experiments and in historical controlled retrospective clinical studies, HMP has been demonstrated to provide better outcomes with regard to early graft function. The effects of preservation methods and cold storage solutions

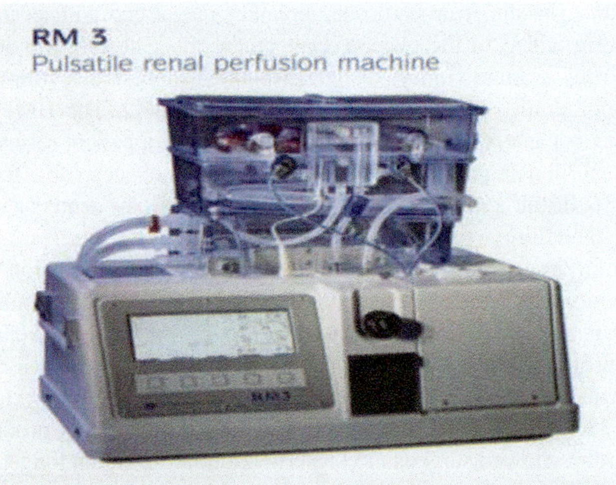

Fig. 15.2 RM 3 renal preservation system, pulsatile preservation technology built by Waters Medical Systems

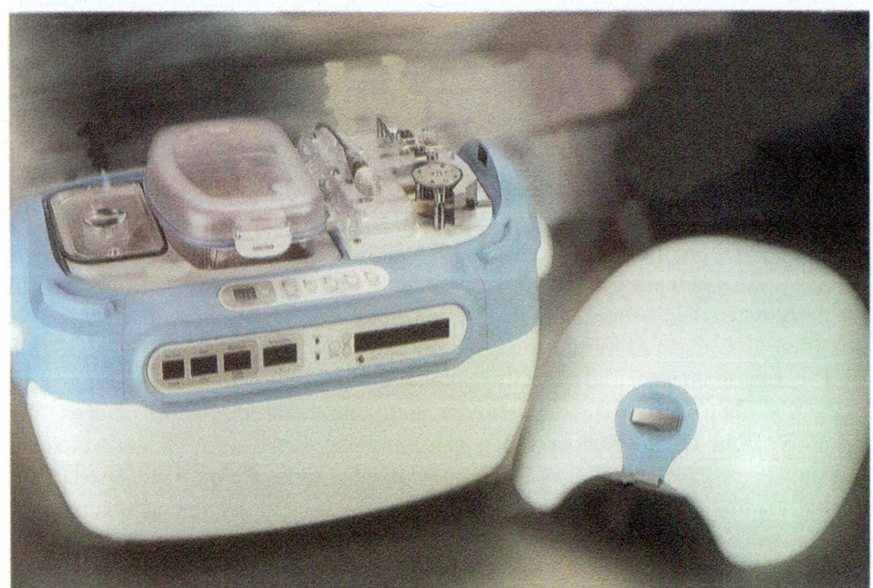

Fig. 15.3 The LifePort kidney transporter (organ recovery system), pulsatile perfusion of a single kidney

on the outcome of more than 17,000 first cadaver kidney transplants were studied from data reported to the UNOS Scientific Renal Transplant Registry and to the UCLA Transplant Registry between 1987 and 1991. The early graft function was better in pump-preserved than cold-stored kidneys (84 % vs. 73 % at 1 week, and

87 % vs. 80 % at discharge) [15]. Medez et al. [16] showed that 65 % of HMP kidneys had immediate function (IF) compared to 34 % of those treated with SCS. In addition, there was a significant increase in the rate of acute tubular necrosis (ATN) if SCS exceeded 24 to 30 h, an effect not seen in HMP organs. Belzer et al. [17] reported only 18 % ATN for HMP in DCD kidneys compared to reported rates 70 % for SCS in DCD kidneys. Ajitani et al. [18] found that dialysis was required post-transplantation in 63 % of patients after SC and 17 % after HMP. Despite the promising evidence, a number of prospective and retrospective studies comparing machine perfusion preservation with cold storage for DCD kidneys have not shown a benefit. Daemen et al. [19] found that the delayed graft function (DGF) and PNF rates for machine-perfused DCD kidneys were higher than those of cold-stored DCD kidneys. However, there was a lower rate of DGF in perfused DCD kidneys. Matsuno et al. [20] used paired kidneys from 13 controlled DCD and randomly allocated them to cold storage or mechanical perfusion. The immediate function was 35 % in the mechanical perfusion group compared to 8 % in the cold storage group, with 1-month graft survival of 100 % for mechanical perfusion and 77 % for cold storage. Sellers et al. [21] studied HMP ($n=568$) and SCS ($n=268$) and found that the HMP group, although having worse donor and recipient characteristics, had a statistically lower incidence DGF compared to the SCS group. Another study compared the use of HMP and SCS before transplantation and showed that, despite a longer cold ischemia time and worse donor hemodynamics in the HMP group, the 5-year graft survival was better in the HMP than in SCS-stored kidneys (68.2 % vs. 54.2 %) [22]. Shah et al. showed a better survival for pulsatile perfusion over SCS, with rates of 95 % and 88 % (graft) and 98 % and 90 % (patient), respectively. The incidence of DGF was 5 % and 35 %, whereas post-transplant dialysis was required in 5 % and 30 % of the pulsatile perfusion and cold storage cases, respectively [23]. However, in most studies, no prospective randomization was performed, and the patient numbers were not large enough. The effectiveness and advantage of the use for ECD and DCD kidneys has been mixed and center-dependent. Recently, Wight et al. reported an excellent meta-analysis based on the results of the current literature concerning HMP versus SCS, clearly demonstrating a 20 % reduction in DGF with HMP [24]. Matsuoka et al. reported that the three-year graft survival of ECD kidneys preserved with MP or SCS with pulsatile perfusion was similar to cold storage kidneys. The incidence of DGF in HMP was significantly lower than that of SCS (26 % vs. 36 %). Despite having a greater number of risk factors for reduced graft viability, the ECD-HMP kidneys had similar graft survival to the ECD-SCS kidneys [25]. The international multicenter trial for HMP in kidney transplantation is a well-designed prospective randomized trial of paired kidneys: one preserved with HMP and the contralateral one preserved with SCS. The study examined 672 renal transplants performed in Europe. Machine preservation significantly reduced the risk of DGF function, as well as significantly improving the rate of the decrease in the serum creatinine level, and reduced the duration of DGF. The risk of DGF was significantly reduced by HMP compared to cold storage (26.5 % vs. 20.8 %; $p=0.05$). Moreover, in recipients who developed delayed graft function, the six-month graft survival was better when kidneys were machine perfused (87 % vs.

76 %, $p=0.05$). The one-year graft survival was improved with the use of HMP from 90 % in the SCS group to 94 % [26]. As part of this study, Treckmann analyzed the possible effects of machine perfusion versus cold storage on DGF and early graft survival in expanded criteria donors [27]. However, Charautrer et al. pointed out that the preservation solutions used were different in the two arms of the studies. The UW or HTK solution was used for SCS, whereas the kidney preservation solution-1 (KPS-1) was used for machine perfusion [28]. Moers et al. extended the follow-up period to evaluate the three-year graft survival. Three years after transplantation, the survival of kidneys donated after brain death remained significantly better after machine perfusion than after SCS, especially in the case of kidneys recovered from patients meeting the expanded criteria donor [29]. On the other hand, Watson et al. reported the results of a multicenter trial of HMP versus SCS. Although their design was similar to that of Moers et al., their findings did not support the conclusions of that study in a specific group of high-risk donors (DCD). No advantage of either of the two preservation methods was observed. This different conclusion may be due to differences in both the donor warm ischemic time (DWIT) and total cold ischemic time (TCIT) between the two studies and in the different immunosuppression strategies used. One additional difficulty in assessing these two preservation methods is the lack of a standardized definition for DGF. DGF is based on the postoperative use of dialysis, which is subjective [30]. Little is known about the cost-effectiveness of various organ preservation methods.

Buchanan et al. analyzed United States Renal Data System (USRDS) data and examined total Medicare payments for transplant hospitalization. HMP utilization was associated with a $2,130 reduction in hospitalization costs. HMP utilization was also associated with lower DGF. Thus, HMP utilization is correlated with lower costs for the associated induction in DGF [31]. Garefield et al. reported machine perfusion is a more cost-effective option than cold storage involving either standard criteria donor (SCD) ($92,561 vs. $104,118) or ECD ($106,012 vs. $114,530) kidneys at 1-year post-transplant [32]. Groen et al. performed an economic evaluation of HMP versus SCS in a multicenter randomized clinical trial (RCT).The short-term evaluation showed that HMP reduced the risk of delayed graft function and graft failure at lower cost than SCS. They use Markov model and revealed cost savings of $86,750 per life-year gained in favor of HMP [33]. In summary, the preservation method or solution can affect the injury and results for the grafts. Any improvement in the preservation of grafts represents a valuable advance toward enlarging the total number of viable donor organs available for transplantation. A more widely accepted method to maintain donor organ viability during the preservation should be developed using continuous machine perfusion.

15.4 Viability Test

An advantage of using machine perfusion is that it enables the performance of viability tests on the kidneys while they are stored. Preservation by machine enables surgeons to judge the acceptability of the graft by registering the flow and pressure characteristics and to analyze the enzymes in the perfusate.

Table 15.2 Early graft function and perfusion states

	n	ATN (days)	IF (%)	PNF (%)	Best Cr (mg/dL)	Flow	Resistance
Group 1	35	12.0±9.7	3 (8.6)	9 (25.7)	1.9±1.2	0.50±0.11	89.80±43.40
Group 2	30	8.6±9/0	5 (16.7)	2 (6.7)	1.5±0.7	0.77±0.08	50.01±18.65
Group 3	23	8.7±12.6	7 (30.4)	0	1.3±1.7	1.12±0.14	37.20±10.94

Group 1, 0.40–0.65 (mL/min/g); group 2, 0.65–0.90 (mL/min/g); group 3, more than 0.90 (mL/min/g)
ATN acute tubular necrosis, *IF* immediate function, *PNF* primary nonfunction, *Cr* creatinine, Flow: perfusion
Flow (mL/min/g), resistance: renal resistance (mmHg/min/g)

15.4.1 α-Glutathione S-Transferase

Koostra's group reported that the level of α-glutathione S-transferase in the perfusate was found to strongly correlate with the warm ischemic time and used it to distinguish nonfunctioning from functioning grafts [34]. However, such biomarkers should be measured rapidly at the bedside for clinical use.

15.4.2 Perfusate Lactate Dehydrogenase

The perfusate lactate dehydrogenase (LDH) [35] levels have been shown to be directly related to the degree of ischemia [36] and are an indicator of preservation damage [37]. The levels are easily assayed, but LDH is relatively nonspecific.

15.4.3 Pressure, Flow, and Resistance During Machine Preservation

Measurement of the pressure, flow, and resistance parameters during machine preservation is a promising method for assessing viability, because ischemic injury causes disturbances in the microcirculation, which leads to high intrarenal resistance and low flow during machine perfusion. Matsuno et al. [38, 39] found that the perfusate flow was a reliable indicator of viability based on the early functional recovery of the kidney (Table 15.2). They discarded all grafts if the flow was less than 0.4 mL/min/g with a concurrent rising perfusion pressure pattern (Figs. 15.4 and 15.5). Using these criteria, grafts with a warm ischemic time of 140 min and terminal certainties of 4.6 and 5.6 mg/dL were successfully transplanted. They reported that kidneys with a machine perfusion flow of 0.40–0.65 mL/min/g machine perfusion flow were considered to be acceptable; however, a high rate of PNF and severe DGF occurred postoperatively when such grafts were used. A preservation time of more than 16 h significantly correlated with a high rate of PNF.

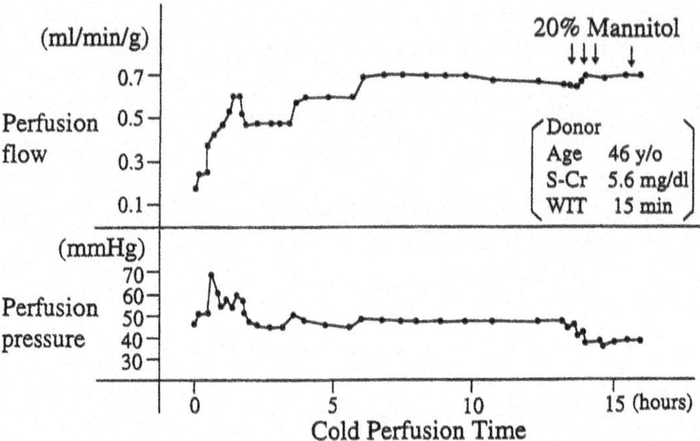

Fig. 15.4 Sequential changes in perfusion of kidney, acceptable for transplantation. Perfusion flow demonstrated more than 0.4 mL/min/g

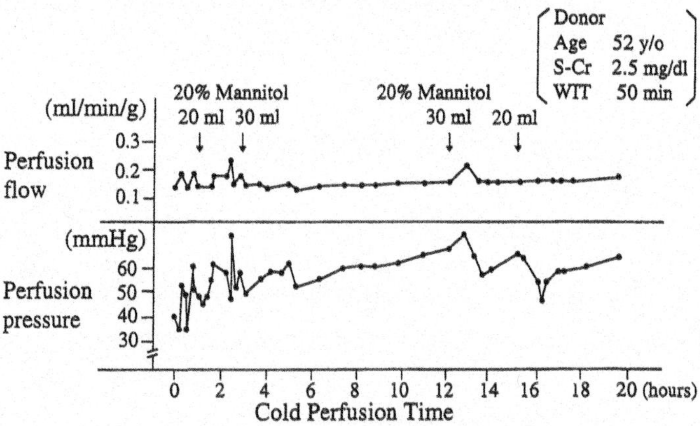

Fig. 15.5 Sequential changes in perfusion data of kidney discarded for transplantation. Perfusion flow and pressure demonstrated less than 0.4 mL/min/g and increase, respectively

Tesi et al. reported that the use of pulsatile perfusion for kidney preservation provided an opportunity to quantitatively evaluate the suitability of an organ for transplantation. In their criteria, a kidney was considered to be acceptable for transplantation if the flow was more than 70 mL/min or the renal resistance (mean pressure/flow) was less than 0.4. They discarded 15 % of kidneys in their group [39]. Balupuri et al. [40] suggested accepting only those kidneys with a flow rate of no less than 50 mL/min/100 g at a perfusion pressure of 60 mmHg. Their results were so encouraging that they suggested that not using machine perfusion for NHBD was difficult to justify. Polyak et al. [41] used papaverine, prostaglandin E1, trifluoperazine, and verapamil during perfusion in an attempt to manipulate kidneys with low flow and high resistance. Unresponsiveness to treatment may indicate a poor-quality kidney. Schold et al. analyzed and reported by the data SRTR in United States from 1994 to 2003 that reduced DGF and significantly lower discard rate of ECDs preserved with machine perfusion suggest an important utility of HMP in renal transplantation [42]. Sung et al. analyzed the factors associated with ECD kidney discard by the Scientific Registry of Transplant recipients (SRTs)/Organ Procurement and Transplant Recipients (OPTN) data [43]. Of the 12,536 recovered ECD kidneys, 5,139 (41 %) were discarded. Among the pumped kidneys, those with a resistance of 1.26–0.38 and >0.38 mmHg/mL/min were discarded more than those with a resistance of 0.18–0.25 mmHg/mL/min, respectively. The biopsy findings and machine perfusion are important correlates with ECD kidney discard, and there are corresponding associations with graft failure [44]. Nyberg et al. proposed quantitative approach to assess donor organs for cadaver renal transplantation by scoring system. They studied 34,324 patients who received diseased renal transplants between 1994 and 1999 and were reported to the UNOS, SRTR. A scoring system was developed from five donor variables (age, history of hypertension, creatinine clearance before procurement, cause of death, HLA mismatch). The influence of donor score on renal function and graft survival was most severe above 20 points. Their scoring system is useful in predicting outcomes after renal transplantation and in identifying kidneys most likely to benefit from HMP [45, 46]. However, one of the difficulties of viability assessment is that the cold conditions of the kidneys downregulate their metabolic activity and make them difficult to interpret. If oxidative metabolism is restarted by cold perfusion in a more physiological setting, then the parameters may be more meaningful.

15.4.4 Normothermic Preservation

It is recognized that preservation injury is an important factor in not only the short-term but also the long-term outcome of transplantation and that the success rates are directly related to the duration of cold ischemia. The grafts from marginal donors are characterized by particularly poor tolerance to the various injuries that occur during the process of preservation and transplantation. Although cooling reduces the metabolic rate of biological tissue, there is still damage even at the freezing temperature and the continued cellular processes lead to the depletion of ATP and accumulation of metabolic waste products. When an organ is rewarmed and reperfused with oxygenated blood, the rapid metabolism within an organ depleted of energy stores leads to the complex ischemia-reperfusion, causing cellular injury by lipid peroxidation and other pathways. The use of marginal donor organs, and particularly, organs from DCD, accelerates these problems of preservation and ischemia-reperfusion injury. It is certain that the use of hypothermic machine perfusion improves the immediate function of DGF, but does not enable sufficiently normal cellular metabolic function or prevent the depletion of energy stores or the deleterious direct effects of cooling. Thus, cold preservation has been considered important for transplantation for many years, but cold is now considered to be a limiting factor in the preservation of marginal donor organs. The principle of normothermic perfusion is to recreate the physiological environment by maintaining a normal temperature and providing the essential substrates for cellular metabolism, oxygenation, and nutrition. In addition to a reduction in ischemia-reperfusion injury, a further potential advantage of normothermic perfusion is the assessment of viability: Because the organ is metabolically active, it is possible to measure its function and to predict the post-transplant outcome [46]. Valero et al. reported short- and long-term function of kidney procured from non-heart-beating donors by means of normothermic recirculation. As a result, incidence of DGF and PNF was significantly lower in kidneys perfused with normothermic perfusion than those with in situ perfusion cooling or total body cooling. However, ethical concern exists when death may be pronounced [47].

Additional benefits may include the use of therapeutic gene therapy during transplantation: normothermic perfusion may provide an ideal environment for local gene delivery, perhaps to further protect against ischemia-reperfusion injury [48].

15.5 Basic Research

Belzer's group developed a synthetic machine perfusion solution, which was found capable of preserving canine kidneys for 3–5 days [49, 50]. This solution eventually contained hydroxyethyl starch, calcium, adenine, and ribose as substrates for ATP synthesis, gluconate to prevent hypothermia-induced cell swelling, and glutathione as an antioxidant. This solution referred to as University of Wisconsin (UW) gluconate, or Belzer machine perfusion solution, replaced previous cryoprecipitated plasma. The UW machine perfusion solution has been used as the "gold" standard machine perfusion solution. The Groningen group reported that low-pressure HMP was found to better preserve the viability of kidneys, resulting in less proximal tubular damage and better functional recovery after transplantation [51]. La Manna et al. [52] were able to show that the use of HMP in kidney autotransplantation reduced the levels of perforin expressed, as well as increasing the amount of cellular ATP, compared with SCS. Reduced reperfusion injury in tubular cells was also described when HMP and SCS with various preservation solutions were compared in a porcine model [53]. The improved histological integrity was related to improved perfusion of the renal cortex microcirculation with the removing of red cells and metabolic products. These benefits have been shown in canine autotransplantation and an isolated perfused kidney model [54, 55]. The Nicholson group demonstrated that HMP reduced the level of preservation injury compared with SCS preservation with HTK and UW solution for porcine kidneys with 10 min of WIT followed by 18 h of SCS, resulting in improved renal and tubular function and less cell inflammation during reperfusion [56, 57].

Rojas-Pena et al. used a porcine model to determine the utility of perfusion with oxygenated blood under normothermic conditions. The authors were able to demonstrate the benefits produced by 90 min of in situ extracorporeal support (ECS) after 30 min of warm ischemia compared to a rapid recovery technique.

The authors demonstrated significant differences in the hemodynamic parameters and markers of renal function [58]. Brasile demonstrated the potential of subnormothermic perfusion to improve the quality of organs damaged by warm ischemia [59]. This so-called metabolic support system used oxygenated culture medium-like perfusion solution at 32 °C to improve the viability of the kidney graft compared with hypothermic perfusion storage after 48 h [60].

In summary, machine perfusion preservation may be beneficial, especially for ECD and DCD kidneys. Overall, it has been suggested that machine perfusion preservation reduces the cost of DCD programs because of the better initial organ function, shorter hospital stay, and need for fewer hemodialysis sessions. On the other hand, recent studies have focused on normothermic preservation, wherein the organ is kept in a physiological environment by maintaining a normal temperature and providing the essential substrates for cellular metabolism, oxygenation, and nutrition. This area of research has led to the development of a tissue culture—like preservation solution with added perfluorocarbon. It includes amino acids, lipids, carbohydrates, proteins, trophic factors, vasodilators, and adenine compound substrates and is adjusted to normal pH. The histological grading of acute tubular necrosis suggested that this warm perfusion may be a valuable tool. However, normothermic perfusion is complex, and multiorgan procurement is generally associated with cooling, followed by cold preservation, in the usual clinical setting. The use of normothermic preservation may therefore not be accepted by procurement teams; however, experimental and early clinical results suggest that this technology may prove to be a significant step in the evolution of organ transplantation when used for marginal donors.

References

1. Lin EC, Terasaki PL. Clinical transplants. In: Terasaki PL, editor. Eary graft function. Los Angeles: UCLA Tissue Typing Laboratory; 1992. p. 401.
2. Sellers MT, Callid MH, Hadson SL, et al. Improved outcomes cadaveric renal allograft with pulsatile preservation. Clin Transplant. 2009;14:543.
3. Hoffman RM, Stratta RJ, D'Alessandro AM, et al. Combined cold storage-perfusion with a new synthetic perfusate. Transplantation. 1989;47:32–7.
4. Yuan X, Thervath AJ, Ge X, et al. Machine perfusion or cold in organ transplantation: indication, mechanisms, and future perspectives. Transpl Int. 2010;23:561–70.
5. Belzer FO, Park HY, Vetto RM. Factors influencing and blood flow during isolated perfusion. Surg Forum. 1964;15:222–4.
6. Belzer FO, Ashbly HY, Husang JS, et al. Etiology of rising perfusion pressure in isolated organ perfusion. Ann Surg. 1968;168(3):382–91.
7. Belzer FO, Asbly BS, Dunphy JE, et al. 24 hour and 72 hour preservation of canine kidneys. Lancet. 1967;2(7515):536–8.
8. Belzer FO, Asbly BS, Gulyassy PI, et al. Successful seventeen-hour preservation and transplantation of human-cadaver kidney. N Eng J Med. 1968;278(1):608–10.
9. Belzer FO, Outhard JH. Principles of solid-organ preservation by cold storage. Transplantation. 1988;45(4):673–676.
10. Baumgariner D, Southard DE, Najarian JS. Studies on segmental pancreas autotransplants in dogs: technique and preservation. Transplant Proc. 1980;12(4 Suppl 2):163–71.

11. Claes G, Blohne I. Experimental and clinical results of continuous albumin perfusion of the kidneys. London: Churchill Livingstone; 1973.
12. Daemen J, Oomen A, Jansen M, et al. Glutathione transferase S- transferase as predictor of functional outcome in transplantation of machine preserved non-heart-beating donor kidneys. Transplantation. 1997;63:89–93.
13. Grundmann R, Raab M, Meusel E, et al. Analysis of the optimal perfusion pressure and flow rate of the renal vascular resistance and oxygen consumption in the hypothermic perfused kidney. Surgery. 1975;77(3):451–61.
14. Hennry SD, Guarera JV. Prospective effects of hypothermic ex vivo perfusion on ischemia/perfusion injury and transplant outcomes. Transplant Previews. 2012;26:163–75.
15. Koyama H, Checka JM, Terasaki PI. A comparison of cadaver donor kidney storage methods: Pump perfusion and cold storage solutions. Clin Transplant. 1993;7:199–203.
16. Medez RG, Koussa N, et al. Preservation effect on oligo-anuria in the cyclosporine era; a prospective trial with 26 paired cadaveric renal allografts. Transplant Proc. 1987;19:2047–50.
17. Southard JH, Belzer FO. New concepts in organ preservation. Clin Transplant. 1997;7134–137.
18. Ajitani MR, Cutler JA, Det Valle CJ, et al. Single-donor cold storage versus machine perfusion in cadaver kidney transplantation. Transplantation. 1985;46:659–61.
19. Daemen JHC, de Vries B, Oomen APA, et al. Effect of machine perfusion preservation on delayed graft function in non-heart beating donor kidneys-Early results. Transpl Int. 1997;10:317–22.
20. Matsuno N, Sakurai E, Tamaki I, et al. Importance of machine perfusion flow in kidney transplantation. Transplant Proc. 1994;26(4):2421–2.
21. Kwiatkowski A, Wazola N, Kosieradzki M, et al. Machine perfusion preservation improves renal allograft survival. Am J Transplant. 2007;7:1942–7.
22. Singh RP, Farney AC, Rojers J, et al. Kidney transplantation from donation after cardiac death donors: lack of impact of delayed graft function on post-transplant outcomes. Clin Transplant. 2011;25:255–64.
23. Sigh RP, Farney AC, Rojers J, et al. Kidney transplantation from donation after cardiac death donors: lack of impact of delayed graft function on post-transplant outcomes. Clin Transplant. 2011;25:258–64.
24. Wight JP, Chilkott JB, Holmes MW, et al. Pulsatile machine perfusion vs cold storage of kidneys for transplantation: a rapid and systemic review. Clin Transplant. 2003;17:293–303.
25. Mtasuoka L, Shah T, Aswad S, et al. Pulsatile perfusion reduces the incidence of delayed graft function in expanded criteria donor kidney transplantation. Am J Transplant. 2006;6:1473–8.
26. Moers C, Smits JM, Maathuis MH, et al. Machine perfusion o cold storage in diseased donor kidney transplantation. N Eng J Med. 2009;360(1):78–80.
27. Treckmann J, Moers C, Smits JM, et al. Machine perfusion in clinical trials: machine vs solution effects. Transplant Int. 2012;25:e69–70.
28. Charautrer N, Thuillier R, Barrou B, et al. Machine perfusion in clinical trials: the preservation solution bias. Transplant Int. 2011;24:e81–2.
29. Moers C, Pirenne J, Paul A, et al. Machine perfusion or cold storage in deceased-donor kidney transplantation. N Engl Med. 2012;366:770–1.
30. Watson C, Wells A, Roberts R, et al. Cold machine perfusion versus static storage of kidneys donated after cardiac death. A UK multicenter randomized controlled trial. Am J Transplant. 2010;10:1991–9.
31. Buchanan PM, Lentine KL, Burroughs TE, et al. Association of lower cost of pulsatile machine perfusion in renal transplantation from expanded criteria donors. Am J Transplant. 2008;8:2391–401.
32. Garfield SS, Poret AW, Evans RW. The cost effectiveness of organ preservation methods in renal transplantation: US projections based on the machine preservation trial. Transplant Proc. 2009;41(9):3531–5.
33. Groen H, Moers C, Smits JM, et al. Cost effectiveness of hypothermic machine preservation versus static cold storage in renal transplantation. Am J Transplant. 2012;12:1824–30.

34. Balupuri S, Buckley P, Mohamed M, et al. Assessment of non-heart-beating donor (NHBD) kidneys for viability on machine perfusion. Clin Chem Lab Med. 2000;38(11):1103–6.
35. Codd JE, Garvin PJ, Morgan R, et al. Allograft viability determined by enzyme analysis. Transplantation. 1979;28:447–50.
36. Kohn M, Ross H. Lactate dehydrogenase output of the excised kidney as index of acute ischemic renal damage. Transplantation. 1971;11:461–4.
37. Liebau G, Kose HJ, Fischbach H, et al. Simple tests of viability of the hypothermic pulsatile perfused dog kidney. Surgery. 1971;70(39):459–66.
38. Matsuno N, Sakurai E, Uchiyama M, et al. Role of machine perfusion preservation in non-heart beating donors. Clin Transplant. 1998;1211–14.
39. Matsuno N, Konnnno O, Mejit A, et al. Application of machine perfusion preservation as a viability test for marginal kidney graft. Transplantation. 2006;82(11):1425–8.
40. Tesi RI, Elkhammas EA, Davis EA, et al. Pulsatile kidney perfusion for evaluation of high-risk kidney donors safely expands the donor pool. Clin Transplant. 1994;8:114–8.
41. Balupuri S, Buckley P, Snowden C, et al. The trouble with kidneys derived from the non-heart beating source. A single center 10 year experience. Transplantation. 2000;69:842–6.
42. Polyak MR, Arbrnoton B, Stubenbord WT, et al. The influence of pulsatile preservation on renal transplantation in the 1990. Transplantation. 2000;69(2):249–58.
43. Sung RS, Christensen LL, Leichtman AB, et al. Determinants of discard of expanded criteria donor kidneys. Impact of biopsy and machine perfusion. Am J Transplant. 2008;8:783–92.
44. Schold JD, Kaolan B, Howard RJ, et al. Are we frozen in time? Analysis of the utilization and efficacy of pulsatile perfusion in renal transplantation. Am J Transplant. 2005;5:1681–3.
45. Nyberg SL, Matas A, Kremers W, et al. Improved scoring system to assess adult donors for cadaver renal transplantation. Am J Transplant. 2003;3:715–21.
46. Nyberg SL, Baskin-Bet ES, Kremers W, et al. Improving the prediction of donor kidney quality; deceased donor score and resistive indices. Transplantation. 2005;80(7):925–9.
47. Arcia-Valdecassas JR, Tabet J, Valero R, et al. Liver conditioning after cardiac arrest the use of normothermic recirculation in an experimental animal model. Transpl Int. 1998;11:424–9.
48. Valero R, Cabrer C, Trias E, et al. Normothermic recirculation reduces primary graft dysfunction of kidneys obtained from non-heart-beating donors. Transpl Int. 2000;13:303–10.
49. Samdovici M, Henning RH, van Goor H, et al. Systemic gene therapy with Interleukin-13 attenuates renal ischemia-reperfusion injury. Kidney Int. 2008;73:1364–73.
50. Belzer FO, Glass NR, Sollinger HW, et al. A new perfusate for kidney preservation. Transplantation. 1982;33(3):322–3.
51. Hofmann RM, Southard JH, Luitz M, et al. Synthetic perfusate for kidney preservation. Its use in 72 h preservation of dog kidneys. Arch Surg. 1983;18(8):919–21.
52. Maathuis MH, et al. Improved kidney graft function after preservation using a novel hypothermic machine perfusion device. Ann Surg. 2007;246:982.
53. La Manna G, et al. In vivo autotransplant model of renal preservation cold storage versus machine perfusion in the preservation of ischemia/reperfusion injury. Artif Organs. 2009;33:565–70.
54. Hosgood SA, et al. A comparison of hypothermic machine perfusion versus static cold storage in an experimental model of renal ischemia reperfusion injury. Transplantation. 2010;89:830–7.
55. McAnulty JF, Ploeg RJ, Southard JH, et al. Successful five day perfusion preservation of canine kidney. Transplantation. 1989;47(1):37–41.
56. Ploeg RJ, Vreugdenhil P, Goossens D, et al. Effect of pharmacologic agents on the function of the hypothermically preserved dog kidney during normothermic reperfusion. Surgery. 1988;103:676–83.
57. Hosgood SA, Bagul A, Yang B, et al. The relative effects warm and cold ischemic injury in an experimental model of nonheartbeating donor kidneys. Transplantation. 2008;85(1):88–92.
58. Rojas-Pena A, Reoma JL, Krause E, et al. Extracorporeal support: Improves donor renal graft function after cardiac death. Am J Transplant. 2010;10:1365–74.
59. Brasile L, Stubenitsky BM, Booster M, et al. Overcoming severe renal ischemia the role of ex vivo warm perfusion. Transplantation. 2002;73:890–7.
60. Brasile L, Stubenitsky BM, Booster M, et al. Hypothermia-a limiting factor in using warm ischemically damaged kidneys. Am J Transplant. 2001;1:316–20.

Chapter 16
ECD for Kidney Transplantation

Naoto Matsuno

16.1 Introduction

Despite the increasing number of kidney transplants performed, the waiting list continues to grow. The shortage of kidneys available for transplantation is well documented, and the death rate for kidney transplant candidates on the waiting list is increasing [1–5]. The shortage of donor kidneys has inspired growing interest in recent years in the use of expanded criteria donors (ECDs).

In 2002, the Organ Procurement and Transplantation Network/United Network for Organ Sharing (OPTN/UNOS) adopted a new ECD allocation policy to increase the use of ECD. ECD kidneys are identified as those from a donor who is ≥60 years of age or one who is ≥50 years of age and has two additional risk factors, including a history of hypertension, an elevated terminal creatinine level, or a cerebrovascular cause of death. An analysis by the Scientific Registry of Transplant Recipients (SRTR) demonstrated that ECD kidneys were associated with a 1.7-fold higher risk for graft loss after transplantation compared with kidneys from non-ECD [6]. The policy was developed to identify with the intent of increasing the recovery and utilization rates of available kidneys and improving the efficiency of the kidney allocation process [7].

The recommendations generally reflect the fact that patients with poor prognoses on dialysis often cannot afford an extended waiting period for a standard kidney donation.

The adoption of the ECD policy was followed by an increase in the total number of recoveries but no significant change in the relative risk for graft loss among the recipients. In 2007, there were 15,793 potentially recoverable kidneys for which consent for donation was obtained. Of these, 2,389 (15 %) were recovered.

N. Matsuno (✉)
Division for Innovative Surgery and Transplantation, National Center for Child Health and Development, 2-10-1 Okura, Setagayaku, Tokyo 157-8535, Japan
e-mail: mtnnot@yahoo.co.jp

T. Asano et al. (eds.), *Marginal Donors: Current and Future Status*,
DOI 10.1007/978-4-431-54484-5_16, © Springer Japan 2014

However, the percentage of kidneys that were not recovered has gradually increased from 6.6 % in 1998 to 8.9 % in 2007 [8].

Additionally, the percentage of recovered kidneys that are discarded has increased gradually from 10 % in 1998 to 17 % in 2007. This increase in the discard rate likely reflects more aggressive recruitment of potential donors. On the other hand, there is a trend toward the development of more restrictive donor and recipient selection criteria for ECD, particularly the use of donor kidney biopsy to determine whether a kidney is suitable, which has occasionally led to the use of dual renal transplantation [9].

This review focuses on the use of ECD kidneys and related issues, including the criteria used to define ECD kidneys, the usefulness of donor kidney biopsy, the variability in ECD kidneys, and recipient selection and outcomes.

16.2 Donor Criteria

On October 31, 2002, the OPTN/UNOS Board of Directors adopted a new ECD allocation policy establishing a definition of ECD based on age and three statistically significant risk factors determined by previous SRTR analysis: history of arterial hypertension, serum creatinine level ≥1.5 mg/dL, and death caused by cerebrovascular accident [9, 10]. Consequently, ECDs were defined as any donor aged ≥60 years or any donor aged >50 years with at least two of the cited risk factors. Each of these criteria was defined by a relative risk of graft loss of 1.7 versus a reference group of "ideal donors," i.e., individuals aged 10–39 years, without hypertension, who did not die of cerebrovascular accident, and whose pre-donation serum creatinine levels were ≤1.5 mg/dL [9]. The model consisted of the donor's age, history of hypertension, serum creatinine level, and cause of death. At present, approximately 2,000 ECD and 8,000 standard criteria donor (SCD) kidneys are transplanted annually in the United States. Therefore, the increased use of ECD kidneys has clearly increased the donor pool. Careful analysis of risk factors may identify a subset of ECD that are suitable for transplantation.

Although numerous clinical studies have shown donor age to be a major determinant of graft outcome, other data are conflicting: some reports show similar 1- and 5-year graft function rates between recipients of renal allografts from younger (<55 years) and older (≥55 years) donors [11]. Regarding as the donor ages, the causes of death is also significantly influenced. Although the number of organ donors dying as a consequence of traumatic injuries has decreased, the number of donors with a cardiovascular or cerebrovascular cause of death has increased [1].

The precise relationship between arterial hypertension in the donor and long-term graft survival remains unclear, whereas preexisting chronic hypertension of the recipient is definitely considered a risk factor [12].

The ECD policy model incorporates the donor's age, history of hypertension, serum creatinine level, and cause of death (particularly cerebrovascular death) but does not include a histologic indicator of the structural integrity of the ECD kidney.

Although creatinine clearance and pretransplant biopsy results were examined for significant predictive value for graft survival, the current model was determined to be the optimal predictor [13]. The use of a glomerulosclerosis index or the degree of fibrous intimal thickening at the time of implantation was useful [14].

Useful scores for donor kidneys have been reported since the beginning of the ECD era. The Nyberg [15, 16] score is based on five donor variables: age, hypertension, creatinine clearance, cerebrovascular cause of death, and human leukocyte antigen (HLA) mismatch. These variables are scored to quantify the degrees of risk and the total score used to divide the donors into four classes from A to D. Rao et al. [17] have developed a kidney donor risk index (KDRI). The KDRI incorporates the ECD risk factors as well as a number of other parameters that affect graft survival, including doctor factors such as diabetes, height, weight, donation after cardiac death, and hepatitis C status and transplant factors such as HLA matching and dual-kidney transplantation. The Anglicheau score [18] combines a simplified histological score (glomerulosclerosis, 10 %) with two donor variables, namely, a serum creatinine level >150 μmol/L and hypertension. The authors provided indications for discarding organs, and the use of kidneys from donors with all three features was strongly limited.

The Schold score [14] employs eight parameters: seven donor-related parameters (donor age and race, cause of death, HLA mismatches, and donor history of hypertension or diabetes) and the cold ischemia time (CIT). The score is calculated by summing all of the risk factors and categorizes donors into five grades with sequentially increasing adjusted hazard ratios for graft loss. This score focuses on the association between degrees, graft survival, and the probability of delayed graft function (DGF).

To help standardizing the preimplantation histologic evaluation of older or ECD kidneys, an international panel of pathologists suggested a biopsy-based scoring system for kidneys, with scores ranging from minimum of 0 (no lesions) to a maximum of 12 (marked changes in vessels, glomeruli, tubules, and connective tissue). Kidneys with scores of three or lower are predicted to contain enough viable nephrons to be used for single transplantation. Those with scores of 4, 5, or 6 could be used for dual transplantation on the assumption that the total number of viable nephrons in the two kidneys approaches the number in a single ideal kidney. An additional advantage of preimplantation histologic evaluation is that discarding kidneys on the basis of unacceptably severe histological changes protects the recipients. Kidneys with scores of seven or higher are discarded [19].

Preliminary studies without control groups suggested that kidneys from donors older than 60 but younger than 75 years of age could be considered for single transplants if the average extent of glomerulosclerosis were <15 % or for dual transplantation if it were >15 % but <50 % [20]. Navarro et al. reported that histological analysis of kidney biopsies before transplantation is a useful tool and that single kidney transplantation should not be recommended when the total score (including glomerular global sclerosis, interstitial fibrosis, tubular atrophy, fibrous intimal thickening, and hyaline arteriolar thickening) is >5 [21].

The use of a biopsy-based strategy increased the number of available kidneys which improved the recipients' chances of receiving a graft and shortened the waiting time for kidneys from deceased donors. Some problems do remain to be solved. The preimplantation evaluation of a biopsy specimen should be compatible with the routine activities of organ procurement and allocation; however, practical difficulties in comparing histology samples between different centers may be a limitation on the systematic application of a biopsy-guided strategy for organ selection and allocation.

An additional problem is that no study to date has compared the predictive values of the histology score and donor kidney function which will affect on short- and long-term survival [22, 23].

A large number ($n = 17,514$) of paired ECD kidneys from the same donors were evaluated by the SRTR registry and transplanted between 1995 and 2009. Although a longer CIT is a risk factor for DGF among ECD kidney transplants, it has no effect on graft survival [24].Therefore, reports based on the UNOS data registry compared allograft outcomes between deceased diabetic donors and ECD and found that the diabetic donors had lower sCr and shorter durations of cold ischemia [24]. Recipients of diabetic kidneys were younger and less likely to experience DGF than recipients of ECD kidneys [25].

Unfortunately, at this time, many kidneys from ECD are eventually discarded as unacceptable. Some of these kidneys could be used for dual-kidney transplantation. Although there are many criteria available for the evaluation of ECD organ quality, the prognostic utility of histological versus clinical scoring systems for determining functioned graft survival after kidney transplantation remains an open question.

16.3 Recipient Criteria

For improving the outcome of the use of ECD kidneys is to minimize the waiting time and thus optimize the "quality" of the recipients. The ECD policy may be understood as primarily an objective definition of higher-risk donation that has only secondarily allowed physicians to recommend the use of these organs in seemingly appropriate candidates. One important method for improving the outcome of the use of ECD kidneys is to minimize the waiting time and thus optimize the "quality" of the recipients. The longer the waiting time for deceased donor kidneys, active programs with short waiting times are advised to be more restrictive in their use of ECD, whereas programs with prolonged waiting times may increase their ECD procurement and use. The strong associations of waiting time with pre- and post-transplant mortality are important considerations in these crucial organ-selection decisions [26–28].

The 2002 conference on the waiting list for kidney transplantation suggested that the most appropriate candidates for receiving ECD transplants would be elderly patients, patients with diabetes, patients with limited vascular access, and non-sensitized patients [29]. Since the ECD policy started, the consent process appears to have substantially affected the distribution of these higher-risk donor grafts to elderly recipients. In general, the recommendations reflect the fact that patients with poor prognoses on dialysis often cannot afford extended waiting periods for a standard kidney donation. Although age alone is not considered in allocation policies for adult candidates, elderly candidates may have greater incentive to accept [30, 31].

According to the SRTR report, 81 % of ECD kidney recipients were ≥50 years old, which is an increase from 55 % in 1996[32]. Because the majority of kidney transplant candidates aged ≥60 years in the United States are listed for an ECD kidney transplant, the percentage of recipients older than 60 years had increased from 36.7 % to 49.3 % [25]. Candidates with longer waiting times were not more likely to be listed for ECD kidneys. In fact, the percentage of candidates listed for ECD kidneys was greater in donor service areas with short (<700 days) waiting times than in those with medium (700 to 1,500 days) or longer (>1,500 days) waiting times. As these investigators stated, areas with aggressive organ donation practices, including the use of ECD and DCD kidneys, may have shorter waiting times as a result of their efforts [25].

Schold reported that the main selection criterion for an ECD kidney transplant, except for retransplantation, was age >40 years; this is because the predicted mortality in such patients was lower for ECD kidney transplantation than for remaining on the waiting list for an SCD kidney [33]. Recipients older than 70 years and even those older than 75 years can benefit from ECD kidney transplantation, with lower mortality than patients receiving dialysis while on the waiting list. This benefit is also significant in elderly patients with diabetes and hypertension [34].

Patients with conditions that affect their prognosis after the onset of ESRD (such as diabetes or polycystic kidneys), particularly those who are able to reduce their exposure to dialysis by accepting ECD organs, may be appropriate candidates for ECD kidneys [35]. The longer the waiting time for deceased donor kidneys, the greater the probability that older candidates will die or be removed from the waiting list because of rapidly declining health. Schold et al. showed that life expectancy was greater for recipients aged 18 to 39 years who received SCD kidney transplants after 4 years of dialysis therapy than for those who received ECD kidney transplants after 2 years of dialysis (26.4 vs. 17.6 years), but this was not the case for recipients older than 65 years (5.6 vs. 5.3 years). Patients with diabetes aged 18–39 years who received ECD kidney transplants after waiting for 2 years showed similar life expectancies as those who waited 4 years for SCD kidney transplants (9.6 vs. 9 years) [33]. A total of 16.4 % of the 74,998 kidney transplants performed in the United States were young-to-old (donor aged 15–50 years to recipient aged >60 years) during the period from 1990 to 2002. The graft survival from the young donors exceeded the patient survival of the older recipients and that the allocation of young kidneys to older recipients resulted in the graft loss [36].

Patients listed in programs with prolonged waiting times benefit from receiving ECD kidneys because of the high mortality associated with remaining on dialysis therapy. Age matching of donor kidneys has proven to be of major importance for maximizing the use of deceased donor kidneys. A donor-recipient age ratio >1.10 (donor age of 55 years to recipient age of <50 years) was associated with a threefold higher rate of graft loss [37]. Proper age-matching algorithms increase the overall time for which patients have functioning transplants. Furthermore, avoiding the allocation of young donor kidneys to older recipients, great efforts to improve the outcomes should be continued to substantially increase the overall function time of the transplants.

Although the graft survival is significantly longer for younger grafts, the 10-year death-censored graft survival in patients who received grafts from elderly living donors (>55 years) and did not experience acute rejection was >90 % [15], suggesting the importance of careful patient selection and the influences of such additional immune-mediated events as ischemia-reperfusion injury and acute rejection.

To inform decision-making regarding transplantation in patients aged ≥65 years, the early post-transplant risk for death was evaluated and compared between recipients and wait-listed dialysis patients in the United States between 1995 and 2007 (total $n = 25{,}468$). As for living donor transplantation, this analysis found that living donor transplantation eliminated early post-transplant mortality risk in low- and intermediate-risk patients and markedly reduced it in high-risk patients. This was especially true in comparison with the alternative, namely, remaining on the waiting list for a transplant [38].

In summary, the available data indicate that patients with diabetes, elderly patients, and those with long durations of dialysis therapy appear to achieve the greatest benefit from being listed for an ECD kidney. However, the most important cause of graft loss in these patients is death, particularly of cardiac origin, with a functioning graft, and therefore, special attention must be paid to cardiac assessment [39]. There was report that a 1-year mortality rate of 14.4 % after ECD kidney transplantation in patients aged ≥60 years and any comorbidity increased this rate. The mortality rate was always greater in elderly ECD kidney transplant recipients [40].

16.4 Kidney Biopsy

The current pretransplant evaluation of ECD organs is based on histological, clinical, or mixed criteria. However, the need for a donor kidney biopsy is controversial because the way that ECD kidneys are allocated on the basis of the histology changes makes interpretation of the outcome data difficult and controversial. Some studies considered only, or mainly, the severity of the glomerular changes [41, 42], whereas others identified the vascular pathology as the strongest predictor of recipient graft function [43]. Using the UNOS Registry, Nyberg et al. developed a 39-point score based on 5 donor variables related to creatinine clearance 6 months after transplantation. Glomerulosclerosis affecting ≥20 % of the glomeruli predicted worse 6-year graft survival [16].

Some of the SRTR analyses assessing the potential value of donor kidney biopsy are available, but their results are contradictory. The percentage of glomerulosclerosis correlated with DGF, primary nonfunction, and graft survival [44].

The most recent report showed greater creatinine clearance 1 year after transplantation, but no difference in graft survival, for kidneys with 0–5 % glomerulosclerosis versus those exhibiting greater percentages [45]. However, histological evaluation prior to kidney allocation might improve the graft survival of ECD kidneys. The main limitation of that study is that dual-kidney transplantation was performed in the majority of patients, and transplantation of two ECD kidneys is expected to yield good results [45].

Even more importantly, the histological findings were most likely affected by the different modalities adopted for tissue sampling. The use of frozen rather than permanent sections may save time but has limitations [46], while the use of needle core biopsy as opposed to wedge biopsy may have advantages. The estimation of glomerulosclerosis from subcapsular wedge biopsy specimens may mask the true importance of this parameter.

16.5 Outcomes

Since the ECD allocation policy started, transplant candidates must accept a lower-quality ECD transplant. The analysis of ECD kidney transplantation outcomes is difficult because all aspects tend to be multifactorial and are subject to great variability. One recent analysis using the UNOS database showed 5-year and 10-year graft survival rates of 68.8 % and 50.9 %, respectively, for standard criteria donor (SCD) kidneys ($n = 33{,}118$) and 51.8 % and 32.9 %, respectively, for ECD kidneys ($n = 5{,}943$) [47].

The initial impact of the ECD policy was to reduce waiting times. However, a significant number of the organs initially recovered for transplantation are eventually discarded [30, 48]. This discard rate is probably unnecessarily high. More than a third of discarded kidneys are not used because of biopsy findings [49]. A similar analysis indicated that the use of biopsy is the strongest determinant of the discard rate [30]. Machine perfusion preservation may decrease the discard rate of potential kidney grafts.

The discard rate in each transplant center will influence on the graft survival. DGF remained an independent predictor of poorer outcome in all recipients. A study performed at eight US transplant centers compared the long-term outcomes of 170 kidneys refused by at least two centers and subsequently transplanted with those of 170 transplantations of kidneys accepted by the first center to which they were offered. Although the use of "marginal" kidneys was associated with a higher rate of DGF (63 % vs. 32 %), a higher rate of primary nonfunction (7.7 % vs. 1.8 %), and a lower creatinine clearance rate (33.3 vs. 48.5 mL/min after 5 years), the 5-year patient and graft survival rates were not significantly different (88.2 % vs. 88.9 % and 70.4 % vs. 76.7 %, respectively), justifying the use of this type of kidney. However, in another report older recipients (aged >60 years) who received an ECD kidney with DGF had a 31 % chance of dying within 1 year [49]. Preliminary uncontrolled studies suggest that kidneys from donors aged >60 but <75 years could be considered for single transplants if the mean rate of glomerulosclerosis were <15 % or for a dual transplant if it were >15 % but <50 % [50]. This approach yielded 1-year graft survival rates of 90 % and 95 % in recipients of single and dual transplants, respectively. In another series of 26 patients, kidneys were selected and allocated to either single or dual transplant on the basis of a scoring system including the donor age, serum creatinine level, kidney weight, and degree of glomerulosclerosis. Each parameter considered was scored 0 or 1 according to whether the value was below or above a cutoff level (65 years for age, 1.8 mg/dL for serum creatinine, 30 % for the degree of glomerulosclerosis, and 300 g for the combined weight of both kidneys). A sum of less than 1 resulted in single kidney transplantation, a sum of 2 in dual-kidney transplantation, and a sum of >2 in refusal of the organ. Graft survival after 1 year was similar between single- and dual-transplant recipients (both 92 %) [51, 52].

Further analyses of dual-transplant recipients whose grafts had been evaluated histologically before implantation showed graft survival similar to that for single transplants from younger donors [52]. Most recently, a single-center study showed that the 3- and 5-year graft survival rates of single transplants from low risk, "ideal" donors (89 % and 79 %) were similar to those of single (82 % and 78 %) or dual (88 % and 78 %) transplants from older donors allocated on the basis of the scoring system and donor-calculated creatinine clearance [28]. On the other hand, a prospective, matched-cohort study [53] found that 3-year graft survival in 62 recipients of one or two kidneys from deceased donors aged ≥60 years that were selected and allocated on the basis of the scoring system (94 %) was identical to that in 124 recipients of single grafts from "ideal" donors aged <60 years (94 %) and remarkably superior to that of 124 recipients of single grafts from donors older than 60 that were not evaluated histologically before implantation (77 %) [53]. Navaro reported overall graft survival rates after 1 and 5 years of 31.7 % and 31.7 %, respectively, for transplants with total kidney biopsy scores of >5 versus 96.8 % and 84.7 %, respectively, for those with total scores of ≤3 and 82.5 % and 69.0 %, respectively, for transplants with scores of 4–5 [22]. As a summary, the outcomes of ECD kidney transplantation are difficult to identify. The combination of older kidneys transplanted into less-ideal recipients maximizes the complication rate and is associated with poor outcomes. Some of the concepts in the proposal touch upon the importance of appropriately age-matching organs with recipients, particularly when ECD organs are used. Careful pretransplant selection of the graft is necessary to ensure the best possible outcome.

16.6 Conclusion

The policy was developed to identify higher-risk deceased donor kidneys with the intent of increasing the rates of recovery and utilization of available kidneys and thus improving the efficiency of the allocation process. A greater effort should be made to extend the true benefits of ECD kidney transplantation to more patients, especially in areas with long waiting lists. Biopsy-guided allocation of ECD kidneys may help to improve graft outcomes, particularly at centers with high rates of procurement from older donors. On the other hand, findings of no or minimal histology changes avoid the performance of unnecessary dual transplants from the already limited organ pool. Finally, the encouraging results described above warrant prospective studies to evaluate formally whether the inclusion of a histologic marker of the structural integrity of the kidney in the model for ECD organ procurement and allocation might increase the number of opportunities for successful ECD kidney transplantation in patients in need.

References

1. United Network for Organ Sharing. United Network for Organ Sharing 1999 Annual report of the U.S. Scientific registry for Transplant recipients and the Organ and Transplantation Network, UNOS, Richmond, 1999.
2. Giral-Classe M, Homant M, Cantarovich D, et al. Delayed graft function of more than six days strongly decreases long-term survival of transplanted kidneys. Kidney Int. 1998;54:972.
3. Hariharan S, Johnson CP, Bresnahan BA, et al. Improved graft survival after renal transplantation in the United States, 1988 to 1996. N Engl J Med. 2000;342:605.
4. Chertow G, Brenner BM, Mackenzie HS, Milford EL. Non-immunologic predictors of chronic renal allograft failure: data from the United network of Organ sharing. Kidney Int Suppl. 1995;52:48.
5. Hariharan S, McBride MA, Bennett LE, Cohen EP. Risk factors for renal allograft survival from older cadaver donors. Transplantation. 1997;64:174.
6. Mirza DF, Gunson BK, DaSilva RF, Mayer AD, Bucke JA, McMaster P. Policies in Europe on 'marginal quality' donor livers. Lancet. 1994;1:1480.
7. Detre KM, Lombadero M, Belle S, et al. Influence of donor age on graft survival after liver transplantation- United network for Organ Sharing Registry. Liver Transplant Surg. 1995;1:311.
8. Tuttle-Newhall JE, Krishnan SM, Levy MF, et al. Organ donation and utilization in the United States; 1998–2007. Am J Transplantation. 2009;9:879–93.
9. Port FK, Bragg-Gresham JL, Metzger RA, et al. Donor characteristics associated with reduced graft survival: An approach to expanding the pool of kidney donors. Transplantation. 2002;74:1281–6.
10. Metzger RA, Delmonico FL, Feng S, Port FK, Wynn JJ, Merion RM. Expanded criteria donors for kidney transplantation. Am J Transplant. 2003;125 Suppl 4:3S–114.
11. Lloveras J, Arias M, Andres A, et al. Five-year follow-up of 250 recipients of cadaveric kidney allografts from donors older than 55 years of age. Transplant Proc. 1995;27:981.
12. Frei U, Schindler R, Wieters D, et al. Pre-transplant hypertension: a major risk factor for chronic progressive renal allograft dysfunction. Nephrol Dial Transplant. 1995;10:1206.
13. Schold JD, Kaplan B, Baliga RS, Meier-Kriesche HU. The broad spectrum of quality in deceased donor kidneys. Am J Transplant. 2005;5:757–65.
14. Escofet X, Osman H, Griffiths DF, Woydag S, Adam Jurewicz W. The presence of glomerular sclerosis at time zero has a significant impact on function after cadaveric renal transplantation. Transplantation. 2003;75:344–6.
15. Nyberg SL, Matas AJ, Rogers M, et al. Donor scoring system for cadaveric renal transplantation. Am J Transplant. 2001;1:162–9.
16. Nyberg SL, Matas AJ, Kremers WK, et al. Improved scoring system to assess adult donors for cadaver renal transplantation. Am J Transplant. 2003;3:715–25.

17. Rao PS, Schaubel DE, Guidnrger MK, et al. A comprehensive risk quantification score for discarded donor kidneys: the kidney donor risk index. Transplantation. 2009;88:231–9.
18. Anglicheau D, Loupy A, Lefaucheur C, et al. A simple clinico-histopathological composite scoring system is highly predictive of graft outcomes in marginal donors. Am J Transplant. 2008;8:2325.
19. Remuzzi G, Grinyo J, Ruggenenti P, et al. Early experience with dual kidney transplantation in adults using expanded donor criteria. J Am Soc Nephrol. 1999;1:2591–8.
20. Andres A, Morales JM, Herrer JC, et al. Double versus single renal allografts from aged donor. Transplantation. 2000;69:2000–1.
21. Navaro MD, Lopez-Andreu M, Radrigiez-Benot A, et al. Significance of preimplantation analysis of kidney biopsies from expanded criteria donors in long-term outcome. Transplantation. 2011;91(4):432–9.
22. Sung RS, Christensen LL, Leichtman AB, et al. Determinants of discard of expanded criteria donor kidneys: Impact of biopsy and machine perfusion. Am J Transplant. 2008;8:783–92.
23. Edwards EB, Posner MP, Maluf DG, Kauffman HM. Reasons for non-use of recovered kidneys: the effect of donor glomerulosclerosis and creatinine clearance on graft survival. Transplantation. 2004;77:1411–5.
24. Kayler LK, Agliocca J, Zendejas I, et al. Impact of cold ischemia time on graft survival among ECD transplant recipients. A paired kidney analysis. Am J Transplant. 2011;11:2647–56.
25. Sung RS, Guidinger MK, Leichtman AB, et al. Impact of the expanded criteria donor allocation system on candidates for and recipients of expanded criteria donor kidneys. Transplantation. 2007;84:1138–44.
26. Cosio FG, Alamir A, Yim S, et al. Patient survival after renal transplantation: I. The impact of dialysis pre-transplant. Kidney Int. 1998;53:767–72.
27. Meier-Kriesche HU, Port FK, Ojo AO, et al. The expanded criteria donor policy: an evaluation of program objectives and indirect ramifications. Am J Transplant. 2006;6:1689–95. Expanded Criteria Donor Policy time on renal transplant outcome. Kidney Int. 2000;58:1311–17.
28. Meier-Kriesche HU, Port FK, Rudich SM, Leichtman AB, Kaufman DB, Kaplan B. Effect of waiting time and primary renal disease on mortality after renal transplantation. Transplantation. 2000;69:S261.
29. Nyberg SL, Baskin-Bey ES, Kremers W, Prieto M, Henry ML, Stegall MD. Improving the prediction of donor kidney quality: Deceased donor score and resistive indices. Transplantation. 2005;80:925–9.
30. Sung RS, Christensen LL, Leichtman AB, et al. Determinants of discard of expanded criteria donor kidneys: impact of biopsy and machine perfusion. Am J Transplant. 2008;8:783–92.
31. Muruve NA, Steinbecker KM, Luger AM. Are wedge biopsies of cadaveric kidneys obtained at procurement reliable? Transplantation. 2000;69:2384–8.
32. Andreoni KA, Brayman KL, Guidinger MK, Sommers CM, Sung RS. Kidney and pancreas transplantation in the United States, 1996–2005. Am J Transplant. 2007;7:1359.
33. Schold JD, Meier-Kriesche HU. Which renal transplant candidates should accept marginal kidneys in exchange for a shorter waiting time on dialysis? Clin J Am Soc Nephrol. 2006; 1:532–8.
34. Rao PS, Merion RM, Ashby VB, Port FK, Wolfe RA, Kayler LK. Renal transplantation in elderly patients older than 70 years of age: results from the Scientific Registry of Transplant Recipients. Transplantation. 2007;83:1069–74.
35. Andres A, Morales JM, Herrero JC, et al. Double versus single renal allografts from aged donors [see comment]. Transplantation. 2000;69:2060–6.
36. Meier-Kriesche HU, Sebold JD, Gaston RS, Wadstrom J, Kaplan B. Kidneys from deceased donors: maximizing the value of a scarce resource. Am J Transplant. 2005;5:1725–30.
37. Swanson SJ, Hypolite IO, Agodoa LY, et al. Effect of donor factors on early graft survival in adult cadaveric renal transplantation. Am J Transplant. 2002;2:68–75.
38. Gill JS, Schaeffner E, Chadban S, et al. Quantification of the early risk of death an elderly kidney transplantation recipients. Am J Transplant. 2013;13:427–32.
39. Filmore H. Cardiac assessment for renal transplantation. Am J Transplant. 2006;6:659–65.

40. Kauffman HM, McBride MA, Cors CS, Roza AM, Wynn JJ. Early mortality rates in older kidney recipients with comorbid risk factors. Transplantation. 2007;83:404–10.
41. Pokoma E, Vitko S, Chadimova M, et al. Proportion of glomerulosclerosis in procurement wedge renal biopsy cannot alone discriminate for acceptance of marginal donors. Transplantation. 2000;69:36–43.
42. Pokoma E, Vftko S, Chadimova M, Schiick O. Adverse effect of donor arteriolosclerosis on graft outcome after renal transplantation. Nephrol Dial Transplant. 2000;15:705–10.
43. Lu AD, Desai D, Myers BD, Dafoe DC, Alfrey EJ. Severe glomerular sclerosis is not associated with poor outcome after kidney transplantation. Am J Surg. 2000;180:470–4.
44. Cicciarelli J, Cho Y, Mateo R, et al. Renal biopsy donor group: the influence of glomerulosclerosis on transplant outcomes. Transplant Proc. 2005;37:712–3.
45. Sung RS, Christensen LL, Leichtman AB, et al. Determinants of discard of expanded criteria donor kidneys: impact of biopsy and machine perfusion. Am J Transplant. 2008;8:783–92.
46. Setti G, Sandrini S, Cancarini G, et al. Reliability of clinical parameters for the selection of elderly cadaveric donors. Transplant Proc. 2001;33:1164–5.
47. Merion RM, Ashby VB, Wolfe RA, et al. Deceased-donor characteristics and the survival benefit of kidney transplantation. JAMA. 2005;294:2726–33.
48. Wolfe RA, Roys EC, Merion RM. Trends in organ donation and transplantation in the United States. 1998-. Am J Transplant. 2010;10:961–72.
49. Mezrich JD, Pirsch JD, Fernandez LA, et al. Differential outcomes of expanded criteria donor renal allografts according to recipient age. Clin J Am Sco Nephlorol. 2012;7:1163–71.
50. Sung RS, Guidinger MK, Lake CD, et al. Impact of the expanded criteria donor allocation system on the use of expanded criteria donor kidneys. Transplantation. 2005;79:1257–61.
51. Morris PJ, Johnson RJ, Fuggle SV, Belger MA, Briggs JD. Analysis of factors that affect outcome of primary cadaveric renal transplantation in the UK. Lancet. 1999;1:1147.
52. The Organ Procurement and Transplantation Network. Allocation of Deceased Kidneys. http://www.optn.org/PoliciesandBylaws/policies/pdfs/policy_7.pdf. Accessed 23 Nov 2005.
53. Sola R, Guirado L, Lopez-Navidad A, et al. Renal transplantation with limit donors: to what should the good results obtained be attributed? Transplantation. 1998;66:1169.

Chapter 17
LD for Kidney Transplantation

Yoshihiko Watarai

17.1 Criteria for Living Donation

Among patients with end-stage renal disease, kidney transplantation has been well documented to improve patient survival and quality of life compared with those on the waiting list who did not undergo transplantation [1]. Living transplant has been reported to lead superior short- and long-term outcomes in patients and graft survival comparing the results of deceased donor transplantation in Japan as well as in the USA (Table 17.1, Fig. 17.1).

Among more than 300,000 end-stage renal disease patients in Japan, the number of kidney transplant is limited up to 1,600 per year because of extreme shortage of deceased donor. As a result of this 86.0 % of transplants were consisted with living donors and only 7.1 % of deceased donors were DBD between 2000 and 2009 (129 DBD and 1,684 DCD) (Fig. 17.2). The Japanese Society of Transplantation reported 91.0 % of 5-year graft survivals in living donor transplant vs. 79.1 % in deceased donor transplant, respectively; even most donors were consisted with DCD, which is comparable with the results of decease donor transplant in the USA and Europe [2, 3] (Table 17.1).

Even the living donor transplant is a very special occasion for surgeon to operate on healthy individuals; more transplant programs have increased efforts to expand their living donor programs to close the gap between the number of wait-listed candidates and available organs, even using web site [4, 5].

Stringent criteria for living donor must be defined to protect profit for their physical health and quality of life.

Y. Watarai (✉)
Nagoya Daini Red Cross Hospital, 2-9 Myokencho,
Showa-ku, Nagoya 466-8650, Japan
e-mail: watarai@nagoya2.jrc.or.jp

T. Asano et al. (eds.), *Marginal Donors: Current and Future Status*,
DOI 10.1007/978-4-431-54484-5_17,

Table 17.1 Graft survival after kidney transplantation in Japan

	N	1 year (%)	3 years (%)	5 years (%)	10 years (%)
Graft survival after living donor kidney transplantation					
1990–1994	1,931	92.9	87.1	79.8	64.3
1995–1999	2,037	94.1	90.2	85.7	74.6
2000–2004	2,815	96.8	94.0	91.0	–
2005–2009	4,126	97.3	95.2	–	–
Graft survival after deceased donor kidney transplantation					
1990–1994	985	83.2	74.4	64.3	49.7
1995–1999	690	86.5	78.3	72.2	59.3
2000–2004	594	89.7	84.1	79.1	–
2005–2009	779	91.3	86.6	–	–

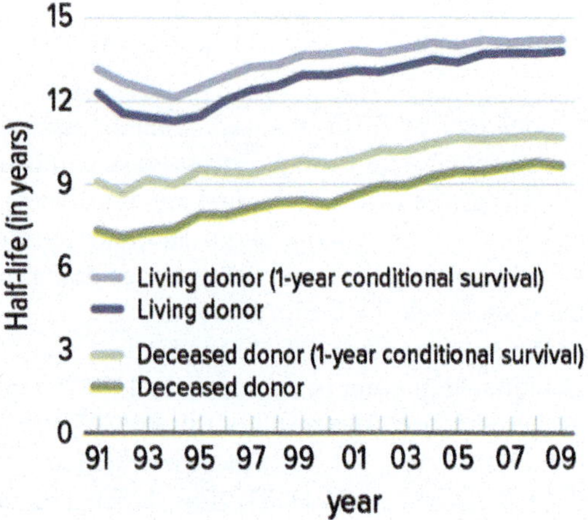

Fig. 17.1 Half-lives for adult kidney transplant recipients. OPTN/SRTR 2011 Annual Report, http://srtr.transplant.hrsa.gov/annual_reports/2011/default.aspx

17.1.1 Initial Screening and Psychological Aspect of Donor Selection

It is critical that donor's decision to donate a kidney for the benefit of another individual is one from their voluntary decision. Most centers demand a donor to be of legal adult age (18 years) and able to provide informed consent in the USA and Europe. Ethics committee in the Japanese Society for Transplantation restricted the donor age of over 20 and donor–recipient relation within the sixth degree consanguinity, spouse, and a relative by affinity within the third degree in principle. Extensive evaluation by psychiatrist and approval from parents and IRB must be achieved for a living donation from 18 to 19 years adolescent.

Donors should be screened that they are highly motivated and willing to take some risk of donor operation without seeking either financial reimbursement or improvement in social status by their donation. Donors should be screened in the absence of family members or recipients that they do not feel overt pressure and undue anxiety.

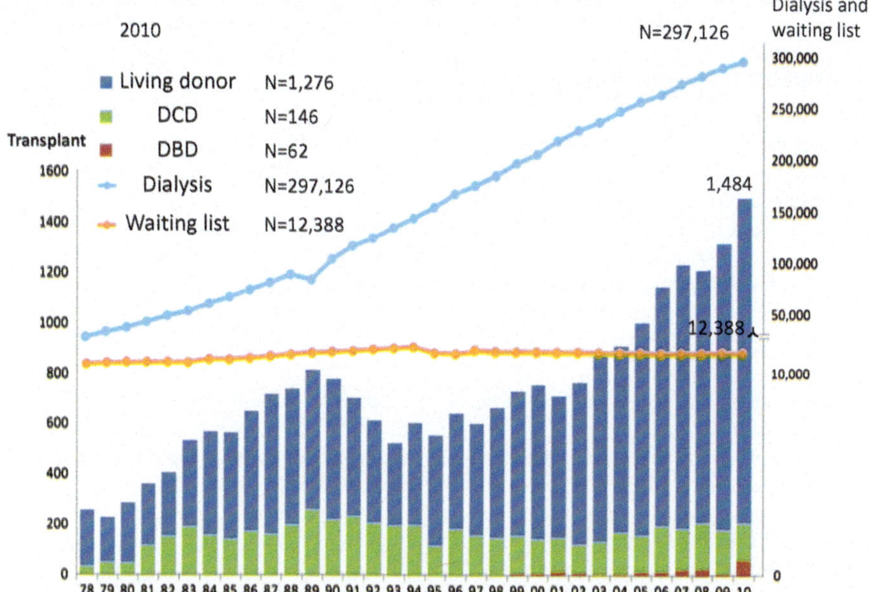

Fig. 17.2 Number of kidney transplant, waiting list, and dialysis patient in Japan

Approach to the potential live donor could be started with web-based application to rule out standard contraindication for donors, but consequently should include an experienced medical team which consisted with transplant surgeons, nephrologists, psychiatrists, social workers, and transplant coordinators.

After screening or evaluation of potential renal donors with experienced transplant team, a significant proportion of prospective living kidney donors have been excluded for medical and psychosocial problems such as obesity, hypertension, nephrolithiasis, positive cytotoxic antibody cross-match result, and abnormal glucose tolerance up to 60 % [4–7].

17.1.2 Medical Evaluation of the Donor

An international consortium of the world's leading kidney transplant physicians and surgeons met in Amsterdam for the International Forum on the Care of the Live Kidney Donor to discuss the standard of care for live donors in 2004. Forum participants included over 100 experts and leaders in transplantation representing more than 40 countries from around the world, including participants from the following continents: Africa, Asia, Australia, Europe, North America, and South America.

With an alliance with the World Health Organization (WHO), the statement of this forum has been proposed as a standard recommendation to the world (Table 17.2) [8, 9].

Table 17.2 Amsterdam forum guidelines

Donor evaluation

Prior to donation, the live kidney donor must receive a complete medical and psychosocial evaluation, receive appropriate informed consent, and be capable of understanding the information presented in that process to make a voluntary decision. All donors should have standard tests performed to assure donor safety

Hypertension

Patients with a BP >140/90 by ABPM are generally not acceptable as donors

BP should preferably be measured by ABPM, particularly among older donors (>50 years) and/or those with high office BP readings

Some patients with easily controlled hypertension, who meet other defined criteria, e.g. >50 years of age, GFR > 80 mL/min, and urinary albumin excretion 30 mg/day may represent a low-risk group for development of kidney disease after donation and may be acceptable as kidney donors

Donors with hypertension should be regularly followed by a physician

Obesity

Patients with a BMI >35 kg/m^2 should be discouraged from donating, especially when other comorbid conditions are present

Obese patients should be encouraged to lose weight prior to kidney donation and should be advised not to donate if they have other associated co-morbid conditions

Obese patients should be informed of both acute and long-term risks, especially when other comorbid conditions are present

Healthy lifestyle education should be available to all living donors

Dyslipidemia

Dyslipidemia should be included along with other risk factors in donor risk assessment, but dyslipidemia alone does not exclude kidney donation

Acceptable donor renal function

All potential kidney donors should have GFR estimated

Creatinine-based methods may be used to estimate the GFR; however, creatinine clearance (as calculated from 24-hour urine collections) may under or overestimate GFR in patients with normal or near normal renal function

Calculated GFR values (MDRD and Cockcroft-Gault) are not standardized in this population and may overestimate GFR

A GFR 80 mL/min or 2SD below normal (based on age, gender, and BSA corrected to 1.73/m^2) generally precludes donation

Urine analysis for protein

A 24-hour urine protein of >300 mg is a contraindication to donation

Microalbuminuria determination may be a more reliable marker of renal disease, but its value as an international standard of evaluation for kidney donors has not been determined

Urine analysis for blood

Patients with persistent microscopic hematuria should not be considered for kidney donation unless urine cytology and a complete urologic workup are performed. If urological malignancy and stone disease are excluded, a kidney biopsy may be indicated to rule out glomerular pathology, such as IgA nephropathy

Diabetes

Individuals with a history of diabetes or fasting blood glucose 126 mg/dL (7.0 nmol/L) on at least two occasions (or 2-hour glucose with OGTT 200 mg/dL (11.1 mmol/L) should not donate

Stone disease

An asymptomatic potential donor with history of a single stone may be suitable for kidney donation if:

- No hypercalciuria, hyperuricemia, or metabolic acidosis
- No cystinuria or hyperoxaluria
- No urinary tract infection
- If multiple stones or nephrocalcinosis are not evident on CT

(continued)

Table 17.2 (continued)

An asymptomatic potential donor with a current single stone may be suitable if:

- The donor meets the criteria shown previously for single stone formers and current stone <1.5 cm in size, or potentially removable during the transplant

Stone formers who should not donate are those with:

- Nephrocalcinosis on X-ray or bilateral stone disease
- Stone types with high recurrence rates, and are difficult to prevent (see text)

Malignancy

A prior history of the following malignancies usually excludes live kidney donation:

- Melanoma, testicular cancer, renal cell carcinoma, choriocarcinoma, hematological malignancy, bronchial cancer, breast cancer, and monoclonal gammopathy

A prior history of malignancy may only be acceptable for donation if:

- Prior treatment of the malignancy does not decrease renal reserve or place the donor at increased risk for ESRD
- Prior treatment of malignancy does not increase the operative risk of nephrectomy
- A prior history of malignancy usually excludes live kidney donation but may be acceptable if: The specific cancer is curable and potential transmission of cancer can reasonably be excluded

Urinary tract infections

The donor urine should be sterile prior to donation; asymptomatic bacteria should be treated per donation

Pyuria and hematuria at the proposed time of donation are contraindications to donation

Unexplained hematuria or pyuria necessitates evaluation for adenovirus, tuberculosis, and cancer. Urinary tuberculosis or cancer is contraindication to donation

Live unrelated donors

The current available data suggest no restriction of live kidney donation based upon the absence of an HLA match. An unrelated donor transplant is equally successful to the outcome achieved by a genetically related family member such as a parent, child, or sibling, who is not HLA identical to the recipient

Determination of cardiovascular risk

The clinical predictors of an increased perioperative cardiovascular risk (for non-cardiac surgery) by the American College of Cardiology/American Hospital Association standards fall into three categories: major, intermediate, minor

All major predictors: unstable coronary syndromes, decompensated heart failure, significant arrhythmias, and severe valvular disease are contraindications to live kidney donation

Most of the intermediate predictors: mild angina, previous myocardial infarction, compensated or prior heart failure, and diabetes mellitus are also contraindications to donation;

Minor predictors: older age, abnormal ECG, rhythm other than sinus, low cardiac functional capacity, and history of stroke or uncontrolled hypertension warrant individual consideration

Assessment of pulmonary issues

A careful history and physical examination are the most important parts of assessing risk

Routine preoperative pulmonary function testing (PFT) is not warranted for potential live kidney donors unless there is an associated risk factor such as chronic lung disease

Increased risk of postoperative pulmonary complication is associated with an FEV1 70 % or FVC 70 % of predicted, or a ratio of FEV1/FVC 65 %

Smoking cessation and alcohol abstinence

Smoking cessation at least 4 weeks prior to donation is advised based on recommendations for patients undergoing elective surgical procedures

Cessation of alcohol abuse defined by DSM-3: 60 g of alcohol/day sustained over 6 months should be avoided for a minimum of 4 weeks to decrease the known risk of postoperative morbidity

BP blood pressure, *ABPM* ambulatory blood pressure monitoring, *GFR* glomerular filtration rate, *BMI* body mass index, *BSA* body surface area, *CT* computed tomography, *ESRD* end-stage renal disease, *HLA* human leukocyte antigen

Although these reports of the Amsterdam forum present a comprehensive review of the international practice of live kidney donation derived from a reflection of published data and physician experience, they are still only guidelines, but not a regulation.

As for the development of medical assessment and treatment for the problems which contraindicate a potential donor, this guideline may be reevaluated to adjust current practice.

Routine medical evaluation of the donor should be started with a history and physical examination and repeated measurement of blood pressure. If there is any history of major illness, including cardiovascular, pulmonary, or liver disease with significant comorbidities, donor candidates are typically excluded.

Routine diagnostic tests for donor candidate include:

1. Urinalysis: Dipstick for protein, blood, and glucose, microscopy, urine culture, and urinary albumin/protein to creatinine ratio
2. Blood tests: Complete blood count, hematological profile, and coagulation screen [international normalized ratio (INR), activated partial thromboplastin time (APTT)]
3. Blood chemistry: Electrolytes, blood urea nitrogen (BUN), creatinine, calcium, phosphate, magnesium, liver function test, and albumin
4. Fasting plasma glucose and glucose tolerance test
5. Lipid profile: Low-density lipoprotein cholesterol (LDL-C), triglyceride (TG), and high-density lipoprotein cholesterol (HDL-C)
6. Tumor marker: Prostate-specific antigen (male, >50 years old)
7. Virology and infectious screening: Hepatitis B and C, syphilis, human immunodeficiency virus and human T-cell leukemia virus, measles, rubella, herpes zoster, Epstein–Barr virus, herpes simplex, and cytomegalovirus
8. Fecal occult blood test and colonoscopy (if positive fecal occult blood test)
9. Cardiopulmonary system: Chest X-ray, electrocardiogram, stress test, and echocardiogram (if indicated)
10. Assessment of renal function: Estimation or measurement of glomerular filtration rate (GFR)
11. Renal imaging: Renal ultrasound and computed tomography with 3D imaging of vasculature

17.1.3 Assessment for Donor Renal Function

Some centers rely on 24-h urine collections for both creatinine clearance and proteinuria. But most centers utilize more accurate assessment of GFR to determine cutoff levels for an acceptable living kidney donor. Although a GFR of 80 ml/min/1.73 m^2 is the typical cutoff value for donation to maintain optimal renal function after nephrectomy, as many as 20 % of US and European transplant centers would accept as low as 60 ml/min [8, 10, 11]. The value of GFR can be age dependent, which declines as individuals age [12].

Classical methods for measurement of GFR by inulin clearance require an intravenous infusion and timed urine collections. It is not always clinically feasible. Excellent alternatives to estimate GFR have been studied using equations based on serum creatinine, sex, age, and ethnicity. The most commonly used formulas are the Cockcroft–Gault and MDRD (Modification of Diet in Renal Disease Study) equation. Those equations were developed and validated from mainly chronic kidney disease subject (CKD) including small population of healthy subjects. The GFR can be overestimated or underestimated in healthy individuals such as donors [13]. Also multilevel ethnic variables have been required for more accurate estimation [14]; a national equation has been developed in Japan [13].

Currently more accurate assessment equations have been developed using age, sex, serum creatinine, and cystatin C as parameters [15, 16]. Those equations will be tested and validated in healthy individuals including living donors as the best alternatives to estimate GFR.

Furthermore, assessment for the functional laterality is another critical issue to preserve better renal function for donor. Nuclear medicine is noninvasive and does not harm renal function to accurately evaluate split renal function using dimercaptosuccinic acid (DMSA), mercaptotriglycine (MAG3), or DTPA, but its use for donor evaluation may enhance a medical economical problem. Previously, CT volumetry has been introduced as an alternative to nuclear medicine and estimated preserved renal function for donors [17].

17.1.3.1 Assessment for Cancer

Kidney donor candidate should be screened for both personal and family history of malignancy. They should be screened with age- and gender-matched tests as recommended by national organization. Active malignancy and infection are usually also contraindications, but may be acceptable if the specific cancer is curable and potential transmission of cancer can reasonably be excluded [6]. Examples include colon cancer (Dukes A, >5 years ago), nonmelanoma skin cancer, or carcinoma in situ of the cervix [18].

17.2 Background: Historical Trials to Extend Living Donor Criteria

17.2.1 Old Donor

The success of LKD transplantation, the organ shortage, and death on the waiting list have opened the window to accept the extended criteria for old live kidney donors [19].

There is no official upper limit for LKD age, but in many publications, a donor is considered old if over 60 or 65 and sometimes over 70.

In the USA living donors older than 65 were 3.6 % in 2000, gradually growing and doubled in 2010 to 7.3 % among all ages [3]. Report from Japanese registry reported by Kitada et al. has revealed that 511 living donors among 1,144 of all donors were at age more than 60 in 2010 which include 93 (8.1 %) in their 70s and 5 in the 80s [20].

Kidney donation from older living donor has two issues to define its underlying problems. One issue is that are the risks for mortality and long-term renal function for the donor small enough? Another issue is whether the results of transplantation are acceptable for the recipients.

17.2.1.1 Mortality and Renal Function for Donors

In a cohort of 80,347 LKD (1994–2004), Segev et al. [21] reported the results according to the age of the donor that the 3-month mortality ranged from 3.0 of 10,000 for LKD between 18 and 39 to 6.6 for those over 60 years and did not change during the last 15 years. With a mean follow-up of 6.3 years (3.2–9.8), mortality was not significantly different when older donors were compared with general population [21]. Another study focused on LKD who were >70 compared their mortality rate with general population found similar mortality rate in both goups up to 10 years of follow-up [19]. Regarding to renal function after donation, older living donors are more likely to develop both lower GFR, less than 60 ml/min/1.73 m^2, and hypertension. But increased risk to develop end-stage renal disease was not found compared to the general population.

17.2.1.2 Outcome of Transplantation from Older Donors

It is clear that the age of the donor has an impact on the transplant outcome. Currently, Lim et al. [22] defined old living donor more than 60 years and recently reported the graft consequences from 346 old living donor (OLD) kidneys among the 6,317 renal transplant recipients using Australia and New Zealand Dialysis and Transplant Registry. Compared with kidneys from standard criteria donor (SCD), OLD kidneys were associated with a greater risk of death-censored graft failure (DCGF; HR 2.00) and an inferior 5-year graft function, although no increase in 5-year mortality. Patient survival was equal, but graft outcomes for recipients of OLD kidneys were inferior to those obtained with YLD and SCD kidneys. This study suggests that OLD kidneys should be utilized cautiously, cognizant of the fact that younger recipients may have a life expectancy in excess of the life of the transplanted kidney.

To evaluate even older donor, Berger et al. [19] have compared the outcome of 219 old donors, defining more than 70 years, with the ones of 16,062 younger

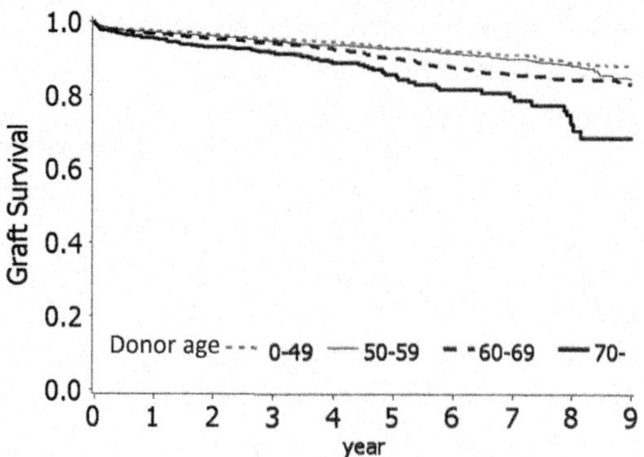

Fig. 17.3 Graft survival after living kidney transplantation after 2000 in Japan (from Japanese registry data). Five-year graft survival reveals more than 90 % with younger donors, and equivalent 5-year graft survival of 85.7 % was achieved with older donors more than 70

donors, defining 50–59 years using the Scientific Registry of Transplant Recipients (SRTR). Among recipients of older live donor allografts, graft loss was significantly higher than matched 50–59-year-old live donor allografts (subhazard ratio [SHR] 1.62), but similar to matched nonextended criteria 50–59-year-old deceased donor allografts. Mortality among living kidney donors aged 70 was not higher, even lower, than the general population. These findings support living donation among older adults more than 70 years, but highlight the advantages of finding a younger donor, particularly for younger recipients.

Kitada et al. based on Japanese registry data have reported excellent 5- and 10-year graft survival in current era with 89.6 % in 5-year and 65.5 % in 10-year graft survivals, even with aged living-donor more than 70 [20] (Fig. 17.3).

In a recent meta-analysis for which the objective was to compare graft survival and graft function in recipients of a kidney from an old (60–85 years) or a young LKD (30–55 years), the donor network reported that graft survival was significantly lower at 5 years when the donor is >60 (72 vs. 80 %, $P<0.05$) [23].

Finally, transplantation from an old living donor appeared to be a reasonably safe procedure for both the donor and the recipient and the age per se is certainly not a contraindication to donation.

17.2.2 Obese Donor

Obesity was defined by a body mass index (BMI) of >30 kg/m^2, and BMI above 35 is generally considered as a relative contraindication for donation. All potential donors should have BMI determined at initial evaluation. Evaluation should also include other comorbidities associated with obesity such as microalbuminuria, impaired GTT, hypertension, hyperlipidemia, cardiovascular disease, sleep apnea, and liver disease.

Obesity should be considered an increased risk for renal disease; however, there is no data on the outcome of such individuals.

Kidney donation from obese donor has two issues to define its underlying concern. One is the risk for morbidity and mortality of donor nephrectomy. Another issue is long-term results of renal function.

Currently systematic meta-analysis regarding perioperative outcome of live donor nephrectomy between donors with high and low BMI revealed that significant differences in favor of low BMI (29.9 and less) donors have been found in operation duration, rise in serum creatinine, and risk ratio for conversion from laparoscopic surgery to open surgery [24]. And higher BMI was associated with both GFR that was lower than 60 ml/min/1.73 m^2 and hypertension, but equivalent prevalence of coexisting conditions compared with BMI matched general population [25].

Thus, a high BMI less than 35 alone is no contraindication for live kidney donation regarding short-term and long-term outcome.

Another concern regarding the acceptance of obese donor is if potential donors with BMI more than 35 are acceptable for donation. Short-term outcome of such individuals with laparoscopic donor nephrectomy has been described with higher incidence of minor postoperative complications, but equivalent rate of major perioperative complications, renal function and microalbuminuria [26, 27].

Thus, obese donors have higher baseline cardiovascular risk and warrant risk reduction for long-term health. While current results with obese donor, BMI less than 35, are encouraging, careful additional study of obese donors with BMI more than 35 is advocated until long-term outcome is available.

17.2.3 Hypertension

Generally, hypertension, resting blood pressure greater than140/90 mmHg, has been considered to be a contraindication in potential renal transplant donors because sequential development of progressive hypertension after uninephrectomy and proteinuria deteriorates renal function [28].

However, several studies have reported long-term follow-up of living donors suggesting a small increase in the risk of hypertension and proteinuria. And the risk of developing renal failure does not appear to be increased [29–31]. Current trends of increasing the number of old and obese donors have also brought the increasing number of potential living donors who also have hypertension.

In general, screening for hypertension in a potential donor includes BP measurement on three separate occasions. But as for a more precise assessment for diagnosing hypertension, BP should preferably be measured by ambulatory blood pressure monitoring (ABPM) according to the guideline by the Joint National Committee (JNC 7).

Most centers follow the indications regarding hypertension for potential donors as indicated in the Amsterdam forum [8]. Patients with a BP > 140/90 mmHg by ABPM are generally not acceptable as donors. Some patients with easily controlled hypertension who meet other defined criteria (e.g., ≥50 years of age, GFR ≥ 80 ml/min, and urinary albumin excretion <30 mg/day) may represent a low-risk group for development of kidney disease after donation and may be acceptable as kidney donors. UK survey of seventy-four medical centers revealed that 64 % of units exclude donors only if they are on more than two antihypertensive drugs.

Textor and colleagues reported a result of a structured program accepting hypertensive donors if kidney function and urine protein were normal [32]. This study, included 148 donors with 24 hypertensive individuals, indicated that donors with moderate, essential hypertension and normal kidney function have no adverse effects regarding blood pressure, GFR, or urinary protein excretion during the first year after living kidney donation. Moreover, blood pressure in hypertensive donors even fell with both nonpharmacologic and drug therapy.

More recently Tent H and colleagues evaluate short-term and 1- and 5-year renal outcome of living kidney donors with preexistent hypertension [33]. Among 47 hypertensive donors and 94 control donors, the predonation difference in blood pressure was lost after donation. Both at 1 and 5 years after donation blood pressure was similar. Renal function was similar at all time points. They defined hypertensive donor as antihypertensive drug use predonation, and donors were found eligible to donate with a well-regulated blood pressure achieved by a maximum of two antihypertensive drugs. Those studies indicate that selected hypertensive patients may be accepted for living kidney donation.

However, previous Japanese study indicates that even pre-hypertension could be a significant predictor of CKD in a general population [34].

Further long-term studies with strict follow-up and medical control of blood pressure are essential to ensure preservation of renal function for living kidney donors with well-regulatd hypertension.

17.2.4 Diabetes Mellitus

When the recipient has diabetes mellitus, the risk of related donors developing diabetes later in life is a major concern. And all potential living kidney donors related to recipients with diabetes have been reported to have a preexisting increased risk of developing diabetes and diabetic nephropathy [35].

All potential living donors should have a fasting plasma glucose estimation to exclude undiagnosed diabetes or glucose intolerance. Most transplantation centers regard established diabetes mellitus as a contraindication to living donation, and many centers exclude individuals deemed as high risk.

Although little is known as to whether single-kidney status would accelerate the progression of diabetic nephropathy, Silveiro and colleagues [36] suggested that nephrectomy in a patient with type 2 diabetes might increase the progression of renal disease and microalbuminuria.

Some centers have been attempting to expand the window for renal donors by advising lifestyle modifications including weight control, diet, exercise, and tobacco and excessive alcohol avoidance to proposed donors with impaired fasting glucose, impaired glucose tolerance, and other risk factors [18]. Okamoto and colleagues

[37] evaluated long-term outcome of living renal donors including 13 diabetic donors among 601, none of these donors developed renal failure. Feasibility to include potential donors with impaired glucose tolerance and controlled diabetes might be evaluated in the near future, but accurate patient selection and systematic counseling of lifestyle modification must be mandatory to avoid a deterioration of renal function after donation.

Individuals with a history of diabetes or fasting blood glucose of ≥126 mg/dl (7.0 mmol/l) on at least two occasions [or 2-h glucose with OGTT≥200 mg/dl (11.1 mmol/l)] should not donate. And patients with significant risk factors for developing type 2 diabetes such as a familial history, a BMI of ≥30 kg/m^2, women with the history of gestational diabetes, and excessive alcohol use should be carefully evaluated as potential renal donors.

17.2.5 Nephrolithiasis

Up to 12 % of men and 5 % of women will develop a symptomatic kidney stone during their lifetime [38]. At a mean follow-up of 7.5 years 27 % of patients experienced symptomatic recurrence [39].

A history of urinary tract stones has been at least a relative contraindication to donation because urinary stones tend to recur and may cause obstruction of a solitary kidney [40]. While the prevalence of asymptomatic solitary nephrolithiasis has increased with the widespread use of screening computerized tomography angiography during renal donor evaluation, the indication for renal donor regarding urinary stone was relaxed previously in the Amsterdam forum [8].

According to the Amsterdam forum, an asymptomatic potential donor with a history of a single stone may be suitable for kidney donation if (1) no hypercalciuria, hyperuricemia, or metabolic acidosis, (2) no cystinuria or hyperoxaluria, (3) no urinary tract infection, and (4) multiple stones or nephrocalcinosis is not evident on computed tomography (CT) scan.

Contraindications to donation in individuals with urinary stones are (1) nephrocalcinosis on X-ray or bilateral stone disease and (2) stone types that have high recurrence rates and are difficult to prevent, such as

1. Cystine stones that have a high rate of recurrence and a need for urologic procedures in the donor.
2. Struvite stones or infection stones that are difficult to eradicate, and thus it is not feasible to transplant a kidney with them into an immunosuppressed patient.
3. Stones associated with inherited or other systemic disorders, such as primary or enteric hyperoxaluria, distal renal tubular acidosis, and sarcoid because of the probability of a high rate of recurrence and the risk of renal insufficiency.
4. Stones in the setting of inflammatory bowel disease with an increased risk of stones particularly after bowel resection, also increased risk of renal insufficiency.
5. Recurrence while on appropriate treatment (i.e., failed therapy).

Asymptomatic potential donor with current single stone may be suitable if:

1. The donor meets the criteria shown previously for single-stone formers and current stone is ≤1.5 cm in size or potentially removable during transplant.

Another important point is the age of the donor. Younger patients have a longer exposure to risk of recurrence. A stone initially detected in a person older than 50 years is unlikely to recur. In contrast, the risk for stone recurrence is higher in donor candidates aged 25–35 years and must be considered during the evaluation process of donors.

It is unknown whether asymptomatic stone disease has similar risk factor and comorbidity associations among persons with asymptomatic vs. symptomatic kidney stones have not been adequately characterized.

Lorenz EC and colleagues reported that among 1957 potential kidney donors, 3 % had past symptomatic stones and 10 % had asymptomatic radiographic stones. And asymptomatic stone formers were not characterized by older age, male gender, hypertension, obesity, metabolic syndrome, abnormal kidney function, hyperuricemia, hypercalcemia, or hypophosphatemia which has been described as the risk factors of symptomatic stone former [41]. These findings suggest that different pathophysiologic mechanisms could be involved in asymptomatic stone formation vs. symptomatic stone passage. And the impacts of asymptomatic stone on remnant kidney function and clinical event may be different from the one of symptomatic stone.

Consequence of kidney transplant after removal of asymptomatic stone has been reported without recurrent stone formation for both donor and recipients up to 5-year follow-up [42–44].

As for assessment of symptomatic stone, ex vivo ureteroscopic treatment can be safely used to remove stones from kidneys before transplantation, without the risk of subjecting the donor to an additional stone-removing procedure.

Based on recent clinical evaluations, it appears that the risk of recurrence and subsequent morbidity in renal donors with a solitary kidney is low but not insignificant. Renal donors and recipients should be educated regarding their unique risk perspectives. Long-term follow-up is mandatory [45].

17.3 Prognosis for Living Donors

17.3.1 Short–Middle-Term Prognosis

Donor mortality after donor surgery is extremely low, but not absent. In 1973, postoperative mortality was estimated at 0.1 % in the USA [46]. In the 1980s, this percentage decreased to 0.04 % [47]. In the 1990s, estimated mortality was 0.03 % [48].

In the 2000s, standard surgery for donor has been shifted from open surgery to laparoscopic procedure. Matas and colleagues [49] surveyed 234 UNOS-listed kidney transplant programs, 171 (73 %) responded, to determine living donor morbidity and mortality in different surgical modalities (open nephrectomy, hand-assisted laparoscopic nephrectomy (LN), and non-hand-assisted LN). Between 1999 and 2001, these centers carried out 10,828 living donor nephrectomies: 52.3 % open, 20.7 % hand-assisted LN, and 27 % non-hand-assisted LN. Two donors (0.02 %) died from surgical complications and one is in a persistent vegetative state (all after LN). Reoperation was necessary in 22 (0.4 %) open, 23 (1.0 %) hand-assisted LN, and 21 (0.9 %) non hand-assisted LN cases ($p=0.001$). Mortality rates of 1 out of 3,000 and complication rate of around 1 % have been reported.

However, current meta-analysis revealed equivalent comorbidity between LN or open nephrectomy for perioperative complications (RR 0.87), reoperations (RR 0.57), early graft loss (RR 0.31), delayed graft function (RR 1.09), acute rejection (RR 1.41), ureteric complications (RR 1.51), kidney function at 1 year (SMD 0.15), or graft loss at 1 year (RR 0.76) [50].

More recent data evaluated mortality risk within 90 days of live kidney donation between 1994 and 2009 [64] from US registry data. There were 25 deaths among 80,347 live kidney donors. Surgical mortality from live kidney donation was 3.1 per 10,000 donors and did not change during the last 15 years despite differences in practice and selection. Surgical mortality was higher in men than in women (5.1 vs. 1.7 per 10,000 donors; risk ratio 3.0), in black vs. white and Hispanic individuals (7.6 vs. 2.6 and 2.0 per 10,000 donors; RR, 3.1), and in donors with hypertension vs. without hypertension (36.7 vs. 1.3 per 10,000 donors; RR, 27.4). However, among a cohort of live kidney donors compared with a healthy matched cohort, the mortality rate was not significantly increased after a median of 6.3 years [21].

Based on OPTN/SRTR 2011 Annual Report, 12 living donors (0.02 %) are dead within 30 days of donation among 62,813 donors between 2002 and 2011 [3]. Among 12 deaths of living donors within 30 days of donation, ten donors died of medical event and two by accident/homicide (Table 17.2).

The Japan Society for Transplantation had reported that there was no perioperative death of living donor up to 2011 [2], but faced 2 perioperative deaths in 2013.

17.3.2 Long-Term Prognosis

Although all transplant programs have a responsibility to follow up living donor during their lifetime with high priority, 40 % of the programs face difficulty achieving it by current survey. Improvements may occur if programs work with donors to develop plans to achieve follow-up, programmatic standards are set for completeness in follow-up data reporting, and sufficient staff resources are available to ensure ongoing postdonation contact [51].

Early excellent study regarding long-term live donor prognosis was published in 1997 by Swedish group. Mortality was calculated from a sample of 430 Swedish donors (which corresponds to >80 % of the donors in this center). The authors describe 41 deaths occurring from 15 months to 31 years after the donation. Once again, for these authors, this mortality rate is 30 % less than the mortality observed in the general Swedish population [52].

Okamoto and colleagues [37] published a Japanese study including 481donors (which corresponds to 80 % of the donors in their center.). Three donors (0.5 %) experienced major perioperative complications, that is, femoral nerve compression, pulmonary thrombosis, and acute renal failure; all of the donors recovered and left the hospital without complications. Three donors developed ESRD to require hemodialysis 79, 99, and 276 months after donation due to chronic glomerulonephritis. Donor survival rates at 5, 10, 20, and 30 years were 98.3 %, 94.7 %, 86.4 %, and 66.2 %, respectively. The survival rate of kidney donors was better than the age- and gender-matched cohort from the general population, and the patterns and causes of death were similar.

The largest study on long-term consequences was published from a Minnesota group evaluating 3,698 kidney donors [25]. They have also evaluated GFR and urinary albumin excretion and assessed the prevalence of hypertension, general health status, and quality of life in 255 donors. ESRD developed in 11 donors, a rate of 180 cases per million persons per year, as compared with a rate of 268 per million persons per year in the general population. At a mean (±SD) of 12.2 ± 9.2 years after donation, survival and the risk of ESRD appear to be similar to those in the general population. Most donors who were studied had a preserved GFR, a normal albumin excretion, and an excellent quality of life.

More recently Mjøen and colleagues [53] reported a Norwegian survey among 2,269 living kidney donors between 1963 and 2007. A median observation time was 14.3 years. Causes of donor's death were similar for donors and controls. By Kaplan–Meier analysis, overall and cardiovascular mortality was lower for previous kidney donors than for matched controls ($P<0.001$ and $P=0.004$, respectively).

As expansion of live donor criteria, precise evaluation of long-term consequences of live donor is warranted. And national registry may play a central role to provide reliable information rather than single institutional evaluation.

References

1. Wolfe R, Ashby V, Milford E. Comparison of mortality in all patients on dialysis, patients on dialysis awaiting transplantation, and recipients of a first cadaveric transplant. N Engl J Med. 1999;341:1725–30.
2. Fact Book 2011. Japanese Society of Transplantation. http://www.asas.or.jp/jst/pdf/factbook/factbook2011.pdf.
3. OPTN/SRTR 2011. Annual report. http://srtr.transplant.hrsa.gov/annual_reports/2011/default.aspx.
4. Rodriguea JR, Cornellb DL, Linc JK, Kapland B, Howarde RJ. Increasing live donor kidney transplantation: a randomized controlled trial of a home-based educational intervention. Am J Transplant. 2007;7:394–401.

5. Moorea DR, Feurera ID, Zavalaa EY, Shaffera D, Karpa S, Hoya H. A web-based application for initial screening of living kidney donors: development, implementation and evaluation. Am J Transplant. 2013;13:450–7.
6. Lapasia JB, Kong S-Y, Busque S, Scandling JD, Chertow GM, Tan JC. Living donor evaluation and exclusion: the Stanford experience. Clin Transplant. 2011;25(5):697–704.
7. McCurdie FJ, Pascoe MD, Broomberg CJ, Kahn D. Outcome of assessment of potential donors for live donor kidney transplants. Transplant Proc. 2005;37:605–6.
8. Delmonico F. A report of the Amsterdam forum on the care of the live kidney donor: data and medical guidelines. Transplantation. 2005;79:53–66.
9. Ethics Committee of the Transplantation Society. The consensus statement of the Amsterdam forum on the care of the live kidney donor. Transplantation. 2004;78:491.
10. Kasiske BL, Bia MJ. The evaluation and selection of living kidney donors. Am J Kidney Dis. 1995;26:387.
11. Gabolde M, Hervé C, Moulin AM. Evaluation, selection, and follow-up of live kidney donors: a review of current practice in French renal transplant centres. Nephrol Dial Transplant. 2001;16(10):2048–52.
12. Imai E, Matsuo S, Makino H, Watanabe T, Akizawa T, Nitta K, Iimuro S, Ohashi Y, Hishida A. Chronic Kidney Disease Japan Cohort study: baseline characteristics and factors associated with causative diseases and renal function. Clin Exp Nephrol. 2010;14(6):558–70. doi:10.1007/s10157-010-0328-6 [Epub 2010 Aug 11].
13. Horio M, Yasuda Y, Kaimori J, Ichimaru N, Isaka Y, Takahara S, Nishi S, Uchida K, Takeda A, Hattori R, Kitada H, Tsuruya K, Imai E, Takahashi K, Watanabe T, Matsuo S. Performance of the Japanese GFR equation in potential kidney donors. Clin Exp Nephrol. 2012;16(3):415–20.
14. Stevens LA, Claybon MA, Schmid CH, Chen J, Horio M, Imai E, Nelson RG, Van Deventer M, Wang HY, Zuo L, Zhang YL, Levey AS. Evaluation of the chronic kidney disease epidemiology collaboration equation for estimating the glomerular filtration rate in multiple ethnicities. Kidney Int. 2011;79(5):555–62. doi:10.1038/ki.2010.462. Epub 2010 Nov 24.
15. Inker LA, Schmid CH, Tighiouart H, The CKD-EPI Investigators, et al. Estimating glomerular filtration rate from serum creatinine and cystatin C. N Engl J Med. 2012;367(1):20–9.
16. Horio M, Imai E, Yasuda Y, Watanabe T, Matsuo S, Collaborators Developing the Japanese Equation for Estimated GFR. GFR estimation using standardized serum cystatin C in Japan. Am J Kidney Dis. 2013;61(2):197–203. doi:10.1053/j.ajkd.2012.07.007. Epub 2012 Aug 11.
17. Yakoubi R, Autorino R, Kassab A, Long JA, Haber GP, Kaouk JH. Does preserved kidney volume predict 1 year donor renal function after laparoscopic living donor nephrectomy? Int J Urol. 2013;20(9):931–4. doi:10.1111/iju.12080 [Epub ahead of print].
18. Caliskan Y, Yildiz A. Evaluation of the medically complex living kidney donor. J Transplant. 2012;2012:6. Article ID 450471.
19. Berger JC, Muzaale AD, James N, Hoque M, Wang JMG, Montgomery RA, Massie AB, Hall EC, Segev DL. Living kidney donors ages 70 and older: recipient and donor outcomes. Clin J Am Soc Nephrol. 2011;6:2887–93.
20. Kitada H, Tanaka M, Tsuruya K. Perspectives of organ transplantation in an aging society: present status and problems of aged renal donor. Isyoku. 2012;47(2&3):166–74.
21. Segev DL, Muzaale AD, Caffo BS, Mehta SH, Singer AL, Taranto SE, McBride MA, Montgomery RA. Perioperative mortality and long-term survival following live kidney donation. JAMA. 2010;303(10):959–66.
22. Lim WH, Clayton P, Wong G, Campbell SB, Cohney S, Russ GR, Chadban SJ, McDonald SP. Outcomes of kidney transplantation from older living donors. Transplantation. 2013;95:106–13.
23. Iordanous Y, Seymour N, Young A, Donor Nephrectomy Outcomes Research (DONOR) Network, et al. Recipient outcomes for expanded criteria living kidney donors: the disconnect-between current evidence and practice. Am J Transplant. 2009;9:1558–73.
24. Lafranca JA, Hagen SM, Dols LF, Arends LR, Weimar W, Ijzermans JN, Dor FJ. Systematic review and meta-analysis of the relation between body mass index and short-term donor outcome of laparoscopic donor nephrectomy. Kidney Int. 2013;83:931–9.

25. Ibrahim HN, Foley R, Tan L, Rogers T, Bailey RF, Guo H, Gross CR, Matas AJ. Long-term consequences of kidney donation. N Engl J Med. 2009;360:459–69.
26. O'Brien B, Mastoridis S, Crane J, Hakim N, Papalois V. Safety of nephrectomy in morbidly obese donors. Exp Clin Transplant. 2012;10(6):579–85.
27. Heimbach JK, Taler SJ, Prieto M, Cosio FG, Textor SC, Kudva YC, Chow GK, Ishitani MB, Larson TS, Stegall MD. Obesity in living kidney donors: clinical characteristics and outcomes in the era of laparoscopic donor nephrectomy. Am J Transplant. 2005;5(5):1057–64.
28. Hakim RM, Goldszer RC, Renner BM. Hypertension and proteinuria: long-term sequelae of uninephrectomy in human kidney. Kidney Int. 1984;25:930.
29. Goldfarb DA, Matin SF, Braun WE, et al. Renal outcome 25 years after donor nephrectomy. J Urol. 2001;166:2043–7.
30. Gossmann J, Wilhelm A, Kachel HG, et al. Long-term consequences of live kidney donation follow-up in 93 % of living kidney donors in a single transplant center. Am J Transplant. 2005;5:2417–24.
31. Boudville N, Prasad GV, Knoll G, et al. Meta-analysis: risk for hypertension in living kidney donors. Ann Intern Med. 2006;145:185–96.
32. Textor SC, Taler SJ, Driscoll N, et al. Blood pressure and renal function after kidney donation from hypertensive living donors. Transplantation. 2004;78:276.
33. Tent H, Sanders JS, Rook M, Hofker HS, Ploeg RJ, Navis G, Van der Heide JJ. Effects of preexistent hypertension on blood pressure and residual renal function after donor nephrectomy. Transplantation. 2012;93:412–7.
34. Kanno A, Kikuya M, Ohkubo T, Hashimoto T, Satoh M, Hirose T, Obara T, Metoki H, Inoue R, Asayama K, Shishido Y, Hoshi H, Nakayama M, Totsune K, Satoh H, Sato H, Imai Y. Pre-hypertension as a significant predictor of chronic kidney disease in a general population: the Ohasama study. Nephrol Dial Transplant. 2012;27(8):3218–23. doi:10.1093/ndt/gfs054. Epub 2012 Apr 17.
35. Simmons D, Searle M. Personal paper: risk of diabetic nephropathy in potential living related kidney donors. Br Med J. 1998;316(7134):846–8.
36. Silveiro SP, Da Costa LA, Beck MO, Gross JL. Urinary albumin excretion rate and glomerular filtration rate in single-kidney type 2 diabetic patients. Diabetes Care. 1998;21(9):1521–4.
37. Okamoto M, Akioka K, Nobori S, Ushigome H, Kozaki K, Kaihara S, Yoshimura N. Short and long-term donor outcomes after kidney donation: analysis of 601 cases over a 35 year period at Japanese single center. Transplantation. 2009;87:419–23.
38. Stamatelou KK, Francis ME, Jones CA, et al. Time trends in reported prevalence of kidney stones in the United States: 1976–1994. Kidney Int. 2003;63:1817–23.
39. Trinchieri A, Ostini F, Nespoli R, Rovera F, Montanari E, Zanetti G. A prospective study of recurrence rate and risk factors for recurrence after a first renal stone. J Urol. 1999;162:27.
40. Kasiske BL, Ravenscraft M, Ramos EL, Gaston RS, Bia MJ, Danovitch GM. The evaluation of living renal transplant donors: clinical practice guidelines. Ad Hoc clinical practice guidelines subcommittee of the patient care and education committee of the American society of transplant physicians. J Am Soc Nephrol. 1996;7:2288.
41. Lorenz EC, Lieske JC, Vrtiska TJ, Krambeck AE, Li X, Bergstralh EJ, Melton 3rd LJ, Rule AD. Clinical characteristics of potential kidney donors with asymptomatic kidney stones. Nephrol Dial Transplant. 2011;26(8):2695–700. doi:10.1093/ndt/gfq769. Epub 2011 Feb 1.
42. Schade GR, Wolf JS, Faerber GJ. Ex-vivo ureteroscopy at the time of live donor nephrectomy. J Endourol. 2011;25(9):1405–9. doi:10.1089/end.2010.0627. Epub 2011 Jun 28; Department of Urology, University of Michigan, Ann Arbor, Michigan, USA.
43. Rashid MG, Konnak JW, Wolf Jr JS, Punch JD, Magee JC, Arenas JD, Faerber GJ. Ex vivo ureteroscopic treatment of calculi in donor kidneys at renal transplantation. J Urol. 2004;171(1):58–60. Source: Department of Urology, University of Michigan Medical Center, Ann Arbor, 48109, USA.
44. Olsburgh J, Thomas K, Wong K, Bultitude M, Glass J, Rottenberg G, Silas L, Hilton R, Koffman G. Incidental renal stones in potential live kidney donors: prevalence, assessment and

donation, including role of ex vivo ureteroscopy. BJU Int. 2013;111(5):784–92. doi:10.1111/j.1464-410X.2012.11572.x. Epub 2012 Oct 30.
45. Strang AM, Lockhart ME, Amling CL, Kolettis PN, Burns JR. Living renal donor allograft lithiasis: a review of stone related morbidity in donors and recipients. J Urol. 2008;179(3):832–6. doi:10.1016/j.juro.2007.10.022. Epub 2008 Jan 25.
46. Ogden DA. Consequences of renal donation in man. Am J Kidney Dis. 1983;2:501–11.
47. Bay WH, Hebert LA. The living donor in kidney transplantation. Ann Intern Med. 1987;106:719–27.
48. Najarian JS, Chavers BM, McHugh LE, et al. 20 years or more of follow-up of living kidney donors. Lancet. 1992;340:807–10.
49. Matas AJ, Bartlettb ST, Leichtmanc AB, Delmonicod FL. Morbidity and mortality after living kidney donation, 1999–2001: survey of United States transplant centers. Am J Transplant. 2003;3:830–4.
50. Wilson CH, Sanni A, Rix DA, Soomro NA. Laparoscopic versus open nephrectomy for live kidney donors. Cochrane Database Syst Rev. 2011;(11):CD006124.
51. Waterman AD, Dew MA, Davis CL, McCabe M, Wainright JL, Forland CL, Bolton L, Cooper M. Living-donor follow-up attitudes and practices in US: kidney and liver donor programs. Transplantation. 2013;95:883–8.
52. Fehrman-Ekholm I, Elinder CG, Stenbeck M, et al. Kidney donors live longer. Transplantation. 1997;64:976–8.
53. Mjøen G, Reisaeter A, Hallan S, Line PD, Hartmann A, Midtvedt K, Foss A, Dahle DO, Holdaas H. Overall and cardiovascular mortality in Norwegian kidney donors compared to the background population. Nephrol Dial Transplant. 2012;27(1):443–7.

Part VII
Pancreas Transplantation

Chapter 18
DCD for Pancreas Transplantation

Toshinori Ito

18.1 Introduction

Before inclusion of the concept of brain death into law in the mid- to late 1970s, all organ transplantations came from cadaveric donors after cardiac death (DCD), i.e., non-heart-beating donors (NHBD). However, the introduction of brain-dead donors (BDD, heart-beating donors) led to better outcomes, as transplant organs were perfused with oxygenated blood right until the time for perfusion and cooling with preservation solution at organ procurement. Thus, DCD were generally no longer utilized, except in Japan.

However, a growing discrepancy between demand for organs and their availability from BDD led to a reevaluation of the use of DCD, and some transplant centers are now trying to use such donors to expand their potential pool of organs.

18.2 Definition of DCD

In relation to organ donation after cardiac death, DCD are classified into the following five categories according to the Maastricht classification [1]: *Category I*, donor dead on arrival to the hospital; *Category II*, a case that was "unable to resuscitate" due to rapid death following cardiac arrest, probably due to myocardial infarction, cerebral bleeding, or injury (unsuccessful resuscitation); *Category III*, a patient in whom cardiac arrest was due to withdrawal or suspension of life-prolonging treatment [awaiting cardiac arrest in patient (withdrawal of support)]; *Category IV*, cardiac arrest after brain stem death; and *Category V*, cardiac arrest

T. Ito (✉)
Departments of Complementary and Alternative Medicine and Gastroenterological Surgery, Graduate School of Medicine, Osaka University, 2-2 Yamada-oka, Suita 565-0871, Japan
e-mail: juki@cam.med.osaka-u.ac.jp

T. Asano et al. (eds.), *Marginal Donors: Current and Future Status*,
DOI 10.1007/978-4-431-54484-5_18,

during hospitalization (cardiac arrest in a hospital inpatient) (amended 2003). Further, *Categories I, II*, and *IV* donors are referred to as uncontrolled DCD, while *Categories III* and *V* donors are referred to as controlled DCD.

18.3 Experimental Study on Warm Ischemia

Concerning pancreatic transplantations (PTx) derived from DCD, Izukura et al. reported on endocrine function using a canine segmental pancreas model subjected to warm ischemia in situ [2]. The schema of this model is shown in Fig. 18.1. In brief, the left lobe of the pancreas was removed after all branches from the splenic artery were ligated and cut. Next, the small vessels between the duodenum and right lobe of the pancreas were also ligated and cut. Thereafter, the right lobe (remaining pancreatic volume >40 %) was perfused only by the superior pancreaticoduodenal (SPD) artery and vein. Subsequently, after heparinization, blood flow into the right pancreatic lobe via the SPD vessels was completely blocked by the application of bulldog clamps for 1, 2, and 3 h at room temperature. Experimental animals were then divided into the following four groups: (1) control (no ischemia); (2) 1-h ischemia; (3) 2-h ischemia; and (4) 3-h ischemia.

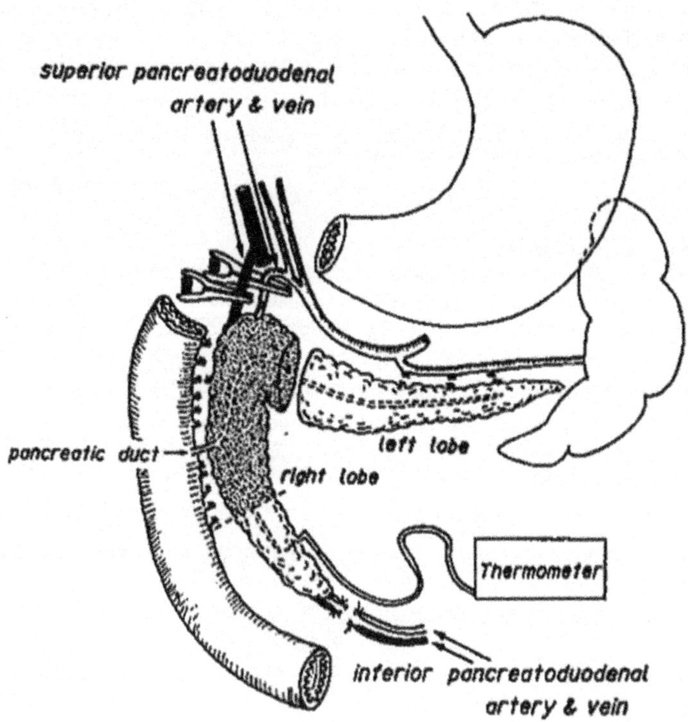

Fig. 18.1 Schema of in situ warm ischemia of canine pancreas [2]

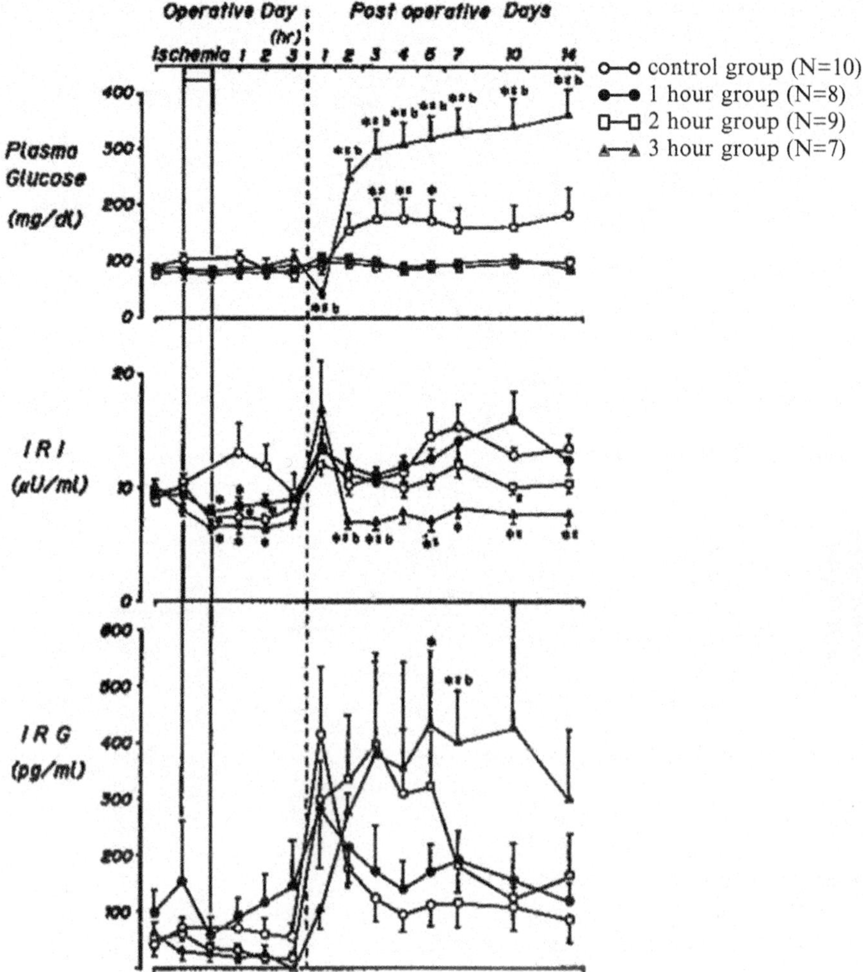

Fig. 18.2 Changes of mean plasma levels of glucose, insulin, and glucagon after warm ischemia in four groups. $^{*}p<0.05$ vs. control group. $\#p<0.05$ vs. group of warm ischemia for 1 h. $^{b}p<0.05$ vs. group of warm ischemia for 2 h [2]

Plasma glucose, insulin (IRI), and glucagon (IGI) were measured after 1, 2, and 3 h of ischemia and daily until 14 days after ischemia, as shown in Fig. 18.2. During the 3 h after declamping, plasma glucose levels did not change significantly in any of the groups. On POD (postoperative day) 1 in the 3-h ischemia group, plasma glucose levels were 45 ± 11 mg/dL, which were significantly lower than in the other three groups. In contrast, plasma glucose levels in the 3-h ischemia group were significantly higher than those in the other three groups after POD 2.

Plasma insulin levels in all the ischemia groups were significantly lower than those in the control group during the first 3 h after declamping, suggesting some disturbance in the secretion or production of insulin in pancreatic β cells.

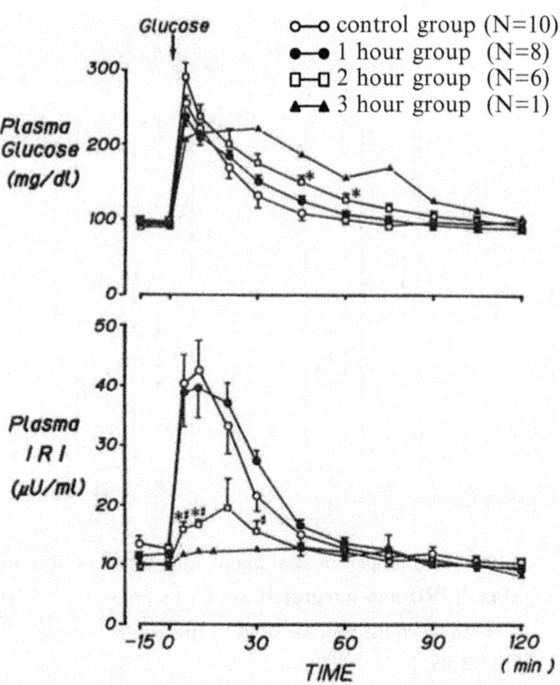

Fig. 18.3 Changes of plasma levels of glucose and insulin after intravenous glucose load. *$p<0.05$ vs. control group. #$p<0.05$ vs. group of warm ischemia for 1 h [2]

Further, the levels in the 3-h ischemia group were significantly lower than those in the other three groups after POD 2. These results indicate that 3-h ischemia resulted in hyperglycemia and hypoinsulinemia, which was derived from dysfunction of pancreatic β cells following ischemia at room temperature. A similar tendency was also observed in the 2-h ischemia model.

Plasma glucagon levels on POD 5 and 7 in the 3-h ischemia group were significantly higher than in the other three groups despite higher plasma glucose levels. A similar tendency was observed in the 2-h ischemia group. These results suggest promotion of glucagon secretion by pancreatic α cells damaged by warm ischemia. Therefore, pancreatic α cell function might be preserved despite warm ischemia for 3 h, compared with β cell function.

An intravenous glucose tolerance test under 24-h starvation was performed on POD 21. The results are shown in Fig. 18.3. In the 2-h ischemia group, plasma glucose levels at 45 and 60 min were significantly higher than those in the control group. Although only one animal was in the 3-h ischemia group, its plasma glucose level peaked at 30 min. Thereafter, the levels slowly decreased. Plasma insulin levels rapidly increased after glucose loading, with a peak at 10 min both in the control and 1-h ischemia groups. However, in the 2-h ischemia group, insulin levels were significantly lower at 5 and 10 min. No change in insulin secretion was observed in the 3-h ischemia group. Insulinogenic indices in the control and 1-, 2-, and 3-h ischemia groups were 0.27±0.06, 0.26±0.03, 0.05±0.01, and 0.02, respectively.

Concerning plasma glucose and insulin levels, this experimental study suggested that even pancreatic grafts perfused after a 1-h warm ischemia period might be tolerated during the first 2 weeks postoperation. Pancreas itself was likely to be more resistant to ischemia than was expected.

18.4 Clinical Outcomes Following Pancreatic Transplantation from DCD

Since no consensus regarding brain death was established in Japan until October 1997, when organ transplantation from BDD became legal, kidney transplantations were performed from DCD or living-related donors and liver transplantation from living-related donors. Unlike Europe and the USA, where controlled DCDs in whom supportive therapy is withdrawn (Category III) are used, Japan utilizes uncontrolled DCD in whom cardiac arrest occurs naturally without withdrawal of support. In such situations, the agonal stage is likely to be much longer.

Thus, 11 cases of PTx were performed using such uncontrolled DCD, mainly at Tokyo Women's Medical University, before the law for organ transplantation was established [3]. Unfortunately, the results were less than satisfactory. Survival rates for pancreatic grafts were 55 %, 46 %, and 36 % for 1, 3, and 5 years, respectively. This was attributed to the viability of pancreatic grafts during the agonal stage prior to procurement. Thus, after enactment of the law, uncontrolled DCDs were generally no longer utilized for PTx in our country.

Due to the concerns regarding post-transplant dysfunction of pancreatic grafts or pancreatitis, PTx using DCD is generally embarked upon with great caution.

Salvalaggio et al. reported the cumulative experience in North America with DCD PTx in 57 simultaneous pancreas and kidney transplants (SPK) [4]. Results showed equivalent 5-year outcomes to BDD PTx, despite more frequent pancreatic thrombosis, delayed kidney graft function, and longer hospital stay in the DCD group. Muthusamy et al. also recently reported a larger number of PTx from controlled DCD [5]. Their study demonstrated comparable results in terms of 1-year pancreatic graft survivals with grafts from DCD (Maastricht III & IV) and BDD. A total number of 1,009 pancreatic grafts (134 from DCD and 875 from BDD) were performed and analyzed in the UK between 2006 and 2010. The criteria of pancreatic donor selection for DCD in this study were as follows: (1) age, 5–60 years; (2) body mass index, <30; (3) absence of contraindications for organ donation (infection, malignancies, etc.); (4) time interval between treatment withdrawal and circulatory arrest, <60 min; and (5) adequate in situ perfusion. A median interval of 13 min elapsed from the time of withdrawal of support to asystole (0–30 min). A median of 5 min (range 0–10 min) elapsed between asystole and initiation of the organ procurement procedure. Overall 1-year pancreatic graft survival was comparable between SPK (88 % of DCD vs. 87 % of BDD) and PA (solitary pancreas transplant) (76 % of DCD vs. 73 % of BDD), with numerically more DCD grafts lost to thrombosis (8 % of DCD vs. 5 % of BDD, $p = \text{NS}$).

These results suggest that controlled DCD like Maastricht Category III are feasible for PTx, with graft and patient outcomes that are similar to those from BDD donors. In terms of current organ shortage, DCD could provide an important additional source for pancreases as well as kidneys. Further investigation, however, will be necessary to predict early postoperative complications in PTx recipients.

References

1. Kootsra G et al. Categories of non-heart beating donors. Transplant Proc. 1995;27:2893–4.
2. Izukura M. An experimental study on the segmental pancreatic transplantation: the influence of warm ischemia on the pancreatic endocrine functions in dogs. Med J Osaka Univ. 1988; 40(3):39–57.
3. Tojimbara S, Teraoka S, Babazono T, et al. Long-term outcome after combined pancreas and kidney transplantation from non-heart cadaver donors. Transplant Proc. 1998;30:3793–4.
4. Salvalaggio PR, Davies DB, Fernandez LA, et al. Outcomes of pancreas transplantation in the United States using cardiac death donors. Am J Transplant. 2006;65(Pt 1):1059–65.
5. Muthusamy ASR, Mumford L, Hudosn A, et al. Pancreas transplantation from donors after circulatory death from the United Kingdom. Am J Transplant. 2012;12:2150–6.

Chapter 19
ECD for Pancreas Transplantation

Toshinori Ito

19.1 Introduction

In terms of absolute shortages of donors, organ transplantation in Japan is in a more serious position than in Europe or the United States. In Japan, a law allowing organ transplantation from brain-dead donors finally came into force in October 1997. The first organ procurement after the enactment of this law was carried out from a deceased donor in February 1999. The heart, liver, and kidneys were successfully transplanted into four recipients. The first pancreas transplantation (PTx) after the law was successfully performed at Osaka University Hospital in April 2000. Since then, however, only 86 cases of procurement occurred over the approximately 13 years from the introduction of the law, because the law was very strict and limited for organ procurement to donors who provided prior written consent. The law was eventually revised to more closely resemble laws in Europe and the United States in July 2010. Since then, procurement numbers have rapidly increased to 118 in 2.5 years. After revision of the law, the number of donations has increased 7.1-fold. The number of PTx was 84 (33.6/year, as of December 31, 2012) after the revision, compared to 64 (5.0/year) before the revision.

Although the number of donors increased, donor shortages and severe environment surrounding donors as described later still exist in our country. Transplant outcomes, however, are comparable to those in Europe and the United States. Most organ transplantations except for small bowel transplantation have been covered by health insurance since April 2006. This is probably due to recognition of the high quality of organ transplantation in Japan.

T. Ito (✉)
The Japan Registry of Pancreas Transplantation, The Japan Society for Pancreas and Islet Transplantation.
Departments of Complementary & Alternative Medicine and Gastroenterological Surgery, Graduate School of Medicine,
Osaka University, 2-2 Yamada-oka, Suita 565-0871, Japan
e-mail: juki@cam.med.osaka-u.ac.jp

T. Asano et al. (eds.), *Marginal Donors: Current and Future Status*,
DOI 10.1007/978-4-431-54484-5_19,

Unlike transplantations of lifesaving organs such as the heart, liver, and lung, PTx is recognized as a treatment mainly focused on quality of life. Recently, however, PTx, particularly simultaneous pancreas and kidney transplantation (SPK), has been reported to improve life expectancy in recipients [1]. With the passage of the waiting period after registration to the Japan Organ Transplant Network (JOTN), both deaths and serious cases of diabetic complications necessitating withdrawal of the registration have increased. Therefore, as potential solutions, so-called marginal donors as well as living donors have been considered in Japan.

This chapter examines the present status and problems of PTx in Japan from the perspective of "marginal donors."

19.2 Definition of a "Marginal Donor"

The term "marginal donor" has not yet been clearly defined but is considered almost equivalent to expanded or extended donors (ECD). According to a report regarding strategies to expand the donor pool by Kapur et al., "marginal donors" are defined as follows [2]: (1) >45 years old; (2) hemodynamically unstable at the time of harvest (usage of high-dose dopamine (>10 μg/kg/min) or at least two vasopressors); and (3) non-heart-beating status. In Kapur's series of PTx, 68 transplants were performed from non-marginal donors, while 69 transplants were from marginal donors according to these criteria. The overall rate of pancreas graft survival was 86 %, with a mean follow-up of 23 months. A total of 22 pancreas grafts were received from donors >45 years old (13 grafts; >50 years old). The actual graft survival rate of the >45-year-old donor group was 86 %. Fifty-one grafts were removed from hemodynamically unstable donors on high-dose vasopressors. The actual graft survival rate in the group was 86 %. Delayed graft function was observed significantly more often among recipients of grafts from donors on high-dose vasopressors, but no significant difference in graft survival was evident between recipients of pancreas grafts from marginal and non-marginal donors.

According to International Pancreas Transplant Registry (IPTR) data, the following variables are associated with increased risk of pancreas allograft thrombosis: (1) donor age over 40 years; (2) cardiovascular or cerebrovascular cause of brain death; and (3) pancreas preservation time more than 24 h [3].

Also, anecdotal experience suggests that (1) donor body weight (BW) >150 % of ideal BW or donor body mass index (BMI) >30 kg/m^2 may be associated with increased risk of pancreas graft loss due to thrombosis, pancreatitis, infection, or primary nonfunction; (2) donor liver biopsy showing greater than 25–30 % macrovesicular steatosis may be associated with a fatty pancreas, leading to increased risk of early graft loss; and (3) fatty infiltration of the pancreas may be associated with increased risk of early graft loss [4].

Donors under cardiac death will be discussed in another chapter.

19.3 Present Status of Donors for PTx in Japan

From October 1999 to the end of 2012, a total of 423 patients with type 1 diabetes (T1D) were registered with the JOTN and 148 cases of PTx were performed. Almost every donor was deceased, with the exception of two non-heart-beating donors. During the waiting period, however, 38 patients died and 33 were withdrawn from registration due to serious diabetic complications, such as cerebral hemorrhage and infarction and myocardial infarction. During the same period, another 26 pancreases were utilized with or without kidneys from living-related donors.

Donor characteristics are shown in Table 19.1. Three obvious differences in donor characteristics exist between Japan and the United States. One is regarding the age of donors, another is the cause of brain death, and the last is the waiting time from registration to transplantation. The mean age of donors was 25.5 years in the United States [5], compared with 43.4 years in Japan. In particular, the population >45 years old accounted for 50.0 % of donors in Japan (6.7 % in the United States), as shown in Fig. 19.1. Next, the most common cause of brain death in the United States was trauma (69.6 %), followed by cerebrovascular accident (CVA, 25.1 %), while the most common causes in Japan were CVA (58.9 %) followed by trauma (18.9 %) (Fig. 19.2). Organs from older donors who have died due to CVA might carry a higher risk of atherosclerotic changes, fatty degeneration, or diabetes. The last issue is about the waiting time until transplantation after registration. In the United States, 65.7 % of patients underwent transplant within 12 months, while most patients (61.5 %) in Japan

Table 19.1 Characteristics of 148 PTx donors

Donor's gender	
Men	80
Women	68
Age at PTx	
10s (%)	5 (3.4)
20s (%)	19 (12.8)
30s (%)	31 (20.9)
40s (%)	38 (25.7)
50s (%)	40 (27.0)
60s (%)	14 (9.5)
70s (%)	1 (0.7)
Cause of death	
CVA (%)	87 (58.8)
Injury (%)	28 (18.9)
Hypoxia (%)	28 (18.9)
AMI (%)	2 (1.4)
Others (%)	3 (2.0)
Resuscitation	
Yes (%)	62 (41.9)
No (%)	86 (58.1)
Marginality	
Yes (%)	108 (73.0)
No (%)	40 (27)

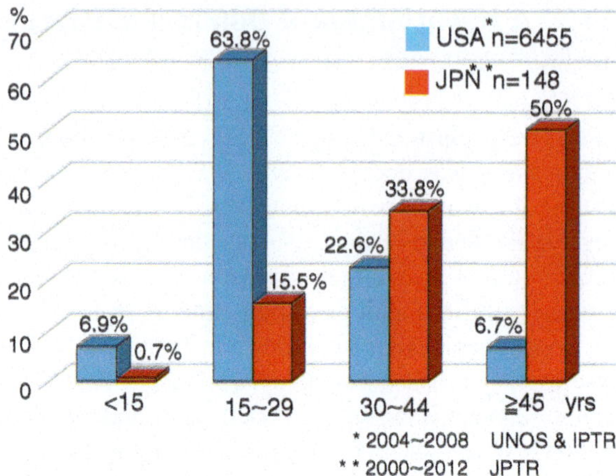

Fig. 19.1 Donor age between the United States and Japan

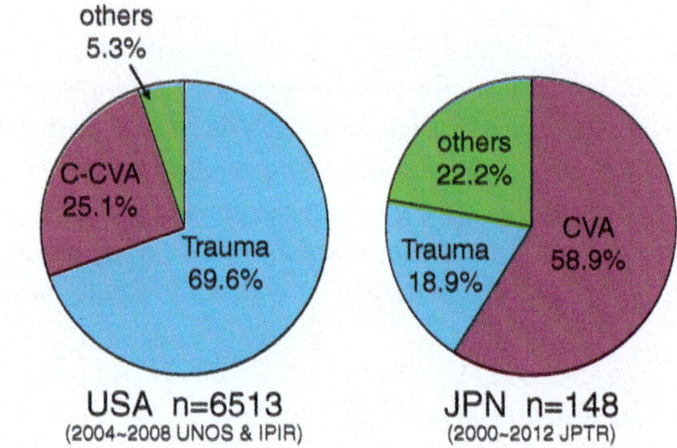

Fig. 19.2 Cause of death between the United States and Japan

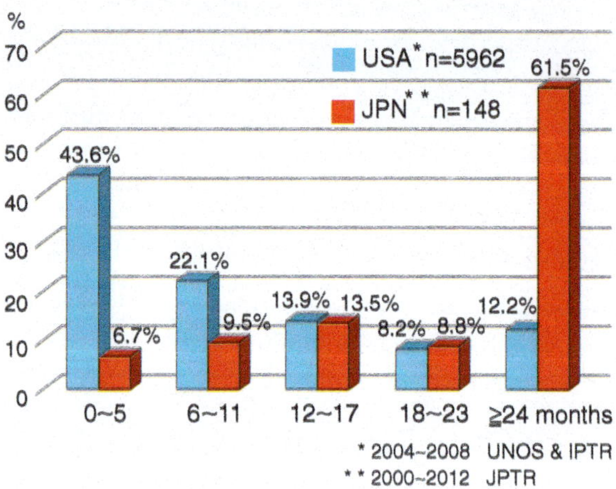

Fig. 19.3 Waiting period for PTx

have to wait >24 months (mean, 1,380 days; Fig. 19.3). Under such circumstances, we Japanese have no choice but to accept marginal donors.

In the present series, 108 donors (73.0 %) meeting at least one of the three conditions in Kapur's criteria were considered as marginal.

During the same period, 176 liver grafts were harvested in our country. Comparing the usage of liver grafts to that of pancreas grafts, the liver to pancreas ratio (L/P ratio) was 1.19. In contrast, ratios in main overseas organ procurement organizations (OPOs) and American OPOs were 7.18 and 3.26, respectively. Pancreas grafts were thus not actively harvested in the United States or other countries. However, there is one transplant center of the University of Wisconsin where selected, less-than-ideal donors are aggressively used, with an L/P ratio of 1.25 [6].

19.4 Outcomes of PTx in Japan

The first case of PTx under brain death was performed at Tsukuba University in 1984, before implementation of the laws regarding organ transplantation [7]. Because no consensus regarding brain death had been established in Japan at that time, 11 cases of PTx were subsequently performed under cardiac death, mainly at Tokyo Women's Medical University [8]. Unfortunately, the results were less than satisfactory. Survival rates for pancreas grafts were 55 %, 46 %, and 36 % for 1, 3, and 5 years, respectively. This was attributed to the viability of pancreatic grafts during the agonal stage prior to procurement.

A total of 148 PTx from 204 organ procurements had been performed as of the end of 2012 after the introduction of laws on organ transplantation. The percentage usage of pancreas grafts was 72.5 %. Characteristics of these transplantations are shown in Table 19.2, revealing similar findings to results from Europe and the United States. In terms of recipient sex, 92 (62.2 %) were females and 56 (37.8 %) were males. Recipient populations in their 40s, 30s, and 50s comprised 66 (44.6 %), 51 (34.5 %), and 23 patients (15.5 %), respectively. Mean duration of diabetes was 27.1 years (range, 6–48 years). However, the mean period of dialysis among SPK patients was relatively longer, at 7.9 years (range, 0–22 years). As described above, the problem is that the waiting time for recipients, which was 1,380 days (range, 45–4,722 days) as of the end of 2012, is getting longer and longer.

Recipients were classified into three categories: spontaneous pancreas and kidney transplantation (SPK); pancreas after kidney transplantation (PAK); and pancreas transplant alone (PTA). As of December 2012, totals of 119 SPK, 20 PAK, and 9 PTA had been performed. Mean total cold ischemic time (TCIT) of the pancreas was 11 h 43 min. Mean TCIT for kidney grafts in SPK patients was 11 h 8 min. Mean number of total HLA-A, -B, and -DR mismatches was 2.61 ± 1.18.

PTx was managed and performed under a cooperative system as an all-Japan team from the beginning in Japan. To increase blood supply to the pancreas head, a donor gastroduodenal artery (GDA) was usually reconstructed with a donor iliac artery (I-graft) (Fig. 19.4). Blood supply to the pancreas head via GDA is usually blocked if the liver is harvested, but if not, blood flow was usually preserved. There are two blood supplies to the pancreas head: one via the GDA from the celiac artery and the other via the inferior pancreaticoduodenal artery (IPD)—first jejunal artery from the superior mesenteric artery (SMA). According to a report by Donatini [9], the main blood flow is supplied from the anterosuperior pancreaticoduodenal artery

Table 19.2 Characteristics of 148 PTx recipients

Recipient's gender	
Men	56
Women	92
Age at PTx	
20s (%)	6 (4.1)
30s (%)	51 (34.5)
40s (%)	66 (44.6)
50s (%)	23 (15.5)
60s (%)	2 (1.3)
Mean duration of DM (years)	32.9 (6–47)
Mean duration of dialysis (years)	7.9 (0–22)
Mean waiting time (days)	1,380 (45–4,722)
TCIT	
Pancreas	11 h 43 min
Kidney	11 h 08 min
Recipient's category	
SPK (%)	119 (80.4)
PAK (%)	20 (13.5)
PTA (%)	9 (6.1)
Immunosuppression	
TAC+ST+MMF+Ab	
TAC+ST+MMF	
CsA+ST+MMF+Ab	
CsA+ST+MMF	
Others	
Tx procedure	
ED (%)	118 (79.7)
BD (%)	30 (20.3)
HLA mismatches	
Mean ± SD	2.61/1.18

TCIT total cold ischemic time, *TAC* tacrolimus, *CsA* ciclosporin, *ST* steroid, *MMF* mycophenolate mofetil, *Ab* antibody, *ED* enteric drainage, *BD* bladder drainage

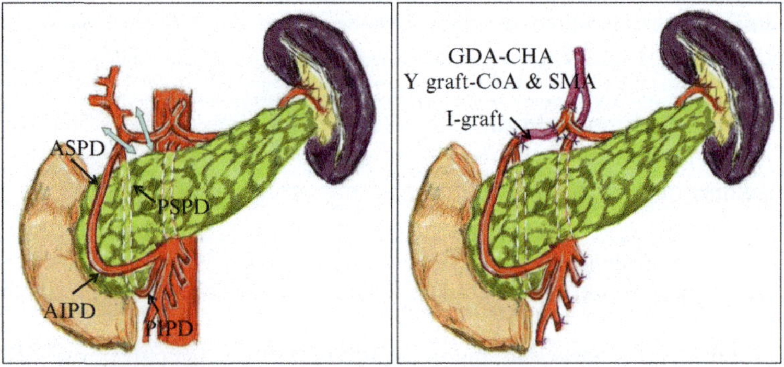

Fig. 19.4 Arterial reconstruction of pancreas graft

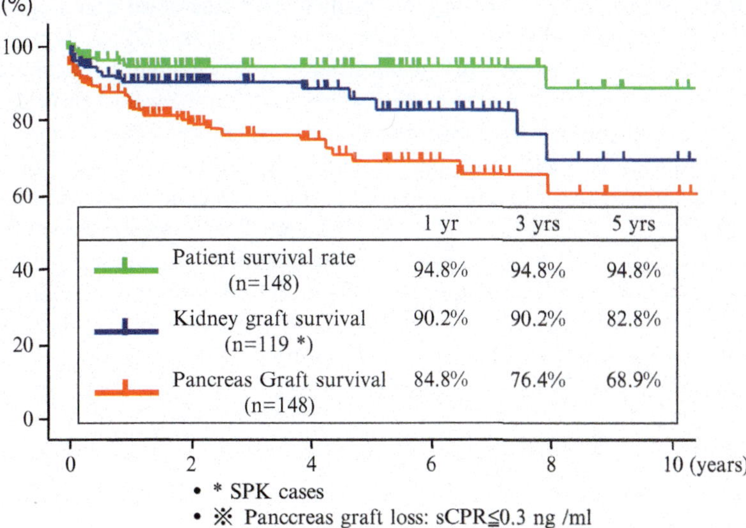

Fig. 19.5 Patient survival and graft survivals of PTx (until December 31, 2012)

(ASPD) via the GDA. Further, regarding communications between the superior and inferior branches of the pancreaticoduodenal artery (PD), there is reportedly communication of 25 % between the ASPD and anteroinferior PD (AIPD) and 75 % between the posterosuperior PD (PSPD) and posteroinferior PD (PIPD). The GDA reconstruction will be useful to increase blood flow to the pancreas, especially in PTx from a marginal donor.

Regarding drainage of pancreatic juice, enteric drainage (79.7 %) was more common than bladder drainage (20.3 %).

In most cases (91.9 %), the immunosuppressive regimen comprised tacrolimus-based quadruple induction therapy. Basiliximab directed against interleukin-2 receptor (CD25) was mostly used as an induction therapy. As an antimetabolite, mycophenolate mofetil was usually used.

Outcomes for 148 PTx are shown in Fig. 19.5. Eight recipients died, due to sepsis ($n=3$), cardiogenic events ($n=3$), graft-versus-host disease (GVHD) ($n=1$), and cerebral bleeding ($n=1$). The patient survival rate was 94.8 % at 1, 3, and 5 years. Nine pancreas grafts were removed in the acute phase, due to thrombus ($n=7$) and perforation ($n=1$) and bleeding ($n=1$) of duodenal grafts. Another 18 pancreases were lost, due to rejection ($n=15$), recurrence of T1D ($n=2$), or graft pancreatitis ($n=1$). Pancreas graft survival rates were 84.8 %, 76.4 %, and 68.9 % at 1, 3, and 5 years, respectively. Pancreas graft loss was defined as a serum C-peptide level <0.3 ng/ml according to high-sensitivity immunoassay. Among SPK recipients, eight kidney grafts were lost and the patients reintroduced onto dialysis due to chronic rejection ($n=7$) or primary nonfunction ($n=1$). Kidney graft survival rates were 90.2 %, 90.2 %, and 82.8 % at 1, 3, and 5 years, respectively.

Next, transplant results were analyzed between marginal cases ($n=108$) and non-marginal cases ($n=40$). Regarding mortality, five marginal recipients (4.6 %)

died, due to sepsis ($n=2$), cardiogenic events ($n=1$), cerebral bleeding ($n=1$), and GVHD ($n=1$), compared to 3 non-marginal recipients (7.5 %; sepsis, $n=1$; cardiogenic event, $n=1$). No significant difference was evident between groups. In terms of pancreas graft function, 23 pancreases (21.3 %) were lost in the marginal group, compared to four pancreases (10.0 %) in the non-marginal group. Pancreas graft survival rates in the marginal group were 80.9 %, 73.2 %, and 66.0 % at 1, 2, and 5 years post-transplantation, respectively. In contrast, survival rates in the non-marginal group were 92.5 %, 85.2 %, and 77.4 %, respectively. Pancreas graft failure tended to be more frequent in the marginal group, but no significant difference existed between groups ($p=0.35$). Similarly, in terms of kidney graft function among SPK recipients, eight kidneys (9.1 %) were lost in the marginal group compared to only one kidney (3.2 %) in the non-marginal group. Again, no significant difference was evident between groups.

19.5 Conclusion

In this study, 73 % of donors for PTx in Japan were marginal because of an absolute shortage of donors. However, transplant outcomes appear comparable to those in Europe and the United States. Pancreas and kidney graft functions in the marginal group tend to be inferior to those in the non-marginal group, but no significant differences are apparent.

Further investigations are necessary to clarify factors in marginal donors that contribute to better or worse outcomes.

Acknowledgement I wish to thank all the members of Practical Committee of 17 Centers (*) for Pancreas Transplantation in Japan, Ms. Y. Saito and Dr. Iwamoto in Japan Diabetes Foundation, and Dr. M. Gotoh, president of Japan Society for Pancreas & Islet Transplantation
(*)
1. Dr. Shimamura, Hokkaido Univ. Hospital
2. Dr. Miyagi, Tohoku Univ. Hospital
3. Dr. Saitoh, Fukushima Medical Univ. Hospital
4. Dr. Kubota, Dokkyo Medical Univ. Hospital
5. Dr. Shimazu, Tokyo Medical Univ. Hospital
6. Dr. Nakajima, Tokyo Women's Univ. Hospital
7. Dr. Wakai, Niigata Univ. Hospital
8. Dr. Akutsu, National Chiba-Higashi Hospital
9. Dr. Narumi, Nagoya Red Cross Hospital
10. Dr. Kenmochi, Fujita Health Univ. Hospital
11. Dr. Dr. Yoshimura, Kyoto Prefectural Medical Univ. Hospital
12. Dr. Iwanaga, Kyoto Univ. Hospital
13. Dr. Nagano, Osaka Univ. Hospital
14. Dr. Matsumoto, Kobe Univ. Hospital
15. Dr. Ohdan, Hiroshima Univ. Hospital
16. Dr. Okano, Kagawa Univ. Hospital
17. Dr. Kitada, Kyushu Univ. Hospital

References

1. Biesenbach G, Konigsrainer A, Gross C, et al. Progression of macrovascular diseases is reduced in type 1 diabetic patients after more than 5 years successful combined pancreas-kidney transplantation in comparison to kidney transplantation alone. Transpl Int. 2005;18:1054–60.
2. Kapur SC, Bonham CA, Dodson SF, et al. Strategies to expand the donor pool for pancreas transplantation. Transplantation. 1999;67:284–90.
3. Gruessner AC, Sutherland DER. Pancreas transplant outcomes for United States cases reported to the United Network for Organ Sharing (UNOS) and non-US cases reported to the international pancreas transplant registry (IPTR) as of October, 2000. In: Cecka JM, Terasaki PI, editors. Clinical transplants 2000. Los Angeles: UCLA Immunogenetics Center; 2001. p. 45–72.
4. Robertson RP, Davis C, Larsen J, et al. Pancreas and islet transplantation for patients with diabetes. Diabetes Care. 2000;23:112–6.
5. Gruessner AC, Sutherland DER. Pancreas transplant outcomes for United States (US) cases as reported to the United Network for organ sharing (UNOS) and the international pancreas transplant registry (IPTR). In: Cecka JM, Terasaki PI, editors. Clinical transplants. Los Angeles: UCLA Tissue Typing Laboratory; 2008. p. 45–56.
6. Krieger NR, Odorico JS, Heisey DM, et al. Underutilization of pancreas donors. Transplantation. 2003;75:1271–6.
7. Fukao T, Ohtsuka M, Iwasaki H, et al. A case of simultaneous whole pancreas and kidney allotransplantation. Jpn J Transplant. 1986;21:331–40.
8. Tojimbara S, Teraoka S, Babazono T, et al. Long-term outcome after combined pancreas and kidney transplantation from non-heart cadaver donors. Transplant Proc. 1998;30:3793–4.
9. Donatini B. A systemic study of the vascularization of the pancreas. Surg Radiol Anat. 1990;12:173–80.

Chapter 20
LD for Pancreas Transplantation

Takashi Kenmochi, Takehide Asano, and Taihei Ito

20.1 Introduction

The first extrarenal organ to be successfully transplanted using living donors was the pancreas. The first pancreas transplantation using a living donor (LDP) was performed on June 20, 1979, at the University of Minnesota [1, 2]. Furthermore, successful simultaneous pancreas and kidney transplantation from a living donor (LDSPK) was started in 1994 also at the University of Minnesota [3]. The outcome of LDPs performed at the University of Minnesota demonstrated that the segmental pancreas was able to normalize plasma glucose levels and realize an insulin independency in the severe diabetic patients. The outcome of the donors was considered to be acceptable when using the stringent donor criteria concerning the endocrine function [4].

Based on a severe shortage of the deceased donors in our country and the satisfactory outcome of LDPs at the University of Minnesota, we have firstly introduced LDP (LDSPK) in our country on January 7, 2004 [5]. Eighteen LDPs (16 LDSPKs) have, so far, been performed in Chiba-East National Hospital. From 2007, we have introduced LDSPK from ABO-incompatible living donors according to our successful desensitization and immunosuppression protocol for ABO-incompatible kidney transplantation and performed, so far, six cases.

In this chapter, we describe the criteria for living donation, historical background, and the prognosis for living donor from our clinical experiences of sixteen LDSPKs.

T. Kenmochi (✉) • T. Ito
Department of Organ Transplant Surgery, Fujita Health University,
1-98 Dengakugakubo, Kutsukake-cho, Toyoake City, Aichi 470-1192, Japan
e-mail: kenmochi@fujita-hu.ac.jp

T. Asano
Department of Surgery and Clinical Research Center, Chiba-East National Hospital,
673 Nitonacho, Chuo-ku, Chiba City, Chiba 260-8712, Japan
e-mail: asano@cehpnet.com

T. Asano et al. (eds.), *Marginal Donors: Current and Future Status*,
DOI 10.1007/978-4-431-54484-5_20, © Springer Japan 2014

20.2 Criteria for Living Donation

Donor safety has been the most important consideration of the enforcement of LDSPK. The criteria of the living donor for pancreas transplantation had been made by transplant surgeon, diabetologist, nephrologist, nurse, and transplant coordinator as shown in Table 20.1. We have referred to the stringent Minnesota criteria and modified it according to the lower ability to secrete insulin from the islet in Japanese.

As the tools for endocrinologic evaluation, we use 75 g oral glucose tolerance test (OGTT), intravenous glucose tolerance test (IVGTT), and HbA1c level. In 75 g OGTT, all of the plasma glucose levels at 0, 30, 60, 90, 120, and 180 min after oral glucose intake must be less than 180 mg/dL. In IVGTT, we use the CS1 that is calculated by the sum of C-peptide secretion rate from 0 to 5 min after glucose injection in IVGTT. Tokuyama et al. demonstrated that the sum of C-peptide secretion rate directly correlates with the β-cell function and CS1 expresses the first phase of insulin release [6]. The upper limit of hemoglobin A1c (HbA1c) was determined to be 5.5 % (JDS), which was equal to 5.9 % (NGSP).

Negative anti-GAD antibody and anti-IA2 antibody were also included in the criteria. Since obesity is the major risk factor of developing diabetes, the body mass index (BMI) of the donor was strictly limited to less than 25 kg/m^2.

Contraindications of the donor were almost similar to those in other living donor organ transplantations. We perform ^{11}C-methionine positron emission tomography (PET) and PET-CT for the evaluation of the pancreatic function [7] in addition to the conventional imaging diagnostic tools including CT scan, MRI, MRCP, and ultrasonography for the evaluation of the anatomy of the pancreas and the vessels.

Table 20.1 The criteria of the donor for living pancreas transplantation (Organ Transplant Team, Chiba-East National Hospital 2007.4)

1. Age: ≤65 years (desirable)
2. No family history except for the recipient
3. Normal endocrine function
   1. 75 g OGTT: normal pattern (all plasma glucose levels <180 mg/dL)
   2. IVGTT: normal CS1[a]
   3. HbA1c (JDS): ≤5.5 %
4. Negative anti-GAD and IA-2 antibodies
5. BMI[b]: <25
   - Contraindications
     1. Active infectious disease
     2. HIV(+), HTLV-1(+), HBs antigen(+), HCV antibody(+)
     3. Malignancy
     4. Abnormal anatomy of the pancreas
     5. Alcoholism

[a]*CS1* the first phase C-peptide secretion calculated from the sum of C-peptide secretion rate from 0 to 5 min after glucose injection

[b]*BMI* body mass index

Table 20.2 The criteria of the endocrine function of the donor for living pancreas transplantation (from the guideline for LDP. The Japan Society for Transplantation 2010.6)

The donor candidate must fulfill all the following items
1. 75 g OGTT: normal pattern (all plasma glucose levels <180 mg/dL)
2. 75 g OGTT: insulinogenic index; ≥0.4; HOMA-β; ≥40 %
3. HbA1c: <5.5 % (<5.9 % NGSP)
4. HOMA-R: <2.5

Subsequently, the Japan Society for Transplantation finally made the guideline for LDP on June 2010 that was prepared according to the criteria and the postoperative outcome of the donor who underwent LDPs in our institution [8]. In this guideline, the criteria of the endocrine function of the donor for LDP were decided as shown in Table 20.2.

20.3 Historical Background

LDP was first introduced at the University of Minnesota in 1979 [2]. Initially, they performed LDP only in recipients without uremia (LDPTA) or recipients who had received a kidney graft from the same donor (LDPAK) [1]. Thereafter, they performed the first successful LDSPK in March 1994 [3], and 20 LDSPKs had been done by March 1997 [4]. The 1-year survival of the patient, kidney graft, and pancreas graft were 100 %, 100 %, and 78 %, respectively, which were higher than those of pancreas transplants from deceased donors at that time. The 1-year survival of the pancreas graft, then, had improved to 87 % in 2001 by analyzing 32 recipients of LDSPK [9, 10]. Those results clearly demonstrated that the segmental pancreas was able to normalize the glucose metabolism of severe diabetic patient. Based on the shortage of deceased donors in Japan and the excellent outcome obtained at the University of Minnesota, the first LDSPK in Japan was performed for a type 1 diabetic patient with ESRD from her father on January 7, 2004 [5, 11].

Kendall et al. reported the evaluation of the impact of distal pancreatectomy (donor operation) on metabolic function of 28 donors [12]. In this report, all donors demonstrated an increase in serum glucose levels and a reduced level of insulin at 1 year after surgery. Moreover, 25 % of the donors displayed abnormal glucose curves on 75 g OGTT. All donors had a significant reduction in stimulated insulin and glucagon secretion [13]. From these investigations, the University of Minnesota developed stringent endocrinologic criteria to select living donors for LDP more safely (Table 20.3) [14]. However, the author mentioned that these criteria could not necessarily guarantee the safety of the donors.

In addition to conventional OGTT, we used a minimal model analysis as an important index for endocrinologic evaluation for the LDP donors [6]. This method is able to estimate more detail in endocrine function, especially first phase insulin release.

Table 20.3 Exclusion criteria for living hemipancreas donors at the University of Minnesota

Historical and clinical criteria

1. History of type 2 diabetes in any first-degree relative (parent, sibling, child)
2. Personal history of gestational diabetes
3. Additional first-degree relative with type 1 diabetes (other than proposed recipient)
4. Body mass index greater than 27 kg/m^2
5. Age greater than 50 years
6. Age of the donor within 10 years of age at which type 1 diabetes was diagnosed in the proposed recipient
7. Clinical evidence of diseases associated with insulin resistance (e.g., polycystic ovarian syndrome, hypertension)
8. Personal history of an autoimmune endocrine disorder involving the thyroid, adrenal pituitary, gonads
9. History of or active diseases of the exocrine pancreas (e.g., active or chronic pancreatitis)
10. Active or uncontrolled psychiatric disorders
11. Heavy smoking, alcoholism, or excessive alcohol use
12. Hypertension, cardiac disease
13. Active infections or malignant disorders

Metabolic criteria

1. Any glucose value above 150 mg/dL during standard oral glucose tolerance tests
2. Hemoglobin A1c greater than 6 %
3. Glucose disposal rate calculated from data collected during intravenous glucose tolerance tests less than 1.0 %
4. Presence of elevated titer of islet cell autoantibodies or anti-GAD antibodies
5. Acute insulin response to intravenous glucose or intravenous arginine of less than 300 % of basal
6. Glucose potentiation of arginine-induced insulin secretion of less than 300 % of basal

20.4 Prognosis for Living Donor

Procurement of the distal pancreas from a living donor was performed according to the procedure of the Minnesota Group as previously reported [1]. In LDSPK, under an open laparotomy, the left kidney was first excised followed by a distal pancreatectomy with a splenectomy. In recent eight donors, however, hand-assisted laparoscopic surgery (HALS) was introduced as a less invasive procedure for a simultaneous nephrectomy and distal pancreatectomy (Fig. 20.1).

In the recipient, the kidney transplantation was performed in the standard fashion as previously described in detail, with vascular anastomoses to the left external iliac vessels and an ureterocystostomy. The segmental pancreatic graft was revascularized by anastomosing the donor splenic artery and vein to the right iliac artery and vein of the recipient. A pancreaticocystostomy was performed using the two-layer technique including the anastomosis between the pancreatic duct and the mucosa of the urinary bladder to drain the pancreatic juice of the graft (Fig. 20.2).

An induction of immunosuppression was achieved by a quadruple therapy using tacrolimus, basiliximab, mycophenolate mofetil (MMF), and prednisone. The maintenance of immunosuppression was performed by a triple therapy with tacrolimus, MMF, and prednisone. Desensitization for the patients from ABO-incompatible

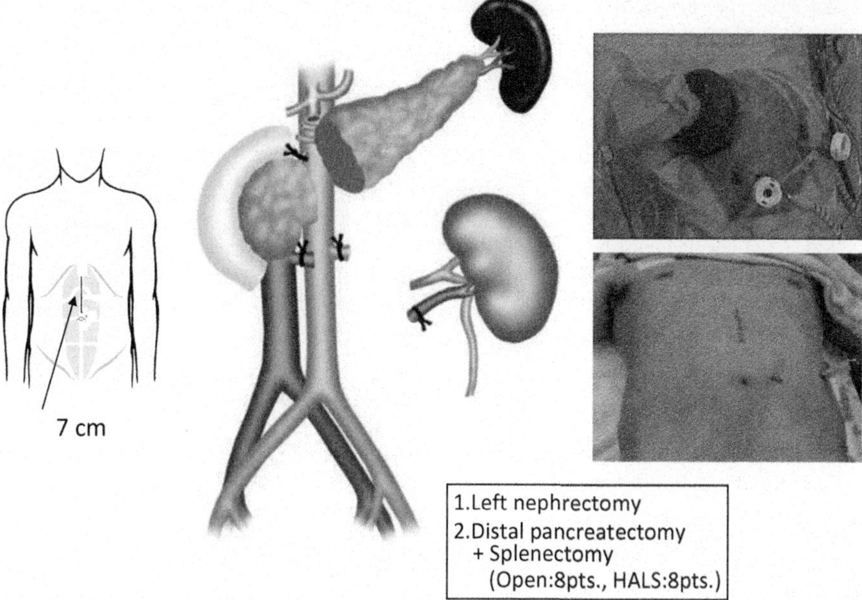

Fig. 20.1 Operation method of LDSPK donor. Department of Surgery, Chiba-East National Hospital 2004.1–2012.8

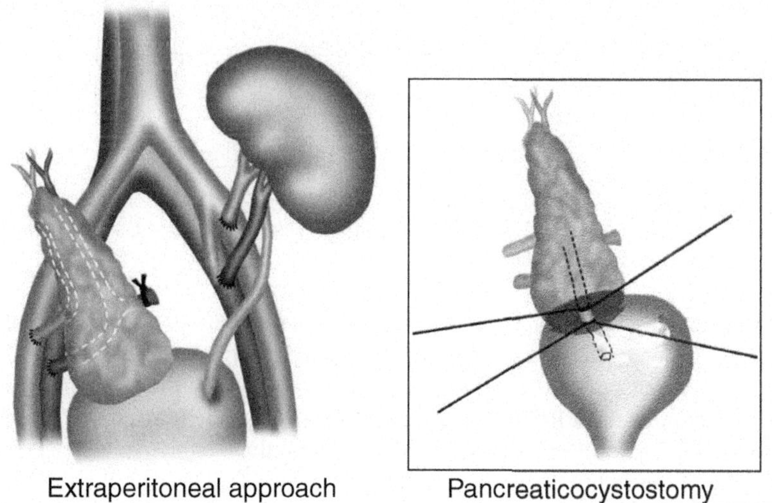

Fig. 20.2 Operation method of LDSPK recipient. Department of Surgery, Chiba-East National Hospital 2004.1–2012.8

donors was achieved according to a protocol for an ABO-incompatible kidney transplantation, including administration of MMF for 4 weeks before transplantation, a splenectomy at 14 days, double-filtered plasmapheresis (DFPP) at 6, 4, and 2 days, and plasma exchange (PE) at 1 day.

Table 20.4 The characteristics of the recipients and donors of pancreas transplantation from a living donor (Department of Surgery, Chiba-East National Hospital. 2004–2012)

Recipients	
Patient number	16
Age (years)	34.2 ± 5.7 (25–48)
Gender (male/female)	6/10
Onset of DM[a] (years old)	13.1 ± 7.2 (0.9–34)
Duration of DM (years)	22.1 ± 4.8 (14–31)
Amount of insulin (units/day)	37.1 ± 13.5 (4 times daily or CSII)
Stimulated C-peptide (ng/mL)	<0.03
Hypoglycemic unawareness	Frequent
Anti-GAD or IA-2 abs[b]	Positive, 9; negative, 7
M value	70.1 ± 15.4
ESRD[c]	HD[d], 14; preemptive, 2
Donors	
Patient number	16
Age (years)	53.9 ± 11.8 (28–66)
Gender (male/female)	6 (3 fathers, 3 brothers)/10 (9 mothers, 1 sister)
ABO blood type	8 identical, 2 compatible, 6 incompatible
75 g OGTT[e]	Normal pattern
IVGTT[f] (CS1[g])	6.86 ± 1.71 ng/mL/5 min
HbA1C (%)	5.12 ± 0.26
HOMA-β	84.6 ± 56.0
Insulinogenic index	1.07 ± 0.65
HOMA-R	1.20 ± 0.62
Body mass index	22.8 ± 1.89

[a]*DM* diabetes mellitus
[b]*ab* antibodies
[c]*ESRD* end-stage renal disease
[d]*HD* hemodialysis
[e]*75 g OGTT* 75 gram oral glucose tolerance test
[f]*IVGTT* intravenous glucose tolerance test
[g]*CS1* the first phase C-peptide secretion calculated from the sum of C-peptide secretion rate from 0 to 5 min after glucose injection

Anticoagulation therapy was started at the time of the operation using heparin (200 units/h), and 10,000–20,000 units were continuously given intravenously for 10 days after transplantation. Six-hundred milligram of gabexate mesilate was continuously administrated for 7 days to inhibit the graft pancreatitis, and 100 units of octreotide were given every 12 h for 5 days to inhibit the secretion of pancreatic juice from the graft. In addition, we also administered antibacterial prophylaxis with piperacillin for a week, antifungal prophylaxis with fluconazole for a week, and anti-cytomegalovirus (CMV) prophylaxis with ganciclovir for 10 days. Insulin was continuously given intravenously to maintain plasma glucose levels at 100–150 mg/dL.

In our 16 consecutive clinical trials of LDSPK (Table 20.4), all recipients were freed from hemodialysis immediately after LDSPK. Insulin independency was achieved in 14 patients (87.5 %). Two recipients, however, failed to achieve insulin independency. One developed a primary nonfunction of the pancreatic graft and the other underwent graftectomy because of a venous thrombosis (Fig. 20.3).

Fig. 20.3 Outcome of the recipients of LDSPK. Department of Surgery, Chiba-East National Hospital 2004.1–2012.8

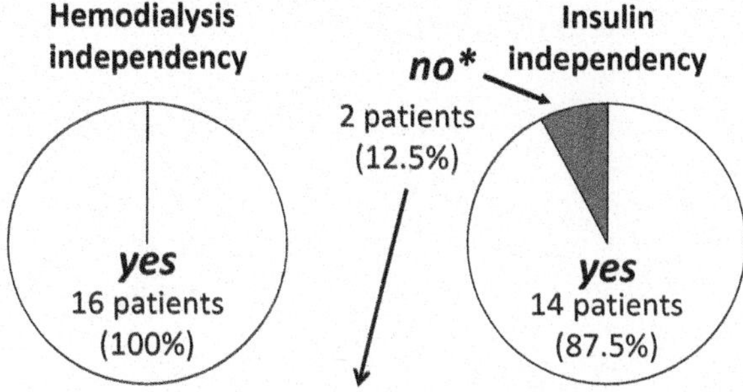

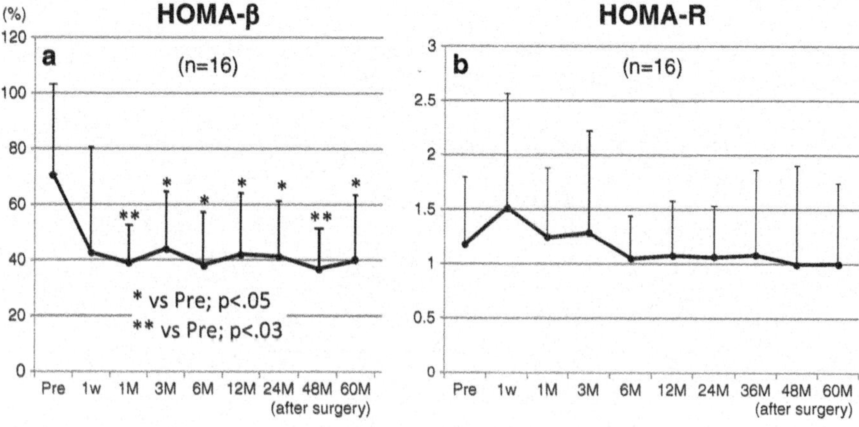

Fig. 20.4 Changes in HOMA-b (**a**), HOMA-R (**b**) of LDSPK donors (5-year follow-up). Department of Diabetology, Chiba-East National Hospital 2004.1–2012.8

All donors were discharged from the hospital at 26.0±6.8 (15–43) days after surgery and immediately returned to their normal life. Although both diabetes and renal dysfunction were not observed in all donors, one donor developed pancreatic pseudocyst at 6 months after surgery with minor symptoms. Liquid content of the cyst was drained into the stomach using gastro-fiberscopy and the cyst completely disappeared without recurrence. Another donor developed grade B pancreatic fistula at 2 weeks after surgery. It was cured, however, by conservative therapy with fasting and the subcutaneous administration of octreotide. Medications including antidiabetic agents and digestives were not needed in any donors after surgery.

Insulin secretion evaluated by HOMA-β immediately decreased after surgery. Significant decrease was detected from 1 month after surgery as compared to preoperative level. Thereafter, HOMA-β was maintained around 40 % during 5 years (Fig. 20.4a). In contrast, insulin resistance evaluated by HOMA-R was gradually decreased after surgery with no significance (Fig. 20.4b). Decline of HOMA-R may cover the deterioration of HOMA-β and prevent donors from developing diabetes.

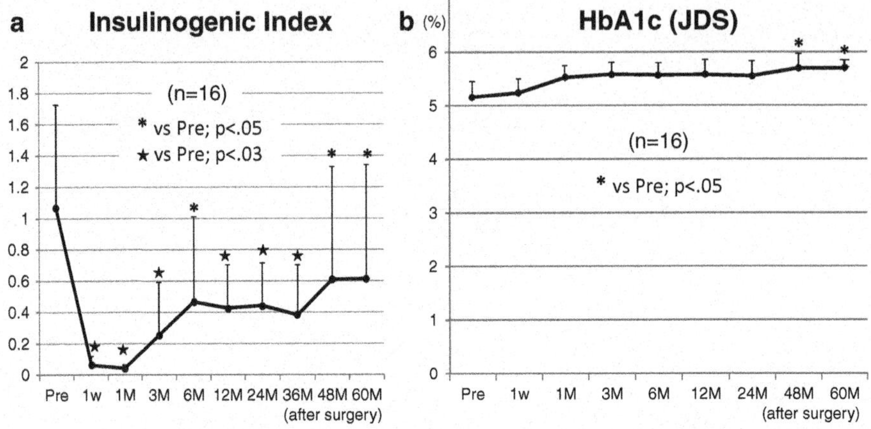

Fig. 20.5 Changes in insulinogenic index (**a**), HbA1c (JDS) (**b**) of LDSPK donors (5-year follow-up). Department of Diabetology, Chiba-East National Hospital 2004.1–2012.8

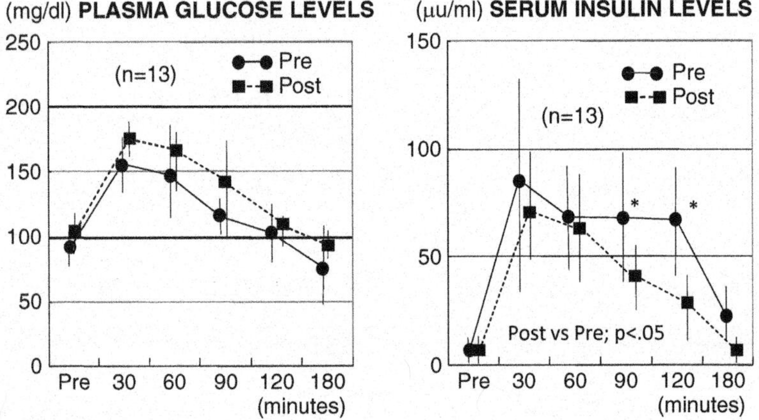

Fig. 20.6 Changes in 75 g OGTT of LDSPK donors (1 year after surgery). Department of Diabetology, Chiba-East National Hospital 2004.1–2012.8

Insulinogenic index calculated from OGTT significantly deteriorated to very low levels during 3 months after surgery. It increased gradually and reached to the level 0.6 at 4 years after surgery. However, insulinogenic index was remained significantly low after surgery as compared to the preoperative levels (Fig. 20.5a). Although HbA1c levels (JDS) were maintained less than 6.0 % in all donors, these levels gradually increased from 5.2 to 5.7 at 4 years, which was significantly higher than the preoperative levels (Fig. 20.5b).

All the donors have not developed diabetes after surgery. Although the glucose curves were normal, significantly decreased insulin secretion was found at 90 and 120 min after glucose challenge in 75 g OGTT which was performed at 1 year after surgery (Fig. 20.6).

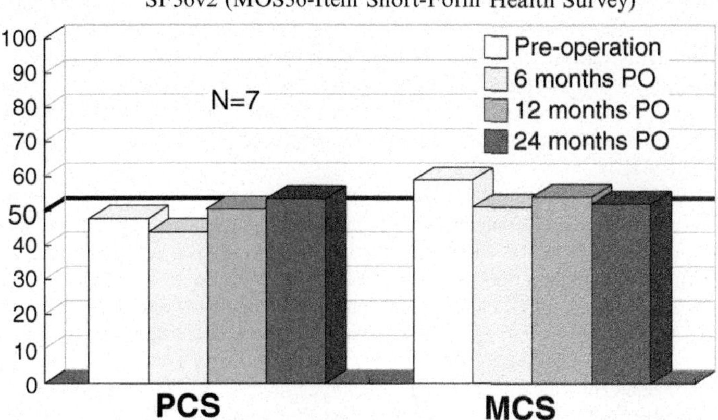

Fig. 20.7 Changes in QOL of LDSPK donors. Department of Surgery, Chiba-East National Hospital 2004.1–2012.8

These results of our investigations concerning the pancreatic endocrine function of the LDP(LDSPK) donors clearly demonstrated that insulin secretion was significantly deteriorated after distal pancreatectomy for donor operation of LDP even though they did not develop diabetes. Development of diabetes, however, was not observed during 5 years after surgery and quality of life, which was evaluated by SF36v2, was well maintained (Fig. 20.7) [15].

References

1. Sutherland DER. Pancreas and islet transplantation. II. Clinical trials. Diabetologia. 1981;20:435–50.
2. Sutherland DER, Goetz FC, Najarian JS. Living-related donor segmental pancreatectomy for transplantation. Transplant Proc. 1980;12:19–25.
3. Gruessner RWG, Sutherland DER. Simultaneous kidney and segmental pancreas transplants from living related donors: the first two successful cases. Transplantation. 1996;61:1265–8.
4. Gruessner RWG, Kendall DM, Drangstveit MB, Gruessner AC, Sutherland DER. Simultaneous pancreas-kidney transplantation from living donors. Ann Surg. 1997;226:471–82.
5. Kenmochi T, Asano T, Maruyama M, Saigo K, Akutsu N, Iwashita C, Ohtsuki K, Suzuki A, Miyazaki M. Living donor pancreas transplantation in Japan. J Hepatobiliary Pancreat Surg. 2010;17(2):101–7.
6. Tokuyama Y, Sakurai K, Yagui K, Hashimoto N, Saito Y, Kanatsuka A. Pathophysiologic phenotypes of Japanese subjects with varying degrees of glucose tolerance: using the combination of C-peptide secretion rate and minimal model analysis. Metabolism. 2001;50:812–8.
7. Otsuki K, Yoshikawa T, Kenmochi T, Maruyama M, Akutsu N, Iwashita C, Ito T, Asano T. Evaluation of segmental pancreatic function using 11C-methionine positron emission tomography for safe living donor operation of pancreas transplantation. Transplant Proc. 2011;43(9):3237–76.
8. The Japan Society for Transplantation. http://www.asas.or.jp/jst/news_top.html

9. Gruessner RWG, Sutherland DER, Drangstveit MB, Bland BJ, Gruessner AC. Pancreas transplants from living donors: short- and long term outcome. Transplant Proc. 2001;33:819–20.
10. Sutherland DER, Gruessner R, Dunn D, Moudry-Munns K, Gruessner A, Najarian JS. Pancreas transplants from living-related donors. Transplant Proc. 1994;26(2):443–5.
11. Kenmochi T, Asano T, Saigo K, Maruyama M, Akutsu N, Iwashita C, et al. The first case of simultaneous pancreas-kidney transplant from living donor in our country. Jpn J Transplant. 2005;40:466–72.
12. Kendall DM, Sutherland DE, Najarian JS, et al. Effects of hemipancreatectomy on insulin secretion and glucagon tolerance in healthy humans. N Engl J Med. 1990;322:898.
13. Seaquist ER, Robertson RP. Effects of hemipancreatectomy on pancreatic alpha and β cell function in healthy human donors. J Clin Invest. 1992;89:1761.
14. Seaquist ER, Gruessner RW. Pancreas transplantation: the donor. Selection criteria for donors. In: Gruessner RW, Benedetti E, editors. Living donor organ transplantation. New York: The McGraw-Hill companies Inc.; 2008.
15. Suzuki A, Kenmochi T, et al. Evaluation of quality of life after simultaneous pancreas and kidney transplantation from living donors using short form 36. Transplant Proc. 2008;40(8):2565–7.

Part VIII
Islet Transplantation

Chapter 21
DCD for Islet Transplantation

Takashi Kenmochi, Takehide Asano, Naotake Akutsu, and Taihei Ito

21.1 Introduction

Pancreatic islet transplantation has the potential to become the most physiologically advantageous and minimally invasive procedure for the treatment of type 1 diabetes mellitus. Since the first clinical islet transplantation was performed at the University of Minnesota in 1974 [1], the results have been far from ideal for more than two decades in spite of an improvement of islet isolation technique by Ricordi et al. [2–4]. The introduction of the Edmonton protocol, with a highly improved rate of insulin independency, encouraged us to promote clinical islet transplantation [5, 6]. In Japan, we organized the Working Group (The Japanese Islet Transplant Registry) in 1997 under the Japanese Society for Pancreas and Islet Transplantation for the purpose of starting clinical islet transplantation. The first issue of the Working Group was to construct a system of clinical islet transplantation in Japan including the registration of the recipients, procurement of the pancreas for islet isolation and transplantation of the isolated islets. In Japan, afterwards, various problems facing to a start of clinical islet transplantation have been discussed and we completed the guideline for clinical islet transplantation in Japan. The Japanese Organ Transplant Law was enforced in 1997 and organ transplantations using brain dead (DBD) donors were finally started. Since the islet transplantation was not included in the Japanese Organ Transplant Law because it was categorized as tissue transplantation, we were able to use the pancreas only from DCD donors for islet transplantation. The first islet isolation from the human pancreas was performed in 2003.9 and the

T. Kenmochi (✉) • T. Ito
Department of Organ Transplant Surgery, Fujita Health University,
1-98 Dengakugakubo, Kutsukake-cho, Toyoake City, Aichi 470-1192, Japan
e-mail: kenmochi@fujita-hu.ac.jp

T. Asano • N. Akutsu
Department of Surgery and Clinical Research Center, Chiba-East National Hospital,
673 Nitonacho, Chuo-ku, Chiba City, Chiba 260-8712, Japan
e-mail: asano@cehpnet.com

T. Asano et al. (eds.), *Marginal Donors: Current and Future Status*,
DOI 10.1007/978-4-431-54484-5_21, © Springer Japan 2014

first islet transplantation was performed in 2004.4 [7–9]. Sixty-five islet isolations and 34 islet transplantations were performed in our country from 2003.9.12 to 2007.3.11 [10].

In this chapter, we describe the current status of clinical islet transplantation using DCD donors in Japan.

21.2 Donor Criteria

Islet transplantation is categorized as tissue transplantation in Japan. Therefore, donor criteria for islet transplantation were based on the guideline issued by Japanese Society of Tissue Transplantation (JSTT) [11], which is shown in Table 21.1. According to the guideline, when a specific disease or state is observed in a donor, retrieval or transplant of tissue from the donor must not be permitted. It is necessary to conduct inspection and palpation of the donor, as detailed as possible. Interview of the donor's next of kin and studying the donor's medical records are also required. The results of a pathological autopsy, if performed, must be reviewed. For all tests performed, conduct the most current methodology. Criteria and methods of tests or examinations must be always updated at a tissue bank (Islet isolation center), in accordance with technical and scientific advancements and new findings in infectious diseases. (It is desirable to involve experts from related

Table 21.1 Exclusion criteria of tissue donors in general (Guideline on the safety, storage, and application of human tissue in medical practice. IV. Criteria for donor screening. Japanese Society of Tissue Transplantation (JSTT)) [11]

- Death from unknown causes
- Documented cases of sepsis or other systemic infectious diseases
- CJD (vCJD) or its suspect of infection
- Malignancy (as for primary brain tumors or solid tumors treated more than 5 years ago, and diagnosed to be cured, judgement may be given by the physicians to procure the tissue)
- Hematologic malignancies, such as leukemia or malignant lymphomas
- Severe metabolic or endocrine disorders. Autoimmune disorders such as hematological diseases or collagen disease
- Syphilis positive
- Hepatitis (HBV positive, HCV positive)
- AIDS (HIV positive)
- Adult T-cell leukemia (ATL), HTLV-1 positive
- Parvovirus B19 positive
- West Nile virus positive
- SARS
- Rabies
- Other patient/donor who corresponds to exclusion criteria set for each tissue

Patients or donors must be negative in interviews and tests (serodiagnosis or NAT) for all these infections and diseases listed above. Where necessary, a patient or donor is to be tested for negative infection of cytomegalovirus and EB virus academic associations in the process of updating the criteria or collecting/evaluating information on infectious diseases, etc.) In accordance with the principle presented in the above notification of the Pharmaceutical and Medical Safety Bureau of MHLW, retrieval of tissue is prohibited when a patient or donor corresponds to any of the following items in Table 21.1.

In addition, the Japanese Islet Transplant Registry determined following four items for donor criteria of islet transplantation: (1) age ≤70 years, (2) warm ischemic time ≤30 min, (3) exclusion criteria of the JSTT guideline (Table 21.1), and (4) recommendation of UW solution or two-layer method (TLM) for preservation.

21.3 Procurement and Preservation of the Pancreas

In Japan, the pancreas from DCD donors are used for islet isolation since the pancreas from DBD donors are usually used for pancreas or pancreas/kidney transplantation according to the Japan Organ Transplant Law. The withdrawal of a respirator is rarely performed even though the donor is diagnosed to be brain dead (Maastricht category 4 [12]). Moreover, the donors usually are not examined to diagnose brain death, and thus, a cannulation into an abdominal aorta with a double-balloon catheter via a femoral artery and a systemic heparinization are not permitted before a cardiac arrest (modified Maastricht category 5 [13]). To shorten warm ischemic time and maintain a viability of the pancreas for islet isolation, we use in situ machine washout (ISMW) technique [14, 15], which was originally developed for the procurement of the kidneys from DCD donors. The efficacy of ISMW on clinical kidney transplantation from DCD donors is described in detail in another chapter. For the procurement of the pancreas from DCD donors, a double-balloon catheter position needs to be changed to perfuse celiac artery and superior mesenteric artery as well as bilateral renal arteries. We usually place the distal balloon in the aorta which is located above the celiac axis and only distal balloon is inflated. X-ray and ultrasound sonography are used for the confirmation of the collect location of the balloon. The University of Wisconsin (UW) solution is most frequently used as the perfusate of ISMW for the procurement of pancreas.

TLM, which was developed by Kuroda Y et al., was frequently used for the preservation of the pancreas before islet isolation. TLM was considered to be advantageous for the preservation of the pancreas for islet isolation, which resulted in higher yield and purity [16–22]. However, Caballero-Corbalán J et al. reported that a TLM had no beneficial effect as compared with the UW solution on human islet isolation and transplantation [23]. Currently, the use of TLM depends on the consideration of each islet isolation and transplantation center.

Procurement of the pancreas from DCD donors is different from that of the DBD donors in Japan. Since pancreatic islet transplantation is categorized as tissue transplantation, the pancreas must be procured after en bloc procurement of bilateral kidneys. Pancreas is procured with or without duodenum from the DCD donor. In back table, pancreas was isolated from the surrounding tissue including the duodenum, spleen, blood vessels, and lymph nodes. When TLM is used for preservation of the pancreatic graft, the graft is moved into TLM container in which oxygenation was already done with 30 min oxygen bubbling. Some institutions perform the ductal injection with UW solution or other solutions into the main pancreatic duct [24–27].

21.4 Quality Control of Islet Transplantation

Quality control (QC) is important for the safe performance of islet transplantation. QC includes infection control and viability assay of the isolated islets. QC committee was placed in the Japanese Islet Transplant Registry, performing QC of all procedures in clinical islet transplantation in Japan [28]. As shown in Table 21.2, infection control is the major issue in QC. In the procurement of the pancreas from DCD donors, donor criteria must be strictly obeyed and past history of the infectious diseases should be carefully checked. Before islet isolation, the checking of the bacterial contamination of the preservation solution must be performed. Islet isolation is permitted to proceed in the authorized islet isolation centers which were acknowledged by the Japanese Society for Pancreas and Islet Transplantation. These centers have GMP-level-regulated cell processing rooms (center) and provide

Table 21.2 Quality control of pancreatic islets of islet transplantation (Committee of Quality Control, The Japanese Islet Transplant Registry, 2006.9) [28]

Quality control of pancreatic islets

1. Infection control
   1. Donor screening and assessment of the infection
   2. Checking of contamination during islet isolation and culture procedure
   3. Checking of endotoxin levels of the media before transplantation
2. Morphological and functional assay of the isolated islets (viability assay)
   1. Microscopic and electron microscopic examination
   2. Trypan blue staining
   3. Static incubation and/or perifusion studies

Algorism of quality control

Procurement team

Procurement of the pancreas: checking of the active infection and past history of the infectious diseases

Islet isolation center

1. GMP level regulated cell processing room must be used (all procedures must be performed in sterile field)
2. Islet isolation: checking of the contamination (preservation solution, isolation media, culture media, etc.), static incubation
3. Cryopreservation of the islets: checking of the contamination (samples of cryopreserved islets), static incubation of samples of cryopreserved islets)

Islet transplantation center

1. Final checking of the contamination and endotoxin level of the islet suspended media

the sterile field on all procedure of islet isolation and islet culture before transplantation. After islet isolation and culture, the media were sampled and checked for bacterial contaminations.

Viability assays of the isolated islets include the results of the isolation such as yield and purity of the islets, volume of the pellet of islets, morphological examination using microscope with dithizone staining, and electron microscope and functional assays.

The Japanese Islet Transplant Registry determined static incubation as the standard method of functional assay of the isolated islets. The technique of the static incubation is shown as follows. Briefly, five aliquots of ten islets were placed into 12-well Transwell microplates with 1 mL RPMI 1640 containing 3.3 mmol/L D-glucose and 0.1 % BSA as the basal medium. After 60 min, the culture Transwells were transferred into new 12-well microplates with RPMI 1640 containing 20 mmol/L D-glucose and 0.1 % BSA (glucose stimulation). After 60 min, the culture Transwells were transferred to new 12-well microplates to add basal medium again for an additional 60 min culture. Each medium was centrifuged and immediately frozen for a later assay of the insulin concentration by ELISA. The stimulation index was calculated by comparing the insulin content in the glucose stimulation medium with the second basal medium.

In addition to the static incubation, we perform the perifusion study to assess the ability of insulin release from the islets. Perifusion study was performed using following technique. Using our original perifusion system, the 50 islets were perifused in a low-glucose medium (Krebs Ringer solution with 3.3 mM D-glucose) for 80 min and then perifused in a high-glucose medium (Krebs Ringer solution with 16.7 mM D-glucose) for 30 min, followed by 60 min perifusion in a low-glucose medium. Stimulation indices were calculated from the ratio of insulin released into the low-glucose medium and the high-glucose medium.

Whether the isolated islets are alive or dead is the first viability assay. Chromogenic dyes such as neutral red or trypan blue are able to visualize live or dead cells. The islet, however, consists of a number of cells; therefore, chromogenic dyes cannot evaluate the islet itself, while fluorescein diacetate (FDA) is used to quantitate the proportion of cells that are intact or that are damaged, which can evaluate the islet more precisely [29]. Live islet is not necessarily able to respond appropriately to glucose stimulation; therefore, in vitro biochemical techniques have predominantly been used to assess islet viability. Insulin release from islets after stimulation with high glucose concentration has commonly been used in static incubation or perifusion study [30–33]. Glucose utilization [32], protein synthesis [34–36], and oxygen utilization [37] have also been used to assess islet function.

In addition to in vitro studies, syngeneic or autologous islet transplantation is preferable to assess islet viability, which simulates the outcome of islet transplantation. Nude (athymic) mice, which were induced with diabetes by intravenous injection with streptozotocin, are commonly used for in vivo assay of human islets [38, 39].

According to the outcome of islet isolation, the Japanese Islet Transplant Registry determined the criteria for fresh islet isolation. When the outcome of the isolation fulfill the criteria ((1) yield ≥5,000 IEQ/kg (recipient body weight); (2) purity

Table 21.3 The rules for recipient selection from the recipient pool in Japan [28]

1. Recipients must be registered to the islet isolation center
2. ABO blood type
3. Second or third transplantation
4. Waiting days

Table 21.4 Indications for the recipient of islet transplantation in Japan [28]

Indications
1. Insulin dependent diabetes mellitus (serum C-peptide level: <0.1 ng/mL)
2. Unstable blood glucose levels even under the treatment by a diabetologist
3. Age: <75 years old (preferable)
4. Sufficient informed consent obtained from the patient, family, and family doctor
Contraindications
1. Severe heart disease or severe liver disease
2. Alcoholism
3. Active infectious disease
4. Malignancy
5. Severe obesity
6. Untreated retinopathy
7. Others

≥30 %; (3) final cell pellet ≤10 ml; (4) viability ≥70 %; and (5) endotoxin ≤5 EU/kg (recipient body weight)), the recipient is selected from the recipient pool by the Japanese Islet Transplant Registry according to the rules for recipient selection (Table 21.3) [28]. The patients were registered to each transplantation center according to the indications of the recipient for islet transplantation in Japan (Table 21.4) [28].

21.5 Outcome of Clinical Islet Transplantation from DCD Donors in Japan

Sixty-five islet isolations were performed at five authorized centers of islet isolation and transplantation from December 2003 to March 2007. Only one isolation (the first isolation in Japan) was performed using the pancreas from DBD donor and the other 64 isolations were performed using DCD donors. Thirty-four successful isolations (53.1 % of 64 isolations from DCD donors) fulfilled the fresh islet transplantation criteria and were transplanted to the 18 patients. The analysis of the factors influencing the results of the islet isolation demonstrated that the donor age and a warm ischemic time did not affect the results. In contrast, duration of low blood pressure of the donor, cold ischemic time, and usage of Kyoto solution for preservation was significantly influenced factors [40]. Multivariate analysis selected usage of Kyoto solution as most important.

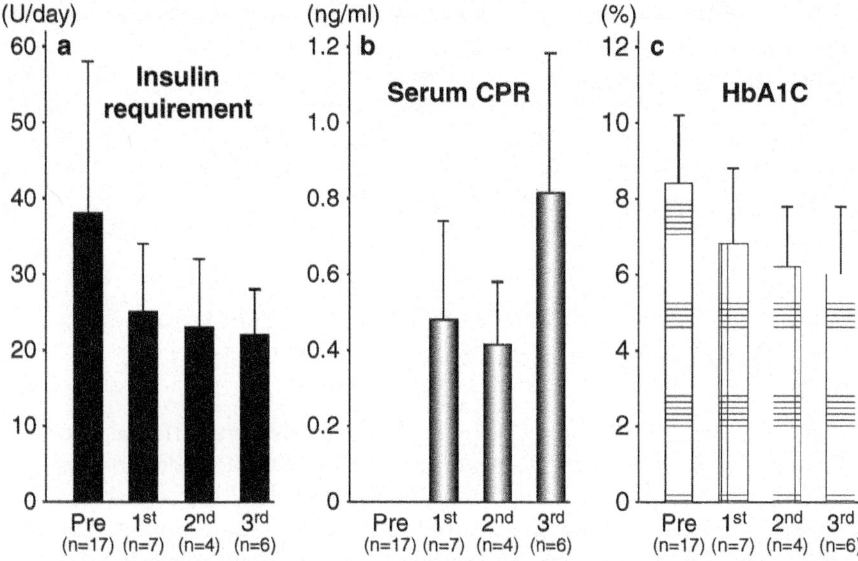

Fig. 21.1 The outcome of clinical islet transplantation in Japan: insulin requirement (**a**) decreased after the first (1st), the second (2nd), and the third (3rd) islet transplantation. Serum C-peptide levels (**b**) became positive after islet transplantation. Especially after the third islet transplantation, serum CPR showed 0.8 + 0.4 ng/mL. Hemoglobin A1C (**c**) decreased after islet transplantation due to the stabilization of blood glucose levels

All 18 recipients were type 1 diabetic patients with the history of diabetes from 6 to 37 years. The age of the recipients ranged from 16 to 61 years (36.2 ± 10.9 years) and the gender was 5 males/13 females. Four patients underwent two sequential islet transplantations and six patients underwent three sequential islet transplantations. Out of four patients who underwent two islet transplantations, one patient showed insulin independency, and two out of six patients who underwent three islet transplantations achieved insulin independency. However, all of these patients returned to insulin dependency from 2 weeks to 6 months after achieving insulin independency. The islet transplantation technique was performed according to the Edmonton Protocol. The isolated islets were transplanted into the portal vein using an angiocatheter via an ultrasonography-guided puncture. A steroid-free immunosuppressive regimen was used with sirolimus, tacrolimus, and anti-CD25 antibody according to the Edmonton Protocol5. As is shown in Fig. 21.1, the serum C-peptide levels were 0.5 ± 0.4 ng/mL after the first, 0.4 ± 0.2 ng/mL after the second, and 0.8 ± 0.4 ng/mL after the third islet transplantation. The positive insulin secretion from the islets, as indicated by the serum C-peptide levels, resulted in the decreased insulin requirement: 39.7 ± 18.0 U/day before, 24.2 ± 110 U/day after the first, 21.4 ± 11.5 U/day after the second, and 21.0 ± 7.7 U/day after the third islet transplantation. In addition, the hemoglobin A1C levels (JDS) decreased from 8.8 ± 1.8 % before transplantation to 7.5 ± 1.4 % after the first, 6.5 ± 1.4 % after the second, and

6.2 ± 1.2 % after the third islet transplantation. All patients obtained stabilized blood glucose levels which resulted in the disappearance of hypoglycemic unawareness19. Overall graft survival defined as C-peptide level more than or equal to 0.3 ng/mL was 76.5 %, 47.1 %, and 33.6 % at 1, 2, and 3 years, respectively, whereas corresponding graft survival after multiple transplantations was 100 %, 80.0 %, and 57.1 %, respectively [40]. Almost all patients showed, however, negative C-peptide level at 5 years after the first islet transplantation.

21.6 Outcome of Clinical Islet Transplantation from DCD Donors in Chiba East National Hospital

From September 2003 to April 2007, 23 islet isolations were performed from the pancreas of non-heart-beating donors in our institution (GMP grade Bio-clean Cell Processing Center (CPC), Clinical Research Center, Chiba-East National Hospital). The age of the donors ranged from 10 to 69 years (37.5 ± 18.0 years), and the gender was 13 males/10 females. The causes of death were cerebrovascular disorder (ten cases), hypoxic encephalopathy (seven cases), trauma (five cases), and one brain tumor. After cardiac arrest, the pancreas were procured using our ISMW technique. In 9 of the 23 donors, permission was not given to insert a catheter into the aorta for systemic heparinization before a cardiac arrest, which resulted in a prolonged warm ischemic period. The pancreas were preserved using a TLM or a simple cold storage in UW solution and were transported to our CPC.

The islet isolation was performed according to the Edmonton Protocol with some modifications [41–48]. Briefly, the pancreas was distended with a cold Liberase solution (Liberase HI, Roche Diagnostics™, IN) by a ductal injection. Thereafter, the distended pancreas were cut into several pieces and put into a Ricordi chamber and digested using a closed automated system at 37 °C. The shaking of the Ricordi chamber was performed either by hand or by a shaking apparatus. The pancreatic digests were collected in a flask on ice and were purified on a Euro-Ficoll discontinuous solution using a COBE 2991 cell processor. When the results of the isolation fulfilled the criteria for fresh islet transplantation in Japan, the islets were immediately transplanted to the recipient.

Our technique of islet transplantation is the same procedure as in the Edmonton Protocol. The immunosuppression protocol was achieved by a triple therapy using sirolimus, tacrolimus, and anti-CD25 antibody. Four patients underwent six islet transplantations. All patients were type 1 diabetic patients (one male, three females) complaining of frequent hypoglycemic unawareness and showing an undetectable serum C-peptide levels (<0.03 ng/mL). The patient ages ranged from 16 to 33 years old. Two patients underwent two sequential islet transplantations.

The islet yield was 400–491,040 IEQ (mean 148,511) and the final purity was 1–70% (mean, 35.3). The stimulation index of static incubation was 1.38–11.69. Six isolations were used for transplantation because they fulfilled the Japanese criteria (success rate: 26.1 %). All patients, including two cases of single transplantation,

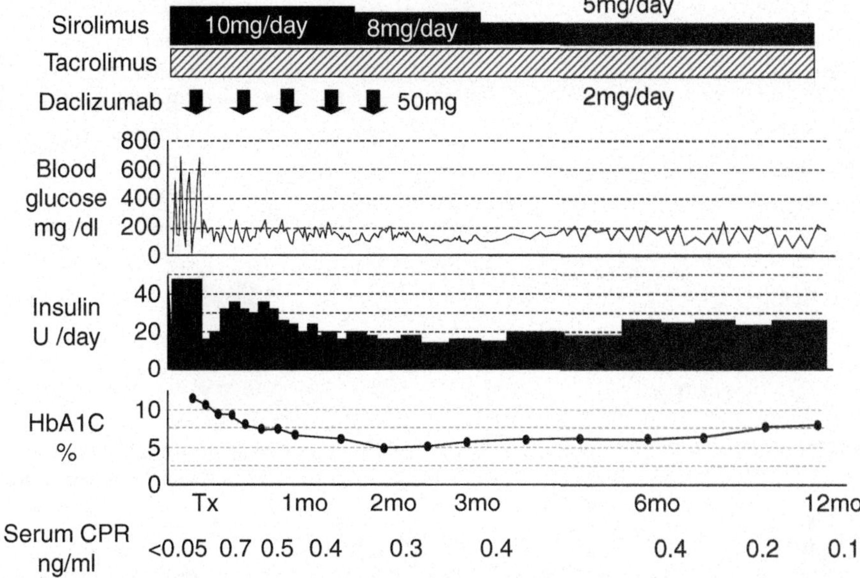

Fig. 21.2 Post-transplant course of the patient #1 (Department of Surgery, Chiba-East National Hospital): stabilization of the blood glucose levels and the decrease of the insulin requirement were obtained due to the positive serum CPR. However, serum CPR decreased gradually after islet transplantation

showed a positive serum C-peptide level (0.4–0.8 ng/mL) immediately after transplantation. Although insulin independency was not achieved, all patients achieved stabilization of blood glucose levels, reduced requirement of insulin, and the disappearance of hypoglycemic unawareness. The hemoglobin A1C levels (JDS) were significantly decreased from 9.4 ± 3.1 % to 6.4 ± 0.6 % at 4 months after transplantation. Although stomatitis and diarrhea, which were considered as the side effects of sirolimus, were observed in two patients, severe complications did not occur. In patient #1, the serum C-peptide levels decreased gradually after transplantation (Fig. 21.2). Blood glucose levels were, however, again stabilized after the second islet transplantation (Fig. 21.3). However, all four patients showed negative C-peptide levels at 5 years after the first islet transplantation.

21.7 Conclusions

Islet transplantation employing DCD can ameliorate severe hypoglycemic episodes, significantly improve HbA1c levels, sustain significant levels of C-peptide, and achieve insulin independence after multiple transplantations. Thus, DCD can be an important resource for islet transplantation if used under strict releasing criteria and

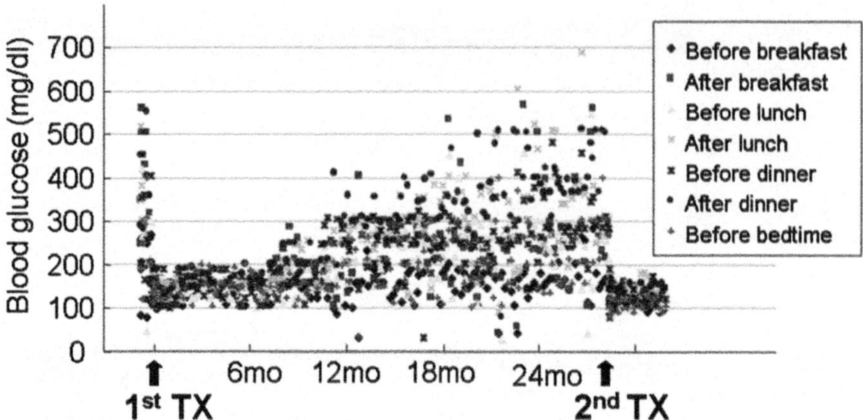

Fig. 21.3 Changes in blood glucose levels after islet transplantation in the patient #1: control of blood glucose levels became poor 12 months after transplantation. However, blood glucose levels were again stabilized by second islet transplantation

in multiple transplantations, particularly in countries where heart-beating donors are not readily available.

However, the outcome of clinical islet transplantation using Edmonton protocol is not satisfactory results. In particular, long-term islet survival has not been achieved, resulting in poor achievement of insulin independency. Based on these results, the Japanese Islet Transplant Registry currently introduced a newly designed clinical islet transplantation protocol including an immunosuppressive protocol using anti-thymus globulin and anti TNF α, and the use of DBD donors.

References

1. Najarian JS, Sutherland DE, Matas AJ, Steffes MW, Simmons RL, Goetz FC. Human islet transplantation: a preliminary report. Transplant Proc. 1977;9:233–6.
2. International Islet Transplant Registry. Newsletter No. 8. 1999.
3. Ricordi C, Finke EH, Lacy PE. A method for the mass isolation of islets from the adult pig pancreas. Diabetes. 1986;35:649–53.
4. Ricordi C, Lacy PE, Finke EH, Olack BJ, Scharp DW. Automated method for isolation of human pancreatic islets. Diabetes. 1988;37:413–20.
5. Shapiro AM, Lakey JR, Ryan EA, Korbutt GS, Toth E, Warnock GL, et al. Islet transplantation in seven patients with type 1 diabetes mellitus using a glucocorticoid-free immunosuppressive regimen. N Engl J Med. 2000;343:230–8.
6. Ryan EA, Lakey JR, Rajotte RV, Korbutt GS, Kin T, Imes S, et al. Clinical outcomes and insulin secretion after islet transplantation with the Edmonton protocol. Diabetes. 2001;50:710–9.
7. Matsumoto S, Okitsu T, Iwanaga Y, Noguchi H, Nagata H, Yonekawa Y, et al. Successful islet transplantation from nonheartbeating donor pancreata using modified Ricordi islet isolation method. Transplantation. 2006;82:460–5.
8. Matsumoto S, Tanaka K. Pancreatic islet cell transplantation. J Hepatobiliary Pancreat Surg. 2005;12:227–30.

9. Saito T, Ise K, Sato Y, Gotoh M, Matsumoto S, Kenmochi T, et al. The start of an islet transplantation program in Japan. Transplant Proc. 2005;37:3424–6.
10. Kenmochi T, Asano T, Maruyama M, Saigo K, Akutsu N, Iwashita C, Ohtsuki K, Ito T. Clinical islet transplantation in Japan. J Hepatobiliary Pancreat Surg. 2009;16(2):124–30.
11. Japanese Society of Tissue Transplantation (JSTT) ed. Guideline on the safety, storage, and application of human tissue in medical practice. IV. Criteria for donor screening. http://www.jstt.org/htm/guideline/Safety.pdf.
12. Kootstra G, Daemen J, Oomen A. Categories of non-heart-beating donors. Transplant Proc. 1995;27:2893–4.
13. Sanchez-Fructuoso A, et al. Renal transplantation from non-heart-beating donors: a promising alternative to enlarge the donor pool. J Am Soc Nephrol. 2000;11:350–8.
14. Arita S, Asano T, Kenmochi T, Enomoto K, Isono K. An initial wash-out solution for "in situ machine wash-out". Transplant Proc. 1991;23:2589.
15. Asano T, Enomoto K, Ohtsuka M, Goto T, Nakagohri T, Kenmochi T, Ochiai T, Isono K. Usefulness of rapid machine cooling in the procurement of livers. Transplant Proc. 1989;21(1 Pt 2):1307–8.
16. Goto T, Tanioka Y, Sakai T, Terai S, Kamoda Y, Li S, et al. Application of the two-layer method on pancreas digestion results in improved islet yield and maintained viability of isolated islets. Transplantation. 2007;27:754–8.
17. Kin T, Mirbolooki M, Salehi P, Tsukada M, O'Gorman D, Imes S, et al. Islet isolation and transplantation outcomes of pancreas preserved with University of Wisconsin solution versus two-layer method using preoxygenated perfluorocarbon. Transplantation. 2006;82:1286–90.
18. Takahashi T, Tanioka Y, Matsuda T, Toyama H, Kakinoki K, Li S, et al. Impact of the two-layer method on the quality of isolated pancreatic islets. Hepatogastroenterology. 2006;53:179–82.
19. Tanaka T, Suzuki Y, Tanioka Y, Sakai T, Kakinoki K, Goto T, et al. Possibility of islet transplantation from a nonheartbeating donor pancreas resuscitated by the two-layer method. Transplantation. 2005;80:738–42.
20. Tsujimura T, Kuroda Y, Churchill TA, Avila JG, Kin T, Shapiro AM, et al. Short-term storage of the ischemically damaged human pancreas by the two-layer method prior to islet isolation. Cell Transplant. 2004;13:67–73.
21. Tsujimura T, Kuroda Y, Kin T, Avila JG, Rajotte RV, Korbutt GS, et al. Human islet transplantation from pancreases with prolonged cold ischemia using additional preservation by the two-layer (UW solution/perfluorochemical) cold-storage method. Transplantation. 2002; 74:1687–91.
22. Tanioka Y, Sutherland DE, Kuroda Y, Gilmore TR, Asaheim TC, Kronson JW, et al. Excellence of the two-layer method (University of Wisconsin solution/perfluorochemical) in pancreas preservation before islet isolation. Surgery. 1997;122:435–42.
23. Caballero-Corbalán J, Eich T, Lundgren T, Foss A, Felldin M, Källen R, et al. No beneficial effect of two-layer storage compared with UW-storage on human islet isolation and transplantation. Transplantation. 2007;84:864–9.
24. Sawada T, Matsumoto I, Nakano M, Kirchhof N, Sutherland DE, Hering BJ. Improved islet yield and function with ductal injection of University of Wisconsin solution before pancreas preservation. Transplantation. 2003;75(12):1965–9.
25. Matsumoto S, Noguichi H, Shimoda M, Ikemoto T, Naziruddin B, Jackson A, Tamura Y, Olson G, Fujita Y, Chujo D, Takita M, Kobayashi N, Onaca N, Levy M. Seven consecutive successful clinical islet isolations with pancreatic ductal injection. Cell Transplant. 2010;19(3):291–7.
26. Anazawa T, Balamurugan AN, Papas KK, Avgoustiniatos ES, Ferrer J, Matsumoto S, Sutherland DE, Hering BJ. Improved method of porcine pancreas procurement with arterial flush and ductal injection enhances islet isolation outcome. Transplant Proc. 2010; 42(6):2032–5.
27. Shimoda M, Itoh T, Sugimoto K, Iwahashi S, Takita M, Chujo D, Sorelle JA, Naziruddin B, Levy MF, Grayburn PA, Matsumoto S. Improvement of collagenase distribution with the ductal preservation for human islet isolation. Islets. 2012;4(2):130–7.

28. Kenmochi T, Matsumoto S, Tanioka Y, Saito T, Ono J, Okamoto M, et al. Manual for clinical islet transplantation in Japan, 3rd ed. In: Fukushima H, editor. The Japanese Society for Pancreas and Islet Transplantation. Fukushima, Japan; 2006. p. 1–55.
29. Ricordi C, Gray DWR, Hering BJ, et al. Islet isolation assessment in man and large animals. Acta Diabetol Lat. 1990;27:185–95.
30. Gray DWR, McShane P, Grant A, Morris PJ. A method for isolation of islets of Langerhans from the human pancreas. Diabetes. 1984;33:1055–61.
31. Andersson A, Borg H, Groth CG, et al. Survival of isolated human islets of Langerhans maintained in tissue culture. J Clin Invest. 1976;57:1295–301.
32. Ashcroft SJH, Bassett JM, Rndle PJ. Isolation of human pancreatic islets capable of releasing insulin and metabolizing glucose in vitro. Lancet. 1971;1:888–9.
33. Ballinger WF, Lacy PE. Transplantation of intact pancreatic islets in rats. Surgery. 1972; 72:175–86.
34. Sutherland DE, Matas AJ, Steffes MW, Najarian JS. Infant human pancreas. A potential source of islet tissue for transplantation. Diabetes. 1976;25(12):1123–8.
35. Davalli AM, Ricordi C, Socci C, Braghi S, Bertuzzi F, Fattor B, Di Carlo V, Pontiroli AE, Pozza G. Abnormal sensitivity to glucose of human islets cultured in a high glucose medium: partial reversibility after an additional culture in a normal glucose medium. J Clin Endocrinol Metab. 1991;72(1):202–8.
36. Kneteman NM, Rajotte RV. Isolation and cryopreservation of human pancreatic islets. Life Support Syst. 1985;3 Suppl 1:712–8.
37. Scharp DW, Lacy PE, Finke E, Olack B. Low-temperature culture of human islets isolated by the distention method and purified with Ficoll or Percoll gradients. Surgery. 1987;102(5):869–79.
38. Povlsen CO, Skakkebaek NE, Rygaard J, Jensen G. Heterotransplantation of human foetal organs to the mouse mutant nude. Nature. 1974;248(445):247–9.
39. Usadel KH, Schwedes U, Bastert G, Steinau U, Klempa I, Fassbinder W, Schöffling K. Transplantation of human fetal pancreas: experience in thymusaplastic mice and rats and in a diabetic patient. Diabetes. 1980;29 Suppl 1:74–9.
40. Saito T, Gotoh M, Satomi S, Uemoto S, Kenmochi T, Itoh T, Kuroda Y, Yasunami Y, Matsumoto S, Teraoka S, Working Members of the Japanese Pancreas and Islet Transplantation Association. Islet transplantation using donors after cardiac death: report of the Japan islet transplantation registry. Transplantation. 2010;90(7):740–7.
41. Kenmochi T, Asano T, Jingu K, Matsui Y, Maruyama M, Akutsu N, et al. Effectiveness of hydroxyethyl starch (HES) on purification of pancreatic islets. J Surg Res. 2003;111:16–22.
42. Kenmochi T, Asano T, Jingu K, Matsui Y, Maruyama M, Miyauchi H, et al. Purification of pancreatic islets using hydroxyethyl starch-Collins solution. Transplant Proc. 2001;33:670–1.
43. Kenmochi T, Miyamoto M, Une S, Nakagawa Y, Moldovan S, Navarro RA, et al. Improved quality and yield of islets isolated from human pancreata using a two-step digestion method. Pancreas. 2000;20:184–90.
44. Kenmochi T, Asano T, Jingu K, Iwashita C, Miyauchi H, Takahashi S, et al. Development of a fully automated islet digestion system. Transplant Proc. 2000;32:341–3.
45. Mullen Y, Arita S, Kenmochi T, Une S, Smith CV. A two-step digestion process and lap-1 cold preservation solution for human islet isolation. Ann Transplant. 1998;2:40–5.
46. Kenmochi T, Miyamoto M, Sasaki H, Une S, Nakagawa Y, Moldovan S, et al. Lap-1 cold preservation solution for isolation of high-quality human pancreatic islets. Pancreas. 1998; 17:367–77.
47. Iwashita C, Asano T, Kenmochi T, Jingu K, Uematsu T, Nakagohri T, et al. Combined method of mechanical chopper and automated two-step digestion technique for islet isolation from canine pancreas. Transplant Proc. 1996;28:337–8.
48. Jingu K, Asano T, Kenmochi T, Enomoto K, Uematsu T, Nakagohri T, et al. Combined method of mechanical chopper and automated digestion system for islet isolation. Transplant Proc. 1996;26:634–6.

Chapter 22
ECD for Islet Transplantation

Takashi Kenmochi, Takehide Asano, Naotake Akutsu, and Taihei Ito

22.1 Introduction

Pancreatic islet transplantation offers a minimally invasive option for type 1 diabetic patients. Before 2000, less than 10 % of the recipients of islet transplantation achieved insulin independency [1]. The introduction of the Edmonton Protocol, however, with a highly improved rate of insulin independency, encouraged us to promote clinical islet transplantation [2, 3]. In the Edmonton Protocol, brain-dead donors were used for islet isolation, and the donors were selected according to the factors that influence the success of islet isolation [4]. Even using the Edmonton Protocol, the results of clinical islet transplantation including a long-term graft survival were far from ideal and were significantly worse than clinical pancreas transplantation (pancreas transplant alone, PTA). The newly designed protocol from Minnesota University by Hering et al. that includes induction therapy with a T-cell-depleting antibody (anti-thymus globulin, ATG) and an inhibitor of tumor necrosis factor-α (TNF-α) achieved successful islet transplantation from a single donor. Short-term and long-term islet graft survivals were shown which were comparable to those in clinical pancreas transplantation (PTA). These results demonstrated that islet transplantation was expected to take the place of solitary pancreas transplantation for the type 1 diabetic patients without renal dysfunction.

Strict donor criteria are not necessarily needed for islet transplantation because the islets were transplanted after its evaluation after isolation, which is different from pancreas transplantation in which the pancreas is transplanted to the

T. Kenmochi (✉) • T. Ito
Department of Organ Transplant Surgery, Fujita Health University,
1-98 Dengakugakubo, Kutsukake-cho, Toyoake City, Aichi 470-1192, Japan
e-mail: kenmochi@fujita-hu.ac.jp

T. Asano • N. Akutsu
Department of Surgery and Clinical Research Center, Chiba-East National Hospital,
673 Nitonacho, Chuo-ku, Chiba City, Chiba 260-8712, Japan
e-mail: asano@cehpnet.com

T. Asano et al. (eds.), *Marginal Donors: Current and Future Status*,
DOI 10.1007/978-4-431-54484-5_22,

recipients immediately after procurement from the donor. Therefore, extended criteria donor has not been clearly defined in islet transplantation. DBD donors were most frequently used for islet transplantation worldwide. In our country, however, DCD donors were used for islet transplantation because of an ultimate shortage of DBD donors and the regulation under Organ Transplantation Law that was enforced in 1997.

Although a clear definition as an extended criteria donor for islet transplantation has not been determined, the factors that influence the outcome of the islet isolation were investigated in previous papers. In this chapter, the factors that influence the outcome of the islet isolation were introduced and extended criteria donor for islet transplantation is discussed.

22.2 The Factors that Influence the Outcome of the Islet Isolation

The first and the most important step in islet transplantation is the isolation of high-quality islets from the pancreas in a high quantity. The pancreatic islet isolation technique involving ductal distension followed by collagenase digestion was first introduced, in rats, by Lacy and Kostianovsky in 1967 [5]. Despite a vast amount of effort [6–8], successful islet isolation from the pancreas of large animal species had not been achieved until recently. Ricordi et al. introduced a highly automated system for the large-scale isolation of islets from the human or porcine pancreas [9, 10], and the number of clinical islet transplantations has gradually but steadily increased from 1990. Islet isolation technique must be the most important factor that directly affects an outcome of islet isolation. In addition, from the previous reports regarding experimental and clinical islet isolation, the various factors in addition to islet isolation technique were investigated to influence the outcome of islet isolation.

22.2.1 Donor Factors

Lakey et al. demonstrated that old age, high body mass index, low minimum blood glucose level, and short or no duration of cardiac arrest were the significant donor factors that result in the high recovery of islets after isolation using 153 human islet isolations [4]. In addition, duration of cold storage was a significant factor to affect the recovery of the islets. Although the higher the donor age, the higher the success rate of isolation, the stimulation index was higher in the islet isolate from the young-aged donor pancreas. In a recent study with 276 islet isolations, however, donor age was shown to have no correlation with islet yield [11]. Also, the data of the Japanese Islet Transplant Program demonstrated that donor age did not influence the recovery of the islets [12]. Since the islet viability must be better in the pancreas procured from the young donor as well as other organs, the improvement of the islet isolation technique might realize the high yield of the islets from the pancreas of young donors.

While previous papers demonstrated that high BMI (>25 or >30 kg/m^2) was a dominant factor that resulted in the high yield of the islets after isolation [13–15]. The reasons why the donors with increased BMI resulted in a significantly higher recovery of the islets are not clearly explained. In contrast, the donors with increased BMI were reported to be not suitable for pancreas transplantation because of the increased complication including graft pancreatitis, thrombosis, and infection after transplantation [16].

Cause of death is another important factor affecting islet recovery after isolation. The donor whose cause of death is trauma seems to be suitable for donation of the pancreas to achieve successful islet isolation. Since the frequency of trauma as the cause of death of DBD donors is less than 20 % in Japan, which is extremely lower than that in other countries, over 80 % of DBD donors are considered to be marginal donors for both pancreas transplantation and islet transplantation.

22.2.2 Procurement and Preservation Factors

Lakey et al. demonstrated that pancreas procured locally had a significantly higher success rate compared with organs procured distantly. Local procurement and decreased duration of cold storage were factors to achieve successful islet isolation. In Japan, 64 islet isolations were performed from the DCD donors. In DCD donors, we insert a double-balloon catheter from the femoral artery before cardiac arrest to shorten warm ischemic time (see Chap. 21). However, the pancreas sustains ischemic damages before cardiac arrest due to a long-lasting systemic hypotension. When we procure the pancreas for islet isolation, we use in situ machine washout (ISMW) technique [17, 18], which was originally developed for the procurement of kidneys from DCD donors.

Preservation of the pancreas is one of the major issues to achieve successful islet isolation. The University of Wisconsin (UW) solution, which is used widely for organ preservation, was considered to be also effective for the preservation of the pancreas for islet isolation [19, 20]. Furthermore, a two-layer method (TLM) designed by Kuroda et al. using the UW solution and perfluorochemical was another effective alternative as the technique for cold storage of the pancreas prior to islet isolation due to its high yield of the islets [21–27]. In addition, histidine-tryptophan-ketoglutarate (HTK), which has been established as an alternative to the UW solution for abdominal organ preservation, seems to be equally effective in the cold storage of the pancreas prior to islet isolation [28–30]. Noguchi et al. reported that the originally developed M-Kyoto solution was superior to the UW solution and HTK in the cold storage of the pancreas prior to islet isolation [31, 32]. In Japanese experiences, we are using the UW solution or TLM with UW solution or M-Kyoto solution [12].

22.3 Experiences of Islet Isolation in Chiba-East National Hospital

We have experienced 23 human islet isolations from September 2003 to April 2007 (see Chap. 21) [33]. Islet yield was compared depending on the donor factors and procurement/preservation factors (Table 22.1). Although the islet yield decreased when we used the pancreas of the donor with an episode of cardiac arrest before admission to the ICU, a cannulation with a double-balloon catheter to the aorta prior to cardiac arrest and turning off of the respirator did not affect the islet yield. The islet yield isolated from the pancreas of the dead donor due to trauma as the cause of death was much higher than cerebrovascular disease and hypoxic encephalopathy. In our series, donor age did not affect the islet yield. This may be because that

Table 22.1 Final islet yield (IEq) depending on the donor factors and procurement/preservation factors. Islet Isolation Center, Clinical Research Center, Chiba-East National Hospital, 2003.9–2007.4

	Yes	No
Episode of cardiac arrest	122,452	207,318
Cannulation to the aorta	170,233	181,327
Respirator off	166,067	167,150
Cause of death		
Cerebrovascular disease	135,370	
Hypoxic encephalopathy	131,356	
Trauma	307,384	
Age		
<20 years	191,353	
>20 years	157,939	
Duration of anuria		
<4 h	183,742	
>4 h	101,674	
Cold ischemic time		
<6 h	227,726	
>6 h	142,533	
Cold storage		
TLM(UW + PFC)	200,219	
Simple cold storage (UW)	94,248	

trauma is frequent as the cause of death in young-aged donors. Prolonged duration of anuria, which reflects a long-lasting hypotension, was a factor that resulted in decreased islet yield, which may be because of continuous warm ischemic injury to the pancreas. Also, prolonged cold ischemic time was a factor that resulted in decreased islet yield. In our series, the pancreas preserved by TLM with UW solution and perfluorochemical yielded twice as compared to the organ preserved by simple cold storage with UW solution.

Out of 23 isolations, seven isolations fulfilled the criteria of the Japanese Islet Transplant Registry for fresh islet isolation [yield, ≥5,000 IEQ/kg (recipient body weight); purity, ≥30 %; final cell pellet, ≤10 ml; viability, ≥70 %; endotoxin, ≤5 EU/kg (recipient body weight)], and six isolations yielded less than 50,000 IEq. The donor, procurement, and preservation factors were compared between former seven isolations (success group) and latter six isolations (poor group). In the success group, trauma was more frequent as the cause of death, and duration of anuria was shorter as compared to the poor group. All pancreata were preserved using TLM in the success group, while two pancreata out of six were preserved in cold storage with UW solution. In the poor group, two pancreata were preserved more than 8 h (CIT) (Table 22.2).

22.4 Discussion and Conclusion

Extended criteria donor has not been clearly defined for islet transplantation. From the many previous studies on the factors that influence the outcome of islet isolation, young age (<18 years old) and low BMI (<25 kg/m^2) might be nominated for the factors of ECD for islet transplantation. However, these two factors emerged from the data of islet isolation, not from the data of islet transplantation. In other words, an improvement of islet isolation technique can make possible higher yield from the pancreas with these two factors. Looking at the existence of islet isolation process in islet transplantation, the pancreas which is not utilized for pancreas transplantation should be used for islet isolation except for malignancy, systematic infection, and diabetes of the donor.

In Japan, the number of DBD donors has increased since the Organ Transplantation Law was revised in 2010. The number of DBD donors still remains lower as compared to other countries such as the USA and Europe. For the efficient use of pancreas from DBD donors for transplantation into the type 1 diabetic patient, we are starting a newly designed clinical islet transplant program. When the pancreas is not procured for pancreas transplantation with reasons such as old age and high BMI of the donor, the pancreas is procured for islet isolation after enough consent and transplanted into the type 1 diabetic patient who has been registered in the Japanese Islet Registry.

ECD for islet transplantation was not clearly determined currently. Although further clinical and experimental investigations should be needed to define ECD for islet transplantation, the pancreas should be used for islet isolation with enough informed consent from the donor without malignancy, infection, and diabetes for the purpose of efficient use for islet transplantation.

Table 22.2 The donor, procurement, and preservation factors of the success group and poor group. Islet Isolation Center, Clinical Research Center, Chiba-East National Hospital, 2003.9–2007.4

	Isolation #	Age	Cause of death	Episode of cardiac arrest	Duration of anuria (min)	Cannulation to aorta	Respirator	Preservation	WIT (min)	CIT (min)
Success group	1	48	CVD	No	180	No	On	TLM	20	365
	3	17	Trauma	No	0	Yes	On	TLM	5	217
	11	38	CVD	No	240	No	On	TLM	15	256
	17	17	Trauma	No	0	Yes	Off	TLM	3	211
	20	45	Hypoxia	Yes	Unknown	Yes	On	TLM	2	335
	21	28	Trauma	No	Unknown	No	On	TLM	12	314
	23	46	CVD	No	Unknown	Yes	On	TLM	1	242
Poor group	4	44	CVD	No	1,320	No	–	CS	15	540
	10	46	Hypoxia	Yes	0	Yes	Off	TLM	2	318
	14	10	Brain tumor	No	360	Yes	On	TLM	3	303
	15	63	CVD	No	0	No	On	CS	27	285
	18	17	Hypoxia	Yes	2,160	Yes	On	TLM	3	515
	19	49	CVD	No	520	Yes	On	TLM	3	220

CVD cerebrovascular disease, *WIT* warm ischemic time, *CIT* cold ischemic time, *TLM* two-layer method, *CS* cold storage

References

1. Hering BJ, Ricordi C. Islet transplantation for patients with type 1 diabetes. Graft. 1999;2:12–27.
2. Shapiro AM, Lakey JR, Ryan EA, Korbutt GS, Toth E, Warnock GL, et al. Islet transplantation in seven patients with type 1 diabetes mellitus using a glucocorticoid-free immunosuppressive regimen. N Engl J Med. 2000;343:230–8.
3. Ryan EA, Lakey JR, Rajotte RV, Korbutt GS, Kin T, Imes S, et al. Clinical outcomes and insulin secretion after islet transplantation with the Edmonton protocol. Diabetes. 2001;50:710–9.
4. Lakey JR, Warnock GL, Rajotte RV, et al. Variables in organ donors that affect the recovery of human islets of Langerhans. Transplantation. 1996;61:1047–53.
5. Lacy PE, Kostianovsky M. Method for the isolation of intact islets of Langerhans from the rat pancreas. Diabetes. 1967;16:35–9.
6. Lacy PE, Lacy ET, Finke EH, Yasunami Y. An improved method for the isolation of islets from the beef pancreas. Diabetes. 1982;31:109–11.
7. Horaguchi A, Merrell RC. Preparation of viable islet cells from dogs by a new method. Diabetes. 1981;30:455–8.
8. Gray DW, McShane P, Grant A, Morris PJ. A method for isolation of islets of Langerhans from the human pancreas. Diabetes. 1984;33:1055–61.
9. Ricordi C, Finke EH, Lacy PE. A method for the mass isolation of islets from the adult pig pancreas. Diabetes. 1986;35:649–53.
10. Ricordi C, Lacy PE, Finke EH, Olack BJ, Scharp DW. Automated method for isolation of human pancreatic islets. Diabetes. 1988;37:413–20.
11. Wang Y, Daneilson KK, Ropski A, Harvat T, Barbar B, Paushter D, Qi M, Oberholzer J. Systematic analysis of donor and isolation factor's impact on human islet yield and size distribution. Cell Transplant. 2013 Jan 28 [Epub ahead of print].
12. Saito T, Gotoh M, Satomi S, Uemoto S, Kenmochi T, Itoh T, et al. Islet transplantation using donors after cardiac death: report of the Japan islet transplantation registry. Transplantation. 2010;90:740–7.
13. Sakuma Y, Ricordi C, Miki A, Yamamoto T, Pileggi A, Khan A, et al. Factors that affect human islet isolation. Transplant Proc. 2008;40:343–5.
14. Ponte GM, Pileggi A, Messinger S, Alejandro A, Ichii H, Baidal DA, et al. Toward maximizing the success rates of human islet isolation: influence of donor and isolation factors. Cell Transplant. 2007;16:595–607.
15. Nano R, Clissi B, Melzi R, Calori G, Maffi P, Antonioli B, et al. Islet isolation for allotransplantation: variables associated with successful islet yield and graft function. Diabetologia. 2005;48:906–12.
16. Benedetti E, Sileri P. Surgical aspects of pancreas transplantation. Donor. Donor selection and management. In: Gruessner RW, Sutherland DE, editors, Transplantation of the pancreas. New York: Springer; 2003; p. 116.
17. Arita S, Asano T, Kenmochi T, Enomoto K, Isono K. An initial wash-out solution for "in situ machine wash-out". Transplant Proc. 1991;23:2589.
18. Asano T, Enomoto K, Ohtsuka M, Goto T, Nakagohri T, Kenmochi T, et al. Usefulness of rapid machine cooling in the procurement of livers. Transplant Proc. 1989;21:1307–8.
19. Kneteman NM, DeGroot TJ, Warnock GL, Rajotte RV. The evaluation of solutions for pancreas preservation prior to islet isolation. Horm Metab Res Suppl. 1990;25:4–9.
20. Chadwick DR, Robertson GS, Contractor HH, Rose S, Johnson PR, James RF, et al. Storage of pancreatic digest before islet purification. The influence of colloids and the sodium to potassium ratio in University of Wisconsin-based preservation solutions. Transplantation. 1994;58:99–104.

21. Goto T, Tanioka Y, Sakai T, Terai S, Kamoda Y, Li S, et al. Application of the two-layer method on pancreas digestion results in improved islet yield and maintained viability of isolated islets. Transplantation. 2007;27:754–8.
22. Kin T, Mirbolooki M, Salehi P, Tsukada M, O'Gorman D, Imes S, et al. Islet isolation and transplantation outcomes of pancreas preserved with University of Wisconsin solution versus two-layer method using preoxygenated perfluorocarbon. Transplantation. 2006;82:1286–90.
23. Takahashi T, Tanioka Y, Matsuda T, Toyama H, Kakinoki K, Li S, et al. Impact of the two-layer method on the quality of isolated pancreatic islets. Hepatogastroenterology. 2006;53:179–82.
24. Tanaka T, Suzuki Y, Tanioka Y, Sakai T, Kakinoki K, Goto T, et al. Possibility of islet transplantation from a nonheartbeating donor pancreas resuscitated by the two-layer method. Transplantation. 2005;80:738–42.
25. Tsujimura T, Kuroda Y, Churchill TA, Avila JG, Kin T, Shapiro AM, et al. Short-term storage of the ischemically damaged human pancreas by the two-layer method prior to islet isolation. Cell Transplant. 2004;13:67–73.
26. Tsujimura T, Kuroda Y, Kin T, Avila JG, Rajotte RV, Korbutt GS, et al. Human islet transplantation from pancreases with prolonged cold ischemia using additional preservation by the two-layer (UW solution/perfluorochemical) cold-storage method. Transplantation. 2002;74:1687–91.
27. Tanioka Y, Sutherland DE, Kuroda Y, Gilmore TR, Asaheim TC, Kronson JW, et al. Excellence of the two-layer method (University of Wisconsin solution/perfluorochemical) in pancreas preservation before islet isolation. Surgery. 1997;122:435–42.
28. Paushter DH, Qi M, Danielson KK, Harvat TA, Kinzer K, Barbaro B, et al. Histidine-tryptophan-ketoglutarate and university of wisconsin solution demonstrate equal effectiveness in the preservation of human pancreata intended for islet isolation: a large-scale, single-center experience. Cell Transplant. 2013;22:1113–21.
29. Caballero-Corbalán J, Brandhorst H, Malm H, Felldin M, Foss A, Salmela K, et al. Using HTK for prolonged pancreas preservation prior to human islet isolation. J Surg Res. 2012;175:163–8.
30. Salehi P, Hansen MA, Avila JG, Barbaro B, Gangemi A, Romagnoli T, et al. Human islet isolation outcomes from pancreata preserved with histidine-tryptophan ketoglutarate versus University of Wisconsin solution. Transplantation. 2006;82:983–5.
31. Noguchi H, Ueda M, Nakai Y, Iwanaga Y, Okitsu T, Nagata H, et al. Modified two-layer preservation method (M-Kyoto/PFC) improves islet yields in islet isolation. Am J Transplant. 2006;6:496–504.
32. Noguchi H, Ueda M, Hayashi S, Kobayashi N, Nagata H, Iwanaga Y, et al. Comparison of M-Kyoto solution and histidine-tryptophan-ketoglutarate solution with a trypsin inhibitor for pancreas preservation in islet transplantation. Transplantation. 2007;84:655–8.
33. Kenmochi T, Asano T, Maruyama M, Saigo K, Akutsu N, Iwashita C, et al. Clinical islet transplantation in Japan. J Hepatobiliary Pancreat Surg. 2009;16:124–30.

Part IX
Small Intestine Transplantation

Chapter 23
ECD for Small Intestine Transplantation

Takehisa Ueno

23.1 Introduction

The prognosis of intestinal failure has improved dramatically owing to the development of parenteral nutrition (PN). However, PN-related complications, such as central venous catheter infection, venous access thrombosis, and intestinal failure associated with liver disorder, are still major causes of mortality in patients with intestinal failure. However, patients who develop life-threatening complications are considered for intestinal transplantation. Intestinal transplantation, which can significantly improve their prognosis and quality of life, has become an established treatment for intestinal failure [1]. More than 2,300 intestinal transplants have been performed worldwide [2].

Although there are relatively few candidates for intestinal transplantation, the waiting time is relatively long. For candidates wait-listed in 2010, the median time to transplant in the United States was 14.9 months for patients less than 18 years old and 2.8 months for those 18 years or older [3].

Since the intestine is very sensitive to ischemia, hemodynamically stable donors have been traditionally preferred. The shortage of organs has led centers to expand their criteria to accept marginal donors. A combination of multiple marginal factors seems to have an additive effect on graft quality. Clinical and new investigational strategies aimed at manipulating marginal donor organs to improve outcome will be covered, as well as approaches for marginal donor allocation.

In the past, intestinal transplant teams could be selective in choosing donor organs for two reasons; first, the supply of potential intestinal grafts far exceeded the comparatively low demand, and second, there were few if any criteria for defining

T. Ueno (✉)
Pediatric Surgery, Graduate School of Medicine, Osaka University,
2-2 Yamadaoka, Suita, Osaka 565-0871, Japan
e-mail: ueno@pedsurg.med.osaka-u.ac.jp

T. Asano et al. (eds.), *Marginal Donors: Current and Future Status*,
DOI 10.1007/978-4-431-54484-5_23,

Table 23.1 Proposed standard and extended criteria donors

Donor data	SCD	ECD
Age	0–50 years	50–60 years
Donor–recipient size match	DRWR and DRHR compatible	Reduced graft
ICU stay	<1 week	1–2 weeks
BMI	<28	28–30
CPR	<10 min	>10 min
Sodium	<155 mEq/L	155–165 mEq/L
Blood group	Identical	Compatible

CPR cardio pulmonary resuscitation, *DRWR* donor–recipient weight ratio, *DRHR* donor–recipient height ratio, *ICU* intensive care unit

the "marginal" intestinal graft. However, as intestinal transplantation has become increasingly common, the "luxury of selectiveness" in graft procurement has diminished greatly, thereby requiring consideration of extended donor criteria in intestinal transplantation, similar to the evolution of transplantation of other solid organs.

23.1.1 Japanese Experience

We performed a retrospective analysis of 12 deceased donors from whom 12 isolated intestinal grafts were recovered and successfully transplanted in Japan between January 2001 and December 2012. Data were extracted from the anonymized database of the Japan Organ Transplant Network. Data were analyzed for every donor, including recipient demographics and initial graft function (Table 23.1).

23.2 Definition

An accepted definition of marginal intestinal donor has not been definitively established. Among the most prominent donor characteristics that may influence graft survival include older age, cardiopulmonary arrest, viral status, graft size mismatch, and elevated liver function tests (LFTs). More long-term determinants of poor patient and graft survival are crossmatch positivity and donor-specific antigen positivity.

23.3 Viability and Outcome

23.3.1 Donor Age

The ideal donor for intestinal transplantation is younger than 50 years [4–7]. Donors older than 50 years are considered extended criteria donors. Some programs reported marginal donor organs have been used successfully [4, 6].

The Japanese experience has been similar. The mean donor age was 37 years old, with two donors over the age of 50 [8]. Among living donors, the maximum age allowed was 60 years [9]. Marginal donor organs should not be discarded.

23.3.2 *Graft Size Match*

Weight is an important factor in donor selection. The donor should be similar in size or smaller than the recipient since the recipient's abdominal cavity is often small due to extensive resection of the intestines. Graft sizes 25–50 % smaller than the recipient are generally preferred [4, 10–13]. Size reduction or adaptation of the graft may be possible to overcome recipient size mismatch [4, 14, 15]. Larger donor organs may be implanted since children with end-stage liver disease often have abdominal distention. It is also possible to decrease the length of donor bowel in patients receiving an isolated small bowel transplant and decrease the size of the liver graft in those requiring a larger composite graft. Due to shortages in pediatric donors, donor size mismatch is not an absolute exclusion. A high body mass index (BMI) may indicate a high mesenteric fat content, which can cause graft size mismatch with hardness of mesenteric fat in cold solution. A study allows BMI 28 kg/m^2 [16]. General surgical experience indicates that a high BMI (≥30 kg/m^2) may increase the risk of surgical complications.

However, a BMI ≥30 may not affect graft quality, and it is not an absolute contraindication to living donation [9]. There is no data supporting a clear cutoff for donor BMI.

23.3.3 *Cause of Death*

The cause of the donor's death is not related to exclusion criterion [17]. However, death due to abdominal trauma is not preferred because of the potential for intestinal injury or contamination. Direct abdominal injury or severe deceleration trauma should be considered contraindication for intestinal donation. Extra-abdominal trauma is acceptable. In our experience, 75 % of intestinal donation had brain-related causes of death, such as head trauma or cerebrovascular accident [8].

23.3.4 *Cardiopulmonary Arrest*

Previously hemodynamically unstable donors are not preferred because the intestine is very sensitive to ischemia. Consequently, potential donors who are managed on high doses of vasopressors, those with extended periods of hypotension, or those who experienced cardiac arrest or cardiopulmonary resuscitation are excluded. Resuscitation has been associated with overall poor donor quality [18].

Neurogenic and hormonally driven splanchnic vasoconstriction may result in clinically relevant intestinal ischemia. Intestinal ischemia may affect graft viability by breaking down the intestinal mucosal barrier. Ischemia may promote leukocyte migration into the intestinal graft, resulting in early acute rejection and increasing the risk of bacterial translocation and infection.

Outcomes of grafts retrieved from donors with and without cardiac arrest used in isolated intestinal transplant and multivisceral transplant have been compared. The mean duration of cardiac arrest and subsequent cardiopulmonary resuscitation (CPR) was 19.3 ± 12.7 min. Compared with donors who did not undergo CPR, there were no significant differences in outcome parameters such as operative time, blood use, duration of mechanical ventilation, length of hospital stay, time to enteral independence, rejection, enteric bacteremia, and survival [17].

These results were consistent with our experience. All patients who received graft from the cadaveric donor with CPR more than 10 min survived. The duration of the CPR ranged from 35 to 47 min [8].

A donor history of cardiac arrest should not automatically exclude the use of the intestinal graft for transplantation.

23.3.5 Inotropic Support

In addition to potential donors who underwent CPR, donor candidates with high doses of vasopressors are excluded. There is concern that high doses of vasoactive medications may damage organs through visceral vasoconstriction. The United Network for Organ Sharing (UNOS) data has previously shown that donor organs subjected to prolonged hypotension have no significant increase in posttransplantation graft loss.

Fischer-Frohlich et al. reported that 31 % of donors were hemodynamically unstable immediately after hospital admission, but subsequently recovered [16]. Initial hemodynamic instability was treated with vasopressors and inotropic agents (e.g., norepinephrine >0.1 μg/kg/min supplemented by dobutamine >10 μg/kg/min) as well as transfusions as necessary until proper circulation was achieved. While there is concern that high doses of vasoactive medications may damage organs through visceral vasoconstriction, all unstable donors in our series recovered hemodynamically, and their organ function recovered subsequently as well. Short-term use of a high dosage of vasopressors in donors unstable upon hospital admission does not exclude intestinal donation.

In the Japanese experience, the most common cause of death was head trauma. Dopamine was used in ten cases (83 %) as a vasopressor, with a mean maximum dose of 10.7 μg/kg/min. The highest maximum dose was 21.2 μg/kg/min. Three donors required more than 15 μg/kg/min of dopamine. All recipients from donors who received high doses of dopamine survived in our experience [8].

Donors who received high doses of vasopressors are not excluded but are considered marginal donors. The question of which catecholamines, and at what doses, are detrimental to organ procurement remains unanswered.

23.3.6 Viral Status

Donor infection with human immunodeficiency virus (HIV), hepatitis C virus (HCV), or hepatitis B virus (HBV) confirmed by blood tests remains a contraindication to intestinal donation [9].

Cytomegalovirus (CMV)-positive donors should not be considered for CMV-negative recipients because of the significantly higher mortality rate in this group [19]. This guideline should be strictly adhered to in isolated intestinal transplants and whenever possible with other types of grafts.

However, with the development of medications and diagnostic tests for CMV, early diagnosis of CMV infection and prompt preemptive therapy have significantly reduced the risk of CMV disease. Even with the nearly unrestricted use of CMV-positive donors, there have been no CMV-associated deaths among recipients [20].

In Japan, most donors are CMV-positive; however, no CMV-related deaths have been reported.

23.3.7 Intensive Care Unit Stay

Intensive care improves the quality of donor organs [21]. A report recommended that intensive care unit (ICU) stays longer than 1 week should not exclude intestinal donation [17]. In our experience, the mean ICU stay was 8 days, and 6 patients (50 %) stayed longer than 1 week [8]. Long ICU stay is also an acceptable extended criterion. Enteral nutrition should be started as soon as possible after admission to the ICU, as recommended by guidelines for enteral nutrition.

23.3.8 Laboratory Values

The sodium level represented the most important parameter influencing the acceptance of intestinal grafts. Serum sodium should be kept within normal range [6, 7, 21]. However, in our experience the mean sodium level was 145 mEq/L, with three patients with a sodium level greater than 150 mEq/L [8]. Other study allows 155 mEq/L sodium level [16]. Sodium in the range of 155–165 mEq/L should be considered an extended criterion. LFTs may show intestinal ischemia; the LFT trend is important. LFTs trending towards the normal range may indicate recovery, while increasing values may represent intestinal ischemia. Following CPR, aspartate transaminase (AST), alanine transaminase (ALT) twice the upper limit of the reference range, as well as creatinine and bilirubin in the reference range had no impact on the outcome of intestinal transplantation [17]. CRP was elevated in our experience, with a mean value of 18 mg/dL [8].

23.3.9 ABO Compatibility

Identical ABO blood type is preferred [12]. Some centers might occasionally decline offers of intestines from nonidentical ABO compatible donors in favor of waiting for an ABO-identical offer. Pediatric centers, however, receive many fewer offers and thus more frequently accept nonidentical but compatible donor intestines if the donor weight and age are favorable [22].

23.3.10 Human Leukocyte Antigen Typing Crossmatch

Ideally, donors with a positive lymphocytotoxic crossmatch should be avoided; however, there is usually a prolonged wait for crossmatch results, which could endanger the graft by extending the cold ischemia time. Pretransplant donor-specific antigen in the intestinal graft can be a risk factor for immediate (hyperacute) but potentially reversible, antibody-mediated rejection. Thus, pretransplant donor-specific antigen and crossmatch results are critical components to be considered in patients awaiting or undergoing intestinal transplantation [23].

23.4 Basic Research

Graft viability prior to transplantation has an important influence on the outcome. Preservation damage is one of many essential factors that can affect the quality of the intestinal graft.

Intestinal graft quality with University of Wisconsin solution (UW), histidine–tryptophan–ketoglutarate (HTK), Celsior, and Polysol has been compared in rats. HTK and Celsior showed benefits versus UW [24].

To facilitate comparing the results using various solutions, adenosine triphosphate (ATP) precursors such as amino acids are added during preservation in order to improve viability. Acidic end products of the tricarboxylic acid (TCA) cycle like ammonia must be buffered. Regarding amino acid supplementation, only 4 % amino acid concentration showed better results than UW [25].

The intestinal lumen is a target for preservation. During ischemic preservation, tissue edema is believed to originate from the lumen, along with increased permeability. Furthermore, the lumen is potentially contaminated by bacteria. Celsior seems to be the best luminal preservation solution [26].

Rapidly progressing mucosal breakdown limits intestinal preservation time to under 10 h. Recent studies indicate that intraluminal solutions containing polyethylene glycol (PEG) alleviate preservation injury of intestines stored in UW. A customized intraluminal PEG solution reduces intestinal preservation injury by improving several major epithelial characteristics without negatively affecting brush-border enzymes or promoting edema [27].

Hypothermic machine perfusion generates a flow of recirculating cold preservation solution. For the intestine, cold storage is assumed to be superior to hypothermic machine perfusion due to possible pressure-induced vascular injury. However, the comparison of two pulsatile perfusion systems with cold storage and with a combination of 6 h of cold storage plus 18 h of pulsatile perfusion demonstrated a better outcome after machine perfusion preservation in a canine model [28].

Several intricate oxygenation techniques have been attempted. A 2-layer oxygenated perfluorocarbon/UW method was evaluated for canine preservation and intestinal transplantation. All dogs in the 2-layer oxygenated perfluorocarbon/UW group survived. Graft histology and absorption capacity was similar to non-preserved grafts [29].

23.5 Summary

Extended criteria for donation of intestinal transplant grafts include donor age 50–60 years, CPR longer than 10 min, ABO compatible, ICU stay from 1 week up to 2 weeks, high doses of vasopressors, elevated LFTs, sodium level 155–165 mEq/L, and a compatible donor–recipient size match. Any extended criteria donor graft should be considered potentially suitable for the patients on long waiting lists and not be discarded without seeking timely intestinal transplantation.

References

1. Fishbein TM. Intestinal transplantation. N Engl J Med. 2009;361(10):998–1008.
2. Grant D. Small bowel transplant registry. In: 12th international small bowel transplant symposium. Washington, USA. 2011.
3. HRSA. Annual data report 2011.
4. Kato T, Tzakis AG, Selvaggi G, et al. Intestinal and multivisceral transplantation in children. Ann Surg. 2006;243(6):756–64. discussion 764–6.
5. Mangus RS, Fridell JA, Vianna RM, et al. Comparison of histidine-tryptophan-ketoglutarate solution and University of Wisconsin solution in extended criteria liver donors. Liver Transpl. 2008;14(3):365–73.
6. Mazariegos GV, Steffick DE, Horslen S, et al. Intestine transplantation in the United States, 1999–2008. Am J Transplant. 2010;10(4 Pt 2):1020–34.
7. Yersiz H, Renz JF, Hisatake GM, et al. Multivisceral and isolated intestinal procurement techniques. Liver Transpl. 2003;9(8):881–6.
8. Furukawa H. Establishment of educational program for multi-organ procurement from deceased donors. Ministry of Health and Laber Welfare, Japan. 2013.
9. Barr ML, Belghiti J, Villamil FG, et al. A report of the Vancouver Forum on the care of the live organ donor: lung, liver, pancreas, and intestine data and medical guidelines. Transplantation. 2006;81(10):1373–85.
10. Pascher A, Kohler S, Neuhaus P, et al. Present status and future perspectives of intestinal transplantation. Transpl Int. 2008;21(5):401–14.
11. Gondolesi G, Fauda M. Technical refinements in small bowel transplantation. Curr Opin Organ Transplant. 2008;13(3):259–65.

12. Tzakis AG, Kato T, Levi DM, et al. 100 multivisceral transplants at a single center. Ann Surg. 2005;242(4):480–90. discussion 491–3.
13. Abu-Elmagd K, Fung J, Bueno J, et al. Logistics and technique for procurement of intestinal, pancreatic, and hepatic grafts from the same donor. Ann Surg. 2000;232(5):680–7.
14. Benedetti E, Holterman M, Asolati M, et al. Living related segmental bowel transplantation: from experimental to standardized procedure. Ann Surg. 2006;244(5):694–9.
15. de Ville de Goyet J, Mitchell A, Mayer AD, et al. En block combined reduced-liver and small bowel transplants: from large donors to small children. Transplantation. 2000;69(4):555–9.
16. Fischer-Frohlich CL, Konigsrainer A, Schaffer R, et al. Organ donation: when should we consider intestinal donation. Transpl Int. 2012;25(12):1229–40.
17. Matsumoto CS, Kaufman SS, Girlanda R, et al. Utilization of donors who have suffered cardiopulmonary arrest and resuscitation in intestinal transplantation. Transplantation. 2008;86(7):941–6.
18. Keitel E, Michelon T, dos Santos AF, et al. Renal transplants using expanded cadaver donor criteria. Ann Transplant. 2004;9(2):23–4.
19. Furukawa H, Manez R, Kusne S, et al. Cytomegalovirus disease in intestinal transplantation. Transplant Proc. 1995;27(1):1357–8.
20. Abu-Elmagd K, Reyes J, Bond G, et al. Clinical intestinal transplantation: a decade of experience at a single center. Ann Surg. 2001;234(3):404–16. discussion 416–7.
21. Zaroff JG, Rosengard BR, Armstrong WF, et al. Consensus conference report: maximizing use of organs recovered from the cadaver donor: cardiac recommendations, March 28–29, 2001, Crystal City, VA. Circulation. 2002;106(7):836–41.
22. Rushton SN, Hudson AJ, Collett D, et al. Strategies for expanding the UK pool of potential intestinal transplant donors. Transplantation. 2013;95(1):234–9.
23. Ruiz P, Carreno M, Weppler D, et al. Immediate antibody-mediated (hyperacute) rejection in small-bowel transplantation and relationship to cross-match status and donor-specific C4d-binding antibodies: case report. Transplant Proc. 2010;42(1):95–9.
24. Wei L, Hata K, Doorschodt BM, et al. Experimental small bowel preservation using Polysol: a new alternative to University of Wisconsin solution, Celsior and histidine-tryptophan-ketoglutarate solution? World J Gastroenterol. 2007;13(27):3684–91.
25. Olson DW, Fujimoto Y, Madsen KL, et al. Potentiating the benefit of vascular-supplied glutamine during small bowel storage: importance of buffering agent. Transplantation. 2002;73(2):178–85.
26. Leuvenink HG, van Dijk A, Freund RL, et al. Luminal preservation of rat small intestine with University of Wisconsin or Celsior solution. Transplant Proc. 2005;37(1):445–7.
27. Oltean M, Joshi M, Bjorkman E, et al. Intraluminal polyethylene glycol stabilizes tight junctions and improves intestinal preservation in the rat. Am J Transplant. 2012;12(8):2044–51.
28. Zhu JZ, Castillo EG, Salehi P, et al. A novel technique of hypothermic luminal perfusion for small bowel preservation. Transplantation. 2003;76(1):71–6.
29. Tsujimura T, Salehi P, Walker J, et al. Ameliorating small bowel injury using a cavitary two-layer preservation method with perfluorocarbon and a nutrient-rich solution. Am J Transplant. 2004;4(9):1421–8.

Part X
ABO-Incompatible Donor

Chapter 24
ABO-Incompatible Donor

Takashi Kenmochi, Takehide Asano, Naotake Akutsu, and Taihei Ito

24.1 Introduction

Human ABO blood type, which was discovered in 1901 by Landsteiner [1], is a major immunological barrier in organ transplantation because of a development of severe rejection due to the humoral reaction between A or B antigens and anti-A or anti-B antibodies. ABO-incompatible kidney transplantation was first performed in 1952 by Hume et al. for the patient of renal failure [2]. The transplanted kidney, however, did not function at all. Starzl et al. also performed ABO-incompatible kidney transplantation in four patients in 1964 and succeeded long-term graft survival in one patient [3, 4]. However, since a success rate was extremely low, ABO-incompatible kidney transplantation generally ceased to be performed [5]. Thereafter, in 1981, Slapak et al. reported the efficacy of plasmapheresis for the rejection after kidney transplantation with ABO incompatibility [6]. Alexandre et al. first performed ABO-incompatible kidney transplantation using the designed protocol using plasma exchange for pretransplant removal of anti-A and anti-B antibodies and splenectomy for long-term graft survival [7–9].

In Japan, Takahashi et al. have introduced the first ABO-incompatible kidney transplantation in 1989 using double-filtered plasmapheresis (DFPP) with immunoabsorption for the removal of antibodies and splenectomy which resulted in long-term graft survival [10–14]. This clinical success encouraged us to promote ABO-incompatible living kidney transplantation in Japan, and 2,218 patients underwent ABO-incompatible living kidney transplantation from January 1 to December 31 [15].

T. Kenmochi (✉) • T. Ito
Department of Organ Transplant Surgery, Fujita Health University,
1-98 Dengakugakubo, Kutsukake-cho, Toyoake City, Aichi 470-1192, Japan
e-mail: kenmochi@fujita-hu.ac.jp

T. Asano • N. Akutsu
Department of Surgery and Clinical Research Center, Chiba-East National Hospital,
673 Nitonacho, Chuo-ku, Chiba City, Chiba 260-8712, Japan
e-mail: asano@cehpnet.com

T. Asano et al. (eds.), *Marginal Donors: Current and Future Status*,
DOI 10.1007/978-4-431-54484-5_24,

The number of ABO-incompatible living kidney transplantation has increased year and year, and currently, about 25 % of living kidney transplantation is ABO-incompatible transplantation in Japan.

In addition to kidney transplantation, ABO-incompatible transplantation has been introduced into liver transplantation [16] and pancreas transplantation [17] in Japan.

ABO-incompatible donor is considered as an immunologically marginal donor for the recipient. Pretreatment for the recipient, which includes pretransplant immunosuppression and improved desensitization protocol as well as careful monitoring of the antibody titer both before and after transplantation, achieved the improved graft survival that is almost equal to that in ABO-compatible kidney transplantation. Especially in Japan, ABO-incompatible kidney transplantation has become widely adopted due to a severe shortage of deceased donors.

In this chapter, we describe the current status of ABO-incompatible kidney transplantation in Japan and our experiences of simultaneous pancreas and kidney transplantation from ABO-incompatible live donors in a single institution.

24.2 Current Status of ABO-Incompatible Kidney Transplantation in Japan

In Japan, Professor Kota Takahashi of Niigata University performed the first successful ABO-incompatible kidney transplantation in 1989, when he was in Tokyo Women's Medical College, using DFPP with immunoabsorption and splenectomy [10, 18]. He organized Japanese Society for ABO-incompatible transplantation, and registration was started in 1997 [19]. All Japanese data shown here was referenced to the data book edited by Takahashi and Tanaka [15].

The number of institutions which participated in the multicenter study was 189. 119 institutions out of 189 (63 %) performed ABO-incompatible kidney transplantation, and the number of the patients is increasing year and year (Fig. 24.1). Total number of the patients from 1989 to 2011 was 2,218. Out of 2,218 patients, valid data from 2,194 patients were used for the following analysis. Age of the recipient and the donor was 43.1 ± 15.1 and 55.1 ± 10.6 years, respectively. Sixty-two percent of the recipients were male, while 64 % of the donors were female. Relationship between the donors and the recipients was parents and children in 47.3 % and spouse in 41 %, which were dominant (Table 24.1).

Desensitization and antibody removal were achieved by pretransplant (1–4 weeks before transplantation) immunosuppression using a calcineurin inhibitor, an anti-metabolic agent, and a steroid; DFPP and/or plasma exchange; and splenectomy or the administration of rituximab, that is, an anti-CD20 monoclonal antibody. Currently, splenectomy is rarely performed, and an administration of decreased dose of rituximab (100 mg X 2 or 200 mg X 1 before and/or at transplantation) is widely performed in place of splenectomy. Pretransplant antibody titers were reduced less than 16-folds in 65 % of the recipients in IgM and 59 % in IgG. However, the patients underwent transplantation with more than 128-folds in 9 % in

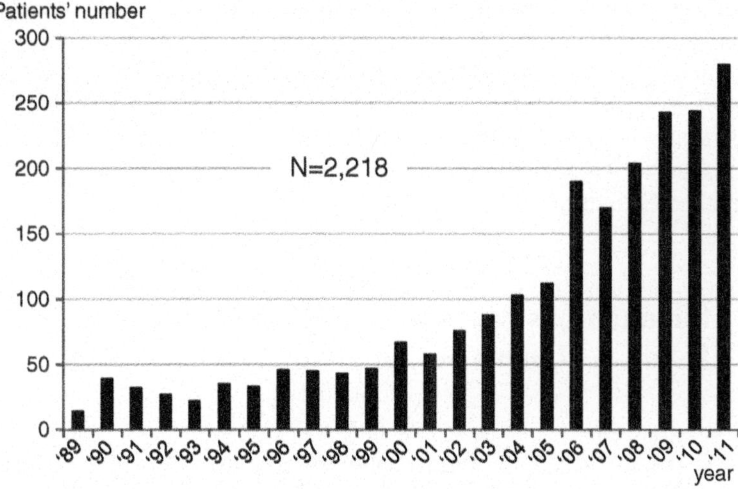

Fig. 24.1 Changes in the number of ABO-incompatible kidney transplantation in Japan. 1989–2011, Japanese ABO-incompatible kidney transplantation registry [15]

Table 24.1 Patients' background of ABO-incompatible kidney transplantation in Japan

Recipients		
Age	43.1 ± 15.1 years old	
Gender	Male 1,356 (62 %)	Female 830 (38 %)
Donors		
Age	55.1 ± 10.6 years old	
Gender	Male 782 (36 %)	Female 1,389 (64 %)
Relationship		
Parents and children (%)	1,039 (47.3)	
Spouse (%)	900 (41.0)	
Siblings (%)	187 (8.5)	
Others (%)	68 (3.1)	
Recipient blood type		
A: 531 (24 %)		
Donor blood type B: 272 (51 %), AB: 267 (49 %)		
B: 525 (24 %)		
Donor blood type A: 315 (60 %), AB: 210 (40 %)		
O: 1,138 (52 %)		
Donor blood type A: 663 (57 %), B: 437 (38 %), AB: 54 (5.0 %)		
HLA-A,B mismatch	2.1 ± 1.1	
HLA-DR mismatch	1.1 + 0.6	

N = 2,194, 1989 ~ 2011, Japanese ABO-incompatible kidney transplantation registry [15]

IgM and 20 % in IgG. Maintenance immunosuppression was achieved by cyclosporine based in 691 patients (32 %) and tacrolimus based in 1,454 (68 %).

Patient survival in total 2,213 patients was 97 % at 1 year, 93 % at 5 years, and 89 % at 10 years. Kidney graft survival was 93 % at 1 year, 85 % at 5 years, and 71 % at 10 years. However, 1,768 patients, who underwent transplantation after 2001, showed the improved results of both patient and graft survival; patient survival was 97 % at 3 years, 95 % at 5 years, and 92 % at 10 years, and graft survival was 94 % at 3 years, 90 % at 5 years, and 84 % at 10 years. These results were comparable to the outcome of ABO-compatible kidney transplantation in Japan. From these results, ABO-incompatible transplantation has become an alternative option as living kidney transplantation.

24.3 Simultaneous Pancreas and Kidney Transplantation from Live Donors in Chiba-East National Hospital

The first extrarenal organ to be successfully transplanted using live donors was the pancreas. The first pancreas transplantation using a live donor was performed on June 20, 1979, at the University of Minnesota [20, 21]. Furthermore, successful simultaneous pancreas and kidney transplantation from a live donor was started in 1994 also at the University of Minnesota [22]. The outcome of the live donor pancreas transplants performed at the University of Minnesota demonstrated that the segmental pancreas was able to normalize plasma glucose levels and realize an insulin independency into the severe diabetic patients. The outcome of the donors was considered to be acceptable when using the stringent donor criteria concerning about the endocrine function [23].

Based on a severe shortage of the deceased donors in our country and the satisfactory outcome of living donor pancreas transplants at the University of Minnesota, we have firstly introduced the living donor pancreas transplant in our country on January 7, 2004 [17]. Eighteen living donor pancreas transplants have, so far, been performed in our institution (Chiba-East National Hospital). From July 5, 2006, we have introduced simultaneous pancreas and kidney transplants from ABO-incompatible living donors according to our desensitization and immunosuppression protocol for ABO-incompatible kidney transplantation and performed, so far, six cases.

In this study, we describe the outcome of six recipients of ABO-incompatible simultaneous pancreas and kidney transplants from live donors in our institution.

24.3.1 Patients and Methods

24.3.1.1 Recipients

Eighteen type 1 diabetic patients underwent living donor pancreas transplants in our institution from January 2004 to June 2012. Sixteen patients (89 %) underwent the simultaneous pancreas and kidney transplant from living donors (LDSPK) because of an end-stage renal disease (ESRD). One patient (5.6 %) underwent pancreas after

Table 24.2 The characteristics of the recipients and donors of ABO-i LDSPK (Department of Surgery, Chiba-East National Hospital. 2004–2013)

Recipients	
Patient number	6
Age (years)	30.8 ± 5.0 (25–40)
Gender (male/female)	2/4
Onset of DM[a] (years old)	9.8 ± 5.5 (0.9–18)
Duration of DM (years)	22.2 ± 5.0 (16–31)
Fasting CPR[b] (ng/mL)	<0.03
Glucagon-stimulated CPR (ng/mL)	<0.03
Amount of insulin (units/day)	29.8 ± 8.4 (4 times daily)
Anti-GAD or IA-2 Abs[c]	Positive: 2, negative: 4
M value	60.6 ± 13.3
ESRD[d]	HD[e]: 5, preemptive: 1
Donors	
Patient number	6
Age (years)	54.5 ± 7.2 (42–63)
Gender (male/female)	1 (brother)/5 (mothers)
75 g-OGTT[f]	Normal pattern
Body mass index	22.9 + 1.87

[a]*DM* diabetes mellitus
[b]*CPR* serum C-peptide
[c]*Abs* antibodies
[d]*ESRD* end-stage renal disease
[e]*HD* hemodialysis
[f]*75 g-OGTT* 75 gram oral glucose tolerance test

kidney transplant from the living donor (LDPAK), and the other one patient (5.6 %) underwent pancreas transplant alone from the living donor (LDPTA). Out of sixteen LDSPK recipients, six patients underwent LDSPK from ABO-incompatible living donors (ABO-i LDSPK).

The characteristics of the ABO-i LDSPK recipients were shown in Table 24.2. All patients were type 1 diabetic patients, and the onset of diabetes has rapidly occurred due to diabetic ketoacidosis. All patients showed a frequent hypoglycemic unawareness despite of four times potent insulin injection therapy depending to the self-measured plasma glucose levels. Unstable plasma glucose levels resulted in the high *M* value level, 60.6 ± 13.3. Both fasting- and glucagon-stimulated serum C-peptide levels were undetectable (<0.03 ng/mL) in all patients.

24.3.1.2 Donors

The donors were one brother and five mothers of the recipients. Ages ranged from 42 to 63 years. A potential donor first must have an interview with the doctors, nurses, transplant coordinators, and medical social workers in our hospital and must provide voluntary consent. Thereafter, the donor must show the negative study in flow cross-match examination between the donor's T lymphocytes and the recipient's serum. All donors must fulfill our criteria for the donor of living pancreas transplant as previously reported [17].

The evaluation of pancreatic endocrine function includes normal data of 75 g oral glucose tolerance test (75 g-OGTT), insulinogenic index, HOMA-β, HOMA-R, and normal level of hemoglobin (Hb)A1C. In addition, the autoantibodies against the islet cell (anti-GAD and anti-IA2 antibodies) must be absent, and body mass index (BMI) must be less than 25 kg/m^2. For the safe procedure of the donor operation, we evaluated the blood vessels of the pancreas and the kidney using a three-dimensional angiography from dynamic CT. In order to evaluate segmental function of the donor pancreas, 11C-methionine positron emission tomography (PET) was also performed [24, 25].

24.3.1.3 Operation Methods

In the donor, under an open laparotomy (first three cases) or under hand-assisted laparoscopic surgery (HALS) (last three cases) [26], the left kidney was first excised followed by a distal pancreatectomy with splenectomy. In the recipient, the kidney was transplanted into the left iliac fossa in extraperitoneal space. Thereafter, the segmental pancreatic graft was transplanted into the right iliac fossa in extraperitoneal space. Bladder drainage of the pancreatic juice was used in all recipients [17].

24.3.1.4 Immunosuppression and Desensitization Protocol

Pretransplant immunosuppression and desensitization protocol includes a suppression of B lymphocytes by 4-week administration of mycophenolate mofetil (MMF), 10-day administration of tacrolimus and prednisolone, and removal of anti-A and anti-B antibodies by administration of rituximab (200 mg/body) (day 14), a double-filtration plasmapheresis (DFPP: days 6, 4, and 2), and a plasma exchange (PEX: day 1). Posttransplant immunosuppression was achieved by a quadruple therapy using MMF, tacrolimus, prednisolone, and basiliximab.

24.3.1.5 Postoperative Care and Monitoring

In the donors, antibiotics were administrated intravenously for 7 days after surgery. Gabexate mesilate (600 mg/day) was given for 7 days for the purpose of inhibition of residual pancreatitis. To assess exocrine and endocrine function of the residual pancreas, serum amylase, lipase, trypsin, and plasma glucose levels were determined daily. In addition, serum C-peptide levels were determined once a week. After discharge, the donors were monitored in the outpatient clinic, and their plasma glucose levels, HbA1C, and serum C-peptide levels were measured at 1 and 3 months and at every year after operation. 75 g-OGTT was performed at 6 months and at every year after surgery.

In the recipients, anticoagulation therapy was started at operation using heparin (200 units/h), and 10,000–20,000 units were continuously given intravenously for 10 days after transplantation. 2,000 mg of gabexate mesilate was continuously administrated for 7 days, and 100 units of octreotide were given at every 12 h for 5 days to inhibit a secretion of pancreatic juice from the graft. The antibacterial prophylaxis consisted of piperacillin for a week, antifungal prophylaxis consisted of fluconazole for a week, and anti-cytomegalovirus (CMV) prophylaxis consisted of ganciclovir for 10 days. Oral intake was started at 7 days after transplantation. During the hospitalization, each recipient was monitored daily for pre- and post-prandial plasma glucose and amylase, blood cell count, electrolytes, serum creatinine, and urinary amylase excretion. All the above parameters were continually monitored in the outpatient clinic. 75 g-OGTT was performed at 1 and 4–6 months and every year after transplantation. Anti-A and anti-B antibodies were measured daily during 2 weeks after transplantation and thereafter once a week during the hospitalization.

Blood flow of both pancreas and kidney grafts was examined daily during 10 days after transplantation using ultrasonography, and plasticity index(PI) and resistive index(RI)were calculated from the wave of pulsed wave Doppler to monitor the arterial and venous thrombosis.

24.3.1.6 Histological Study of the Pancreas and Kidney Grafts

Before transplantation, small specimens were excised from kidney and pancreas grafts, and they were provided for histological study (0 h biopsy). Expression and distribution of blood type A and B antigens were examined by immunochemical staining with type A and B antibodies. In addition, at 1 h after reperfusion, needle biopsy of both kidney and pancreas grafts was performed and provided for histological study (1 h biopsy).

24.3.2 Results

24.3.2.1 Immunological Study for ABO-i LDSPK

ABO blood types of donor and recipient were A to O in three cases, B to O in one case, AB to A in one case, and AB to B in one case. Type A was confirmed to be subtype A1 using an anti-A1 lectin reagent (Ortho-Clinical Diagnostics, Co., Mfg., Tokyo) in all donors. Differences of HLA types between donor and recipient were three mismatches in three cases, two mismatches in one case, one mismatch in one case, and identical in one case. Flow cross-match study showed negative in all cases. Flow PRA study also showed negative activity (<5.0 %) in both classes I and II in all recipients. Anti-A and anti-B antibody titers ranged from 8-folds to 256-folds.

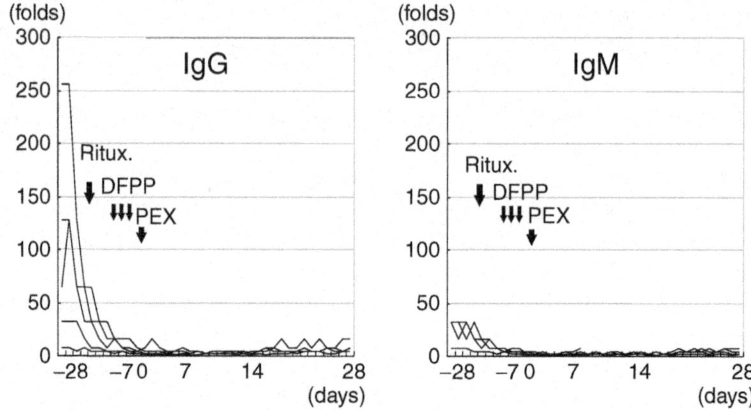

Fig. 24.2 Changes in anti-A and anti-B antibody titers before and after ABO-incompatible simultaneous pancreas and kidney transplantation (*Ritux.* rituximab, *DFPP* double-filtration plasmapheresis, *PEX* plasma exchange)

24.3.2.2 Donor Outcome

No complication including a formation of pancreatic fistula and an intra-abdominal abscess was observed during hospitalization. The donors discharged from the hospital at 21.8 ± 5.1 days after surgery and immediately returned to their social life. One donor developed pancreatic pseudocyst at 6 months after surgery even with a little symptom. We performed the punction from the stomach using gastrofiberscope, and the cyst has completely disappeared and no recurrence was observed thereafter. Development of diabetes was not, so far, observed in all donors during the observation period from 7 to 9.5 years.

24.3.2.3 Recipient Outcome

Anti-A and anti-B antibody titers (IgG, IgM) decreased to less than 16-folds at transplantation day, and those were maintained less than 16-folds at least 1 month after transplantation (Fig. 24.2).

All recipients showed immediate function of kidney graft, and no hemodialysis was needed after transplantation. Serum creatinine levels were maintained from 0.6 to 1.8 mg/dL after transplantation. One patient developed, however, kidney graft failure at 2.5 years after transplantation due to the severe dehydration from the uncontrollable diarrhea.

All recipients achieved insulin independency immediately after transplantation, and no hypoglycemic unawareness was observed among all patients. Fasting plasma glucose levels were stabilized under 100 mg/dL, and positive serum C-peptide levels ranging from 1.2 to 6.8 ng/mL were maintained (Fig. 24.3). The levels of HbA1C decreased to less than 6.0 % within 3 months after transplantation. 75 g-OGTT

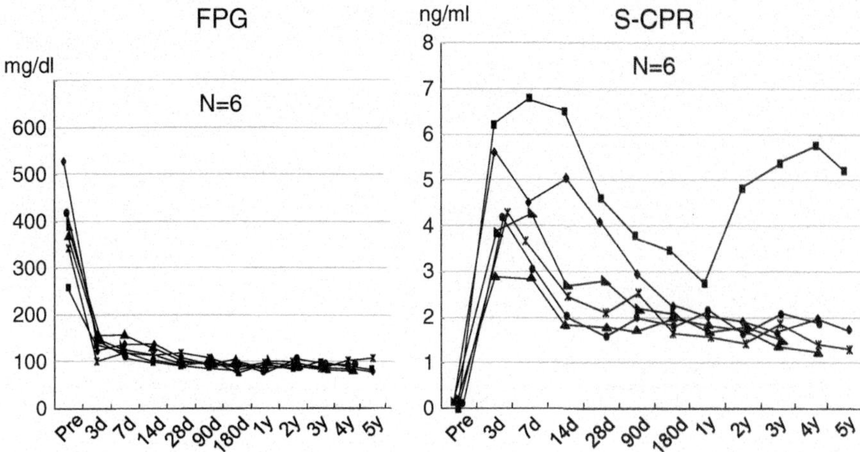

Fig. 24.3 Fasting plasma glucose (*FPG*) and serum C-peptide (*S-CPR*) levels after ABO-incompatible simultaneous pancreas and kidney transplantation

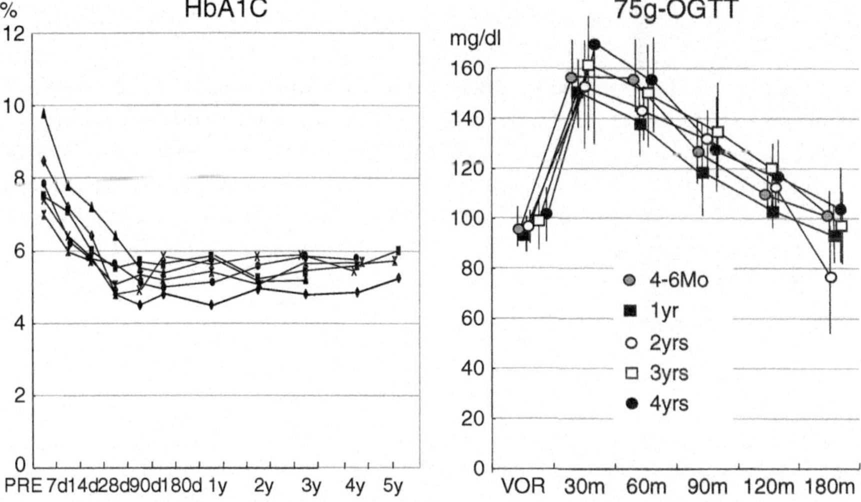

Fig. 24.4 Changes in HbA1C and 75 g-OGTT after ABO-incompatible simultaneous pancreas and kidney transplantation

performed at 4–6 months and 1, 2, 3, and 4 years after transplantation showed the normal pattern (Fig. 24.4).

Although a biopsy-proven acute cellular rejection (ACR) was observed in two patients (33.3 %), the steroid pulse rescue therapy completely eliminated ACR in both patients. Antibody-mediated rejection (AMR) did not occur in all patients. As a surgical complication, the leakage of the pancreatic juice was observed in two patients.

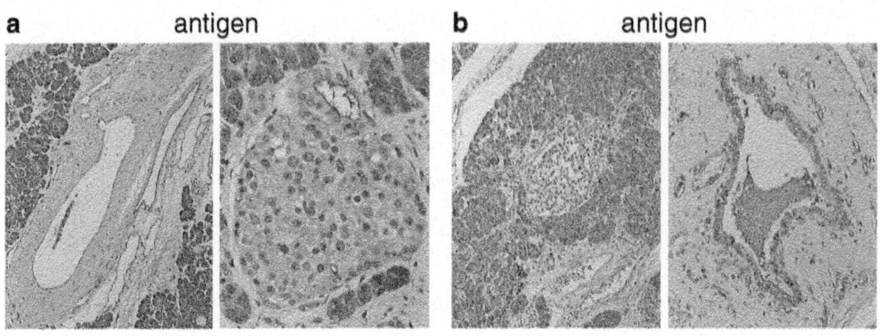

Expression of blood group antigen in human pancreas

	Artery	Vein	Capillary	Acinar cell	Centroacinar cell	Intercalated duct	Interlobular duct	Main duct	Islet
A	+	+	+	+*	−	−	+*	+*	−
B	+	+	+	+*	−	−	+*	+*	−

* focal

Fig. 24.5 Expression and distribution of blood type A and B antigens in the pancreas graft tissue

Conservative therapy including administration of octreotide and percutaneous aspiration of collecting fluid around pancreatic graft was effective on curing the leakage of the pancreatic juice, and both patients did not need an additional surgical treatment. Cytomegalovirus antigenemia was shown to be positive in three patients (50 %) from 30 to 46 days after transplantation, and two patients required an intravenous administration of ganciclovir. The patients discharged from 35 to 125 days after transplantation and returned to their social life.

24.3.2.4 Histological Study of the Pancreas and Kidney Grafts

Both blood type A and B antigens were expressed on acinar cells and main and interlobular pancreatic duct epithelial cells in addition to the vessels' endothelial cells. However, centroacinar cells and intercalated ductal epithelium showed no expression of both antigens. Also, no expression of A and B antigens was observed on islet cells (Fig. 24.5).

In Japan, the number of diabetic patients has increased every year and has reached to over eight million. Although type 1 diabetes is less frequent in our country as compared to the United States and Europe, a quality of life and a prognosis are extremely lower in the type 1 diabetic patients with ESRD. Pancreas transplantation using brain-dead donors has been restarted in 2,000 for those patients. Only 119 pancreas transplants, however, were performed for 11 years because of a severe shortage of deceased donors in our country. Thirty-seven patients on the waiting list of pancreas transplantation, so far, actually died due to the diabetic complications such as hypoglycemic unawareness and cardiovascular diseases [7].

Living donor pancreas transplantation has been introduced at the University of Minnesota in 1979 [8]. Initially, they performed living donor pancreas transplants only in the recipients without uremia (LDPTA) or the recipients who had received the kidney graft from the same donor (LDPAK). Thereafter, they performed the first successful LDSPK in March 1994 [10], and 20 LDSPKs had been done until March 1997 [11]. The 1-year survival rates of the patient, kidney graft, and pancreas graft were 100 %, 100 %, and 78 %, respectively, which were higher than those of pancreas transplants from brain-dead donors at that time [15]. The 1-year survival of the pancreas graft, then, had improved to 87 % in 2001 by analyzing 32 recipients of LDSPK [16]. Those results clearly demonstrated that segmental pancreas was able to normalize the glucose metabolism of severe diabetic patient.

Based on a shortage of the deceased donors in our country and the excellent outcome of the University of Minnesota, we have performed the first LDSPK in Japan for a type 1 diabetic patient with ESRD from her father on January 7, 2004 [12]. Donor safety has been the most important consideration of the enforcement of LDSPK. The criteria of the donor for pancreas transplantation had been made by transplant surgeons, diabetologist, nephrologist, nurses, and transplant coordinators. We have referred to the stringent Minnesota criteria and modified it according to the lower ability to secrete insulin from the islet in Japanese [12].

ABO blood type used to be a major barrier in clinical transplantation. Since ABO-incompatible kidney transplantation has been successfully performed in the world [17] and Japan in 1989 [18], this procedure has become the popular alternative for the living donor kidney transplantation. Because of the severe shortage of cadaveric donors in our country, more than 80 % of the kidney transplantations are from living donors. In addition to the living-related donors, the living-unrelated (spouse) donor has become popular in kidney transplantation in Japan. From these backgrounds, ABO-incompatible kidney transplantation is recently an important option.

In our institution, we performed ABO-incompatible kidney transplantation for 21 patients with an end-stage renal disease from April 2004 to October 2007 [19]. The patient and graft survival rates were highly maintained in the 21 patients who underwent ABO-incompatible kidney transplantation in our institution. These data indicated that the safety and the efficacy of ABO-incompatible kidney transplantation have reached the levels of those in ABO-matched and ABO-compatible kidney transplantation.

From these results of ABO-incompatible kidney transplantation, we have introduced ABO-i LDSPK on July 5, 2006. In the University of Minnesota, three ABO-i pancreas transplantations (two living donor recipients and one deceased donor recipients) were performed [20]. In all the three ABO-i pancreas transplantations, blood type A2 donors were used because of the low expression of A2 (vs. A1) determinants. These three cases demonstrated the excellent pancreas graft function using plasmapheresis and IV Ig. In our series, however, blood types of the donors were A1 incompatible to the recipients in four cases and B incompatible in two cases. Among these six patients, although two patients developed ACR, we have not experienced AMR, and no vessel thrombosis occurred in any patients that indicated that high expression of A1 determinant can be inhibited and may induce accommodation using our desensitization and immunosuppression protocol. Our results clearly demonstrated that ABO-i pancreas transplantation is successfully performed as well as the kidney transplantation even using A1- and B-incompatible donors. Our result is the first report in the world. In the histological study using the biopsied specimens of the pancreas grafts at 0 h after transplantation, blood type A and B antigens were strongly expressed on the acinar cells and pancreatic ductal epithelium in addition to vessels' endothelium. Islet cells did not express these antigens, while, in the kidney grafts, blood type A and B antigens were strongly expressed in distal tubular epithelium as well as vessels' endothelium. Glomerular cells did not express the antigens. Distribution and intensity of A and B antigens may be equal between pancreas and kidney. These results may explain our clinical outcome.

The leakage of pancreatic juice was the most major problem as a surgical complication after living pancreas transplant in our experience. Although two patients out of six developed the leakage of pancreatic juice after transplantation, the leakage disappeared by conservative treatment including aspiration of the fluid and the administration of octreotide, and both patients maintained normal function of pancreatic graft. Other surgical complication was not observed in all patients, which demonstrated the safety seemed to be almost the same as kidney transplantation.

In the series of ABO-i LDSPK in our institution, we obtained the excellent outcome of both the recipients and the donors. Further considerations should be needed to establish this procedure in our country as one of the therapies for severe diabetic patients with ESRD. The most major issue must be the safety of the donor. We have introduced hand-assisted laparoscopic surgery for simultaneous nephrectomy and distal pancreatectomy in recent three donors. Operation was performed mainly according to the previously reported technique [21]. The pancreas, however, was dissected directly from the open 7 cm wound for HandPort System [14]. This procedure is for the purpose of eliminating the loss of pancreas by stapling. The three donors who underwent HALS operation rapidly recovered after operation, and no analgesics were needed in addition to an epidural administration of local anesthetics. The introduction of this procedure may contribute the improvement of the donor safety. In addition, a long-term maintenance of the metabolism of the donor is still an important problem. In our experience, the donors did not develop diabetes for more than 5 years. Increased levels of HbA1C within normal range and decreased insulin release at 90, 120, and 180 min after oral glucose challenge were observed in our studies [12]. Therefore, all donors are carefully followed up by the diabetologist and the nephrologist in addition to the transplant surgeons in our hospital.

24.4 Conclusions

From Japanese experiences of ABO-incompatible kidney transplantation and our experiences of ABO-incompatible pancreas transplantation, ABO-incompatible live donors who are considered to be immunologically marginal donors are able to donate the kidney and the pancreas when the sufficient treatment of pretransplant desensitization is performed to the recipients.

References

1. Tagareli A, Landsteiner K. A hundred years later. Transplantation. 2001;72:3–7.
2. Hume DH, Merril JP, Hiller BF, Thorn GW. Experiences with renal homo-transplantation in the human: report of nine cases. J Clin Invest. 1995;34:327–82.
3. Starzl TE, Marchioro TL, Rifkind D, Holmes JH, Rowlands Jr DT, Waddell WR. Renal homografts in patients with major donor recipient blood group incompatibilities. Surgery. 1964;55:195–200.
4. Starzl TE, Tzakis A, Makowka L, Banner B, Demetrius A, Ramsey G, Duquesnoy R, Griffin M. The definition of ABO factors in transplantation: relation of other humoral antibody states. Transplant Proc. 1987;19:4492–7.
5. Gleason RE, Murray JE. Report from kidney transplant registry: analysis of variables in the function of human kidney transplants. Transplantation. 1967;52:343–59.
6. Slapak M, Naik RB, Lee HA. Renal transplant in a patient with major donor-recipient blood group incompatibility. Reversal of acute rejection by the use of modified plasmapheresis. Transplantation. 1981;31:4–7.
7. Alexandre GP, De Bruyere M, Squifflet JP, Moriau M, Latinne D, Pirson Y. Human ABO incompatible living donor renal homografts. Neth J Med. 1985;28:231–4.
8. Alexandre GP, Squifflet JP, De Bruyère M, Latinne D, Reding R, Gianello P, Carlier M, Pirson Y. Present experiences in a series of 26 ABO-incompatible living donor renal allografts. Transplant Proc. 1987;19(6):4538–42.
9. Alexandre GPJ, Latinne D, Gianello P. Performed cytotoxic antibodies and ABO-incompatible grafts. Clin Transplant. 1991;5:583–93.
10. Takahashi K, Agishi T, Oba S, et al. Extracorporeal plasma treatment for extending indication of kidney transplantation: ABO-incompatible and preformed antibody-positive kidney transplantation, Therapeutic plasmapheresis, vol. IX. Cleveland: ESAO; 1990. p. 61–3.
11. Takahashi K, Tanabe K, Ooba S, Yagisawa T, Nakazawa H, Teraoka S, Hayasaka Y, Kawaguchi H, Ito K, Toma H. Prophylactic use of a new immunosuppressive agent deoxyspergualin in patients with kidney transplantation from ABO-incompatible or preformed antibody positive donors. Transplant Proc. 1991;26:1078–82.
12. Takahashi K, Sonda K, Okuda H, Nakazawa H, Kawaguchi H, Toma H, Agishi T, Ota K, Nakabayashi M, Takeda Y. The first report of a successful delivery in a woman with an ABO-incompatible kidney transplantation. Transplantation. 1993;56:1288–9.
13. Takahashi K, Yagisawa T, Sonda K, Kawaguchi H, Yamaguchi Y, Toma H, Agishi T, Ota K. A ABO-incompatible kidney transplantation in a single-center trial. Transplant Proc. 1993; 25:271–3.
14. Tanabe K, Takahashi K, Sonda K, Tokumoto T, Ishikawa N, Kawai T, Fuchinoue S, Oshima T, Yagisawa T, Nakazawa H, Goya N, Koga S, Kawaguchi H, Ito K, Toma H, Agishi T, Ota K. Long-term results of ABO-incompatible living kidney transplantation: a single-center experience. Transplantation. 1998;65:224–8.
15. Saito K, Takahashi K. Registry 2012 of ABO-incompatible living kidney transplantation in Japan. In: Takahashi K, Tanaka K, editors. The new strategies of ABO incompatible transplantation-2013-(Japanese). Niigata: Japanese Society for ABO-incompatible transplantation; 2013. p. 3–18.
16. Egawa H, Teramukai S, Haga H, Tanabe M, Fukushima M, Shimazu M. Present status of ABO-incompatible living donor liver transplantation in Japan. Hepatology. 2008;47(1):143–52.
17. Kenmochi T, Asano T, Maruyama M, Saigo K, Akutsu N, Iwashita C, Ohtsuki K, Suzuki A, Miyazaki M. Living donor pancreas transplantation in Japan. J Hepatobiliary Pancreat Sci. 2010;17(2):101–7.
18. Takahashi K. ABO-incompatible kidney transplantation. Amsterdam: Elsevier; 2011.
19. Takahashi K, Saito K, Tanabe K, et al. Multicenter cooperative study group. First report of 7-year survey on ABO-incompatible kidney transplantation in Japan. Clin Exp Nephrol. 2001;5:119–25.

20. Sutherland DER. Pancreas and islet transplantation. II. Clinical trials. Diabetologia. 1981; 20:435–50.
21. Sutherland DER, Goetz FC, Najarian JS. Living-related donor segmental pancreatectomy for transplantation. Transplant Proc. 1980;12:19–25.
22. Gruessner RWG, Sutherland DER. Simultaneous kidney and segmental pancreas transplants from living related donors: the first two successful cases. Transplantation. 1996;61:1265–8.
23. Gruessner RWG, Kendall DM, Drangstveit MB, Gruessner AC, Sutherland DER. Simultaneous pancreas-kidney transplantation from living donors. Ann Surg. 1997;226:471–82.
24. Otsuki K, Kenmochi T, Saigo K, Maruyama M, Akutsu N, Iwashita C, Kono T, Okazumi S, Asano T, Yoshikawa K. Evaluation of segmental pancreatic function using 11C-methionine positron emission tomography for safe operation of living donor pancreas transplantation. Transplant Proc. 2008;40:2562–4.
25. Otsuki K, Yoshikawa K, Kenmochi T, Saigo K, Maruyama M, Akutsu N, Iwashita C, Ito T, Kono T, Okazumi S, Asano T. Evaluation of segmental pancreatic function using 11C-methionine positron emission tomography for safe living donor operation of pancreas transplantation. Transplant Proc. 2011;43(9):3273–6.
26. Maruyama M, Kenmochi T, Akutsu N, Saigo K, Iwashita C, Otsuki K, Ito T, Asano T. Laparoscopic-assisted distal pancreatectomy and nephrectomy from a live donor. J Hepatobiliary Pancreat Sci. 2010;17:193–6.

The manufacturer's authorised representative in the EU is Springer Nature Customer Service Centre GmbH, Europaplatz 3, 69115 Heidelberg, Germany. If you have any concerns regarding our products, please contact ProductSafety@springernature.com

Printed and bound by CPI Group (UK) Ltd, Croydon, CR0 4YY
15/07/2026
02167627-0003